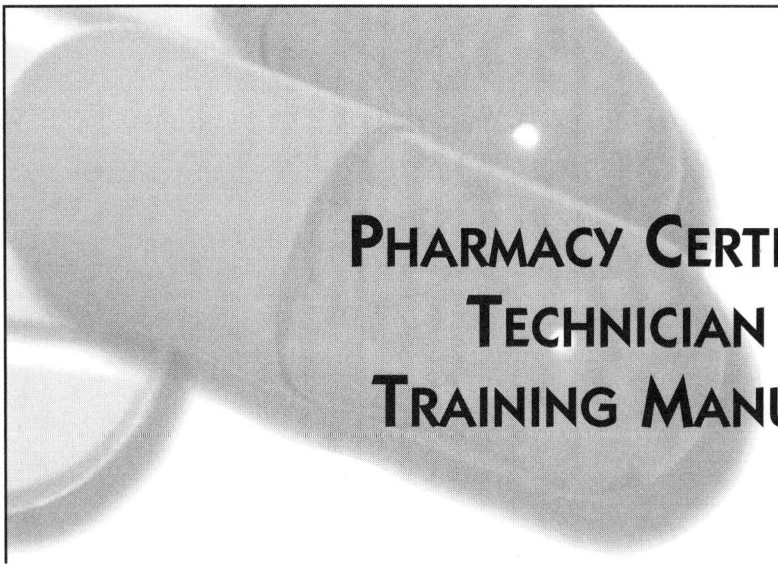

Pharmacy Certified Technician Training Manual

Editors

James M. Lile, Pharm.D.
Clinical Pharmacy Supervisor
MidMichigan Medical Center
Midland, Michigan

Dianne E. Miller, R.Ph.
Associate Executive Director
Michigan Pharmacists Association
Lansing, Michigan

Jennifer L. Pakkala, B.A.
Director of Marketing & Communications
Michigan Pharmacists Association
Lansing, Michigan

8th Edition

Michigan Pharmacists Association
815 N. Washington Ave., Lansing, MI 48906
(517) 484-1466; FAX (517) 484-4893
www.mipharm.com

The *Pharmacy Certified Technician Training Manual* was developed by the Michigan Pharmacists Association with support of the Michigan Society of Pharmacy Technicians.

815 N. Washington Ave., Lansing, MI, 48906

1st Edition, 1981
2nd Edition, 1982
3rd Edition, 1985
4th Edition, 1986
5th Edition, 1990
6th Edition, 1992
6th Edition, second printing, 1993
7th Edition, 1997
8th Edition, 2001

Table of Contents

PART IV: MEDICATION DISTRIBUTION AND CONTROL MEASURES

Chapter

PART V: PROFESSIONAL CONDUCT

Chapter

PART VI: CALCULATIONS

APPENDICES

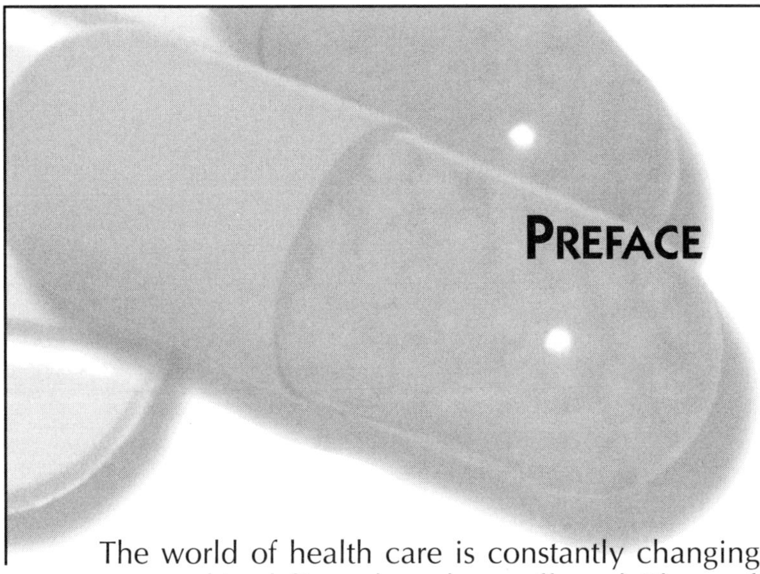

Preface

The world of health care is constantly changing. All components of health care and its delivery have been affected. The profession of pharmacy and that of the pharmacy technician have been impacted by healthcare changes. As managed care and pharmaceutical care both seek to redefine the role of pharmacists, the role and duties of pharmacy technicians continue to change dramatically.

The *Pharmacy Certified Technician Training Manual* is a revised and updated training tool designed to provide pharmacy technicians with practical and useful information for their activities.

This manual is written with the realization that, by the time it is published, certain aspects of health care will already have changed. For this reason, pharmacy technicians are advised to continue to augment the information contained herein with appropriate continuing education, communication, and preceptorship with pharmacists and fellow technicians.

This manual, like its predecessors, is the result of a volunteer committee of contributing authors from around the country. These men and women have pooled their talents and resources to produce an in-depth manual that can be used by both the technician in training and the technician with experience.

ACKNOWLEDGEMENTS

Associate Editors: Pamela L. Farley and Andrea L. Rybicki, B.A.

The Michigan Pharmacists Association wishes to acknowledge the following individuals for their contributions to this manual. Additional acknowledgments are contained within certain chapters of the manual.

Linda M. Branoff, CPhT
Candace J. Fong, Pharm.D.
Stephanie M. Gwin, CPhT
Ann P. Kluck, R.Ph.
Lynn Nowak, R.Ph.
Dick F. Kuschinsky, R.Ph.
Ronald H. Lukasiewicz, M.S.
Franz Neubrecht, Pharm.D.
John C. Polanyi, R.Ph.
Jeff W. Rabinowitz, R.Ph.
Sheldon J. Rich, R.Ph.
Lauren Tackel, R.Ph.

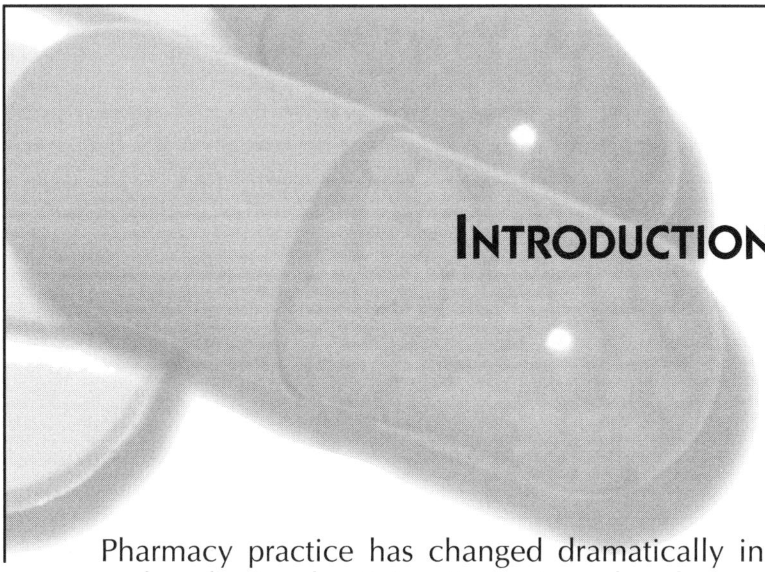

INTRODUCTION

Pharmacy practice has changed dramatically in both personal orientation and professional activity. Once viewed as the curator of medicinal herbs, the pharmacist is now viewed as the healthcare team member responsible for providing the right drug to the right patient at the right time. In many cases, pharmacy professionals have become involved with various patient care functions through clinical pharmacy activities.

Improved healthcare technology and healthcare legislation are the imposing forces that have created significant new demands on the practice of pharmacy. In order to fulfill the new, multifaceted role being demanded by the public and other healthcare professionals, pharmacists now delegate more and more technical functions to supportive personnel. With the assistance and help of well-trained pharmacy technicians, pharmacists are able to devote more time and energy to direct patient care services (pharmaceutical care) and advance their community's public health standards.

Today, technicians perform a variety of duties in many areas of pharmacy practice. Technicians have responsibility to enter data into computers, maintain technology, prepare prescriptions, compound intravenous solutions and solids, screen telephone calls, interact with patients, collect laboratory data, and organize workflow. These and other roles will continue to expand as pharmacy broadens its professional scope.

The Michigan Pharmacists Association (MPA) believes a recognized educational baseline to measure a uniform educational program is essential if technicians are to assume increased responsibilities. For this reason, MPA worked with the American Pharmaceutical Association, the American Society of Health-System Pharmacists, and the Illinois Council of Health-System Pharmacists to create one consolidated, national certification program for pharmacy technicians. MPA also developed and published the *Pharmacy Certified Technician Training Manual* as a tool for education, training, and preparation for pharmacy technician certification and practice.

The conception of this manual can be traced to the Michigan Tripartite Committee on Ancillary Personnel in Pharmacy, which was formed in 1970.

The Tripartite Committee was composed of representatives from the Michigan Board of Pharmacy, the three colleges of pharmacy in Michigan, and the MPA. In the committee's final report, issued in 1973, the members recommended that MPA develop a formal training manual to assist in the delivery of an inservice training program.

In 1979, the MPA Task Force on Pharmacy Supportive Personnel was established. The identical charge of the Task Force was to develop a training program with a training manual, appropriate exams, and guidelines for pharmacy technician practice experience.

Various documents and manuals were reviewed for style and content before any decisions concerning the development of the manual were made. The objective of the task force was to produce a comprehensive, practical manual that would meet pharmacy technicians' present and future educational needs, while being consistent with professional health care and pharmacy standards.

Work on this edition began in August 1999 with the intent of upgrading and revising both the structure and content of the previous edition. We feel we have produced a user-friendly product and look forward to any advice or comments the reader may have to improve our current effort.

How to use this manual

This manual is intended to be used for on-the-job training under the direction of a pharmacist or in an academic environment such as a community college. The importance of having a pharmacist to answer questions and monitor progress cannot be stressed heavily enough. As with most textbooks, this manual only highlights certain information. Therefore, it is important to have an experienced pharmacy professional available to answer questions that might arise.

Before reading Chapter 1, the technician should briefly skim through the manual. Each chapter contains three basic elements: (1) learning objectives at the beginning of each chapter, (2) the main text, and (3) self-assessment questions at the end of each chapter.

The purpose of the learning objectives is to inform the technician as to what must be learned and retained from each chapter. The objectives are a description of a pattern of behavior or performance that the technician should be able to demonstrate. Studying the objectives before reading the main text will allow the technician to become familiar with the main concepts to be mastered.

The main text of each chapter is written in textbook style. At the end of several chapters are references to resources for further research. Questions that arise should be directed to the pharmacist.

Each chapter ends with self-assessment questions to measure comprehension. These questions may also be used by the practicing technician and pharmacist to ascertain whether all objectives are understood and achieved. Answers to the self-assessment questions can be found in Appendix A.

After completion of the manual

Technicians should understand that successfully mastering the learning objectives in this manual achieves only the minimum groundwork of knowledge needed by a good pharmacy technician. The material in this manual should be augmented with extensive work experience and ongoing continuing education. Only through continued learning will the technician be valuable to help fulfill and go beyond the profession's role of providing the right medication to the right patient at the right time.

Technicians who have successfully mastered the learning objectives in this manual may wish to take the national examination for certification administered by the Pharmacy Technician Certification Board (PTCB). The material for this manual is derived from the outline for the exam and should, therefore, be helpful in preparing the technician for the exam.

It is not the intent of the chapter authors, editor, or publisher to train pharmacists with this manual. Use of this manual does not supercede professional judgment or education on the part of the pharmacist.

Completion of the manual alone does not entitle a pharmacy technician to certification. Only upon successful completion of the PTCB exam may a technician be certified and entitled to the designation *CPhT* (certified pharmacy technician).

Part I:
Pharmacy Technician Roles

CHAPTER

1

INTRODUCTION TO HEALTH CARE

Stephanie D. Taylor, R.Ph., Ph.D.

Learning objectives

Upon completion of this chapter, the technician should be able to do the following:

- Describe the trends in national health care expenditures.
- Describe the nature of health insurance coverage in the United States.
- Differentiate between the Medicare and Medicaid healthcare programs.
- Define the types of managed care organizations.
- Define accreditation and relate how it serves a role in the promotion of quality health care.

Introduction

Health care is a major industry employing millions of healthcare providers and support personnel. In the United States, health care is provided through a mixture of public and private plans. Consequently, the financing and delivery of health care is complex and exciting. This chapter provides an overview of the financing and structure of healthcare systems.

Health care delivery systems have undergone radical changes in recent years. With technological advances in diagnosis and treatment, individuals are healthier, and even those with chronic conditions have enhanced quality of life and longevity. However, these advances are not without cost. The promise of affordability and access to modern health care has figured prominently in the presidential campaigns for the last couple of decades. Both state and federal governments spend a significant portion of their annual budgets on healthcare benefits for persons eligible for Medicare, which covers the elderly and disabled, and for Medicaid, which covers persons meeting the low-income eligibility threshold.[1] Furthermore, the private sector is concerned with the high cost of providing employee healthcare benefits.

Chart 1 National health expenditures

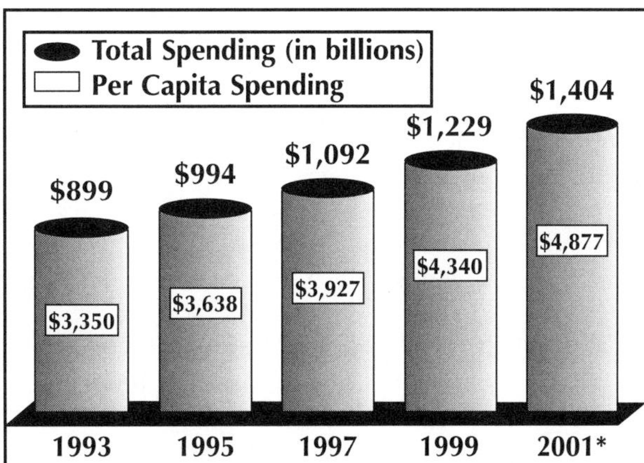

*Estimated value
Source: Health Care Financing Administration, Office of the Actuary.

In 1999, total spending for national health expenditures topped $1.2 trillion, representing a significant increase from 1997.[2] Total national expenditures and the average amount spent on each person are illustrated in Chart 1. For the 285.5 million persons residing in the United States, the average expenditure for health care in 1999 was \$4,340 per person.[3] Of the nation's healthcare dollar, approximately 17 percent of the healthcare dollar is paid for out-of-pocket with the remainder coming from a mix of public (45 percent) and private (38 percent) funds. This means that, on average, each person spent \$222 a year from personal funds to pay for insurance premiums, copayments, and health services used prior to reaching a specified annual deductible. These are cost sharing dollars since the consumer shares the cost of treatment with the insurer. A person's amount of out-of-pocket expenses depends on the type of insurance or the government program.[1,2,3] Sources of payment for health care are displayed in Chart 2.

Chart 2 Nation's 2000 health dollar

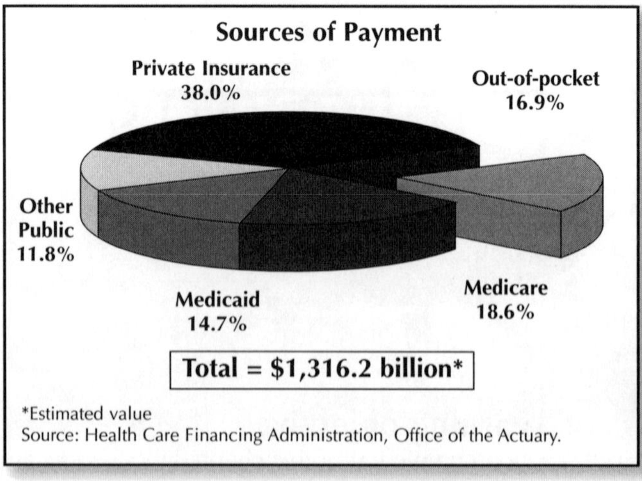

Chart 3 Nation's 2000 health dollar

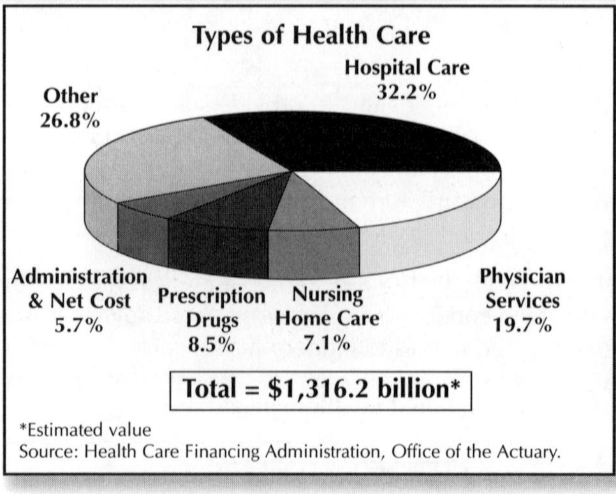

Traditionally, hospital care and physician services account for the majority of healthcare spending (see Chart 3). However, in recent years, the percentage of healthcare expenditures being spent on these services has been declining. There has been an increase in nursing home care, administration costs, prescription drugs, and other healthcare services.[3] An important observation is that 1999 prescription drug expenses per person are \$393 per year.[4] This is a small expense compared to the total \$4,340 spent on all health services. However, on average, consumers spend more than \$100 from personal funds for prescription drugs because insurance plans tend to require the consumer to share these costs. Also, the proportion of persons with insurance for medications is only about two-thirds of all persons. Elderly consumers experience much higher medication costs, estimated to be approximately \$688 in 1996 with \$316 as an out-of-pocket cost.[4] Consequently, there is high criticism over the cost of medications because the industry is profitable, prices increase faster than general inflation and the out-of-pocket share paid by consumers is conspicuous. Increases in expenditures are the sum of prices and use. Recently, price and use have increased and new pharmaceutical treatments tend to be expensive.

Nearly 85 percent of the 285.5 million Americans had some type of insurance in 1998.[5] The proportion of the population enrolled in the various types of health insurance is displayed in Chart 4. The largest shares of public health expenditures are for government's two largest healthcare programs—the Medicare (18.6 percent) and Medicaid (14.7 percent) programs.[1] Together, Medicare and Medicaid financed \$439.1 billion in healthcare services in 2000—more than one-third of the nation's total healthcare bill and almost three-fourths of all public spending on health care.[6]

Chart 4 Primary health insurance: U.S. population, 1998

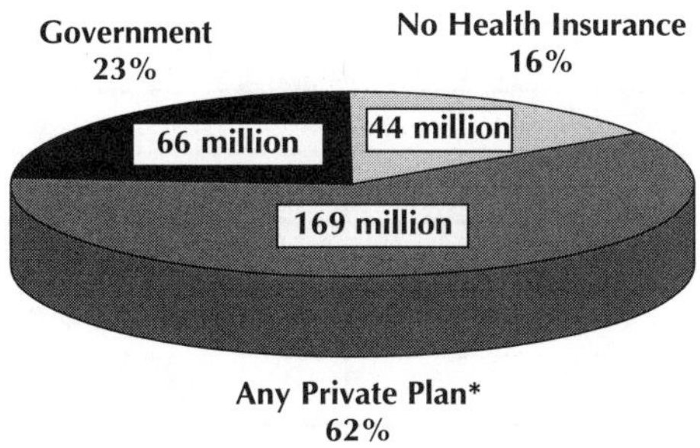

*Total private = 70%, 7.8% of population has Medicare primary coverage with secondary private insurance.

Note: Total does not equal 100% due to individuals enrolled in more than one insurance plan.

Source: Estimated using U.S. Census Bureau. Current Population Survey, March 1999.

Health care for the uninsured and adequate coverage for the underinsured are significant policy issues. Although many people have health insurance, the United States Census Bureau reports that approximately 16.3 percent of the population is without health insurance coverage. Surprisingly, these are not necessarily the poor and unemployed. Employment status of the uninsured is illustrated in Chart 5. There are forty-four million individuals who have no insurance and another 22 million who lack adequate coverage. Approximately one-fourth of the U.S. population (63 million people) will lose health insurance coverage for some period over the next two years.[5,7,8]

Medicare

Medicare is the federal healthcare program for the elderly and disabled, Title XVIII of the Social Security Act, entitled "Health Insurance for the Aged and Disabled." As part of the Social Security Amendments of 1965, the Medicare legislation established a health insurance program for aged persons to complement the retirement, survivors, and disability insurance benefits under Title II of the Social Security Act. When implemented in 1966, Medicare covered only persons age 65 and older. By the end of 1966, 3.7 million persons had received at least some healthcare services covered by Medicare.[9] Enrollment in Medicare is expected to exceed 40.3 million persons in 2001.[2] In 1973, other groups became eligible for Medicare benefits: persons who are entitled to Social Security or Railroad Retirement disability benefits for at least 24 months; persons with end-stage renal disease (ESRD) requiring continual dialysis or a kidney transplant; and certain otherwise non-covered elderly persons who elect to buy into Medicare.[9] Today, Medicare is the nation's largest health insurance program. The program is administered by the Health Care Financing Administration (HCFA—pronounced "hick-fa").

Chart 5 Employment status of uninsured: 1998

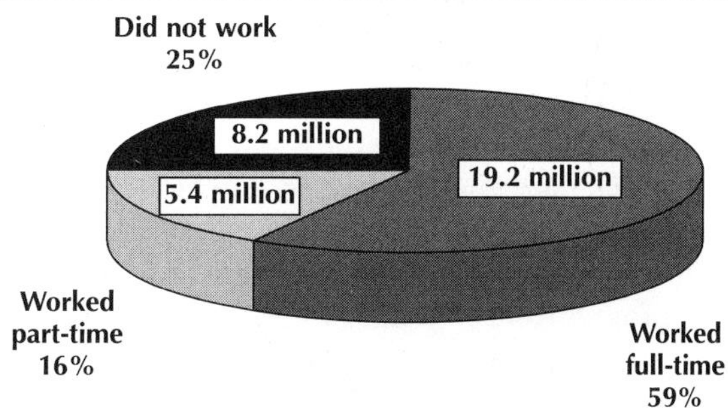

Note: Individuals ages 18-64

Source: Estimated using U.S. Census Bureau. Current Population Survey, March 1999.

Medicare consists of two primary parts: Medicare Part A and an optional Part B. In 2000, approximately 39.5 million persons were enrolled in Part A with 37.8 million also enrolled in optional Part B.[6] A recent addition to Medicare, Part C, was established by the Balanced Budget Act of 1997 (BBA).[9] Specific services and their attendant cost sharing are illustrated in Tables 1 and 2. Non-covered services under Medicare include long-term nursing care or custodial care, and certain other healthcare needs—such as dentures and dental care, eyeglasses, hearing aids, and most prescription drugs.[9] These are not a part of the Medicare program unless they are included in a managed care plan, or are selected as a part of the Medicare+Choice program.[9,10]

Table 1 Medicare Part A: 2000

Services	Benefit	Medicare Pays	You Pay
Hospitalization	First 60 days	All but $776	$776
	61-90 days	All but $194 per day	$194 per day
	91 to 150 days	All but $388 per day	$388 per day
	Beyond 150 days	Nothing	All costs
Skilled Nursing Facility Care	First 20 days	100% of approved amount	Nothing
	Additional 80 days	All but $97 per day	Up to $97 per day
	Beyond 100 days	Nothing	All costs
Home Health	Unlimited as long as enrollee meets Medicare conditions	100% of approved amount; 80% of approved amount for durable medical equipment	Nothing for services, 20% of approved amount for durable medical equipment
Hospice Care	For as long as physician certifies need	All but limited costs for outpatient drugs and 95% for inpatient respite care	A copayment of up to $5 for outpatient drugs and 5% for inpatient respite care
Blood	Unlimited if medically necessary	All but first three pints per calendar year	For first three pints

Source: *Medicare and You 2000, HCFA*

Medicare Part A

Part A, Hospital Insurance (HI), provides coverage of inpatient hospital services, skilled nursing facilities, home health services and hospice care to all persons eligible for Medicare without premium costs. This part of Medicare is financed primarily through a mandatory payroll deduction ("FICA tax"). Almost all employees and self-employed workers in the United States work in employment covered by the Medicare program and pay taxes to support the cost of benefits for elderly and disabled beneficiaries.[9]

Cost sharing is required. For hospital care, the beneficiary's payment share includes an annual deductible. This covers the beneficiary's part of the first 60 days of each stay of inpatient hospital care. If continued inpatient care is needed beyond the 60 days, additional coinsurance payments ($194 per day in 2000) are required through the 90th day of a benefit period.[10] (See Table 1.)

Medicare Part B

Supplementary Medical Insurance (SMI), Part B, assists in paying for the cost of physician services, outpatient hospital services, medical equipment and supplies, and some of the other health services and supplies (excluding most pharmaceuticals). Part B is financed through: (1) premium payments, which are usually deducted from the monthly Social Security benefit checks, and (2) through contributions from general revenue of the U.S. Treasury. Part B benefits may also be "bought" for persons by a third party directly paying the premium on behalf of the enrollee. Beneficiary premiums are currently set at a level that covers 25 percent of the average expenditures for elderly beneficiaries. The beneficiary's payment share includes one annual deductible ($100 for the year 2000), the monthly premiums, and payment. These cost-sharing contributions are required of the beneficiaries for Part B services. For ESRD patients, Medicare Part B covers kidney dialysis and physician charges incurred by the patient and donor during the transplant and follow-up care.[9]

Table 2 Medicare Part B: 2000

Services	Benefit	Medicare Pays	You Pay
Medical and other services	Unlimited if medically necessary	80% of approved amount (after $100 deductible)	$100 deductible plus 20% of approved amount and limited charges above approved amounts, except in the inpatient setting 20% for all outpatient physical, occupational and speech therapy services 50% for most outpatient mental health
Clinical Laboratory Services	Unlimited if necessary	Generally 100% of approved amount	Nothing
Home Health Care	Unlimited as long as enrollee meets Medicare conditions	100% of approved amount, 80% of approved amount for durable medical equipment	Nothing for services 20% of approved amount for durable medical equipment
Outpatient Hospital Service	Unlimited if medically necessary	Medicare payment to hospital based on hospital cost	20% of billed amount (after $100 deductible)
Blood	Unlimited if medically necessary	80% of approved amount (after $100 deductible and starting with fourth pint)	For first three pints, then 20% of approved amount for additional pints (after the deductible)

Source: Medicare and You 2000, HCFA

Medicare Part C

The third part, Medicare+Choice program, known as "Part C," started in January 1999. As part of the program, Medicare beneficiaries who have both Part A and Part B can choose to get their benefits through a variety of risk-based plans. The primary Medicare+Choice plans are: (1) coordinated care plans, which includes Health Maintenance Organizations (HMO), Provider-Sponsored Organizations (PSO) and Preferred Provider Organizations (PPO), and (2) other certified public or private coordinated care plans and entities that meet the approved required standards. The Medicare Part C program (Medicare+Choice) has rather complex financing, depending upon which plan is chosen. Basically, the funding for the Medicare+Choice program comes from the HI and SMI trust funds in proportion to the relative weights of HI and SMI benefits to the total benefits paid by the Medicare program. For Part C, the beneficiary's payment share is based upon the cost-sharing structure of the specific Medicare+Choice plan selected by the beneficiary, as each plan has its own requirements. For Part C, payments to the Medicare+Choice plans are based on a blend of local and national capitated rates. Actual payments to plans vary based on characteristics of the enrolled population.[9]

Medicare managed care

Managed care plans function on a basis different from regular fee-for-service covered under Medicare. Under managed care plans, the Medicare beneficiary selects a specific HMO or other approved plans within a service area for comprehensive healthcare services. It is central to the managed care concept that this selected plan coordinates all of the healthcare services for that person. Managed care plans function on a financial basis that is different from the traditional fee-for-service reimbursements to healthcare providers. Managed care plans receive a per-person payment from Medicare that is predetermined, based on a formula that is established by law and the demographic characteristics of the Medicare beneficiaries enrolled in their plan. Generally, this is a percentage of the average adjusted costs per person (AACPP) for the respective region of the country.[9]

In addition to the regular services covered under Medicare, the managed care plans often cover services such as preventive care, prescription drugs, eyeglasses, dental care, or hearing aids. Electing to participate in a managed care plan may also serve as an alternative to purchasing "Medigap insurance." The term "Medigap" is used to mean private health insurance that, within limits, pays most of the healthcare service charges not covered by Parts A or B of Medicare. Although there are certain restrictions, limitations, and differences from the fee-for-service plans, the managed care plan's fixed monthly premiums and cost-sharing structure help to provide more predictability for out-of-pocket costs for the beneficiaries who do not have Medigap insurance.[9]

Beneficiary payment liabilities

For Parts A and B, beneficiaries are responsible for charges not covered by the Medicare program, and for various cost-sharing aspects of both HI and SMI. These liabilities may be paid: (1) by the Medicare beneficiary, (2) by a third party such as private "Medigap" insurance purchased by the Medicare beneficiary, or (3) by Medicaid, if the person is eligible. These policies—which must meet federally imposed standards—are offered by Blue Cross and Blue Shield, and various commercial health insurance companies.[9]

Medicaid

Medicaid is the largest source of funding for medical and health-related services for America's poorest people. In 2000, it provided healthcare assistance to more than 35.6 million persons, at a cost of $210.8 billion dollars.[6] Title XIX of the Social Security Act is a federal-state matching entitlement program that pays for medical assistance for certain vulnerable and needy individuals and families with low incomes and resources.

Within broad national guidelines established by federal statutes, regulations and policies, each state: (1) establishes its own eligibility standards, (2) determines the type, amount, duration, and scope of services, (3) sets the rate of payment for services, and (4) administers its own program. Medicaid policies for eligibility, services, and payment are complex, and vary considerably even among similar-sized and/or adjacent states. Thus, a person who is eligible for Medicaid in one state might not be eligible in another state; the services provided by one state may differ considerably in amount, duration, or scope from services provided in a similar or neighboring state. In addition, Medicaid eligibility and/or services within a state can change during the year.[9]

Medicaid does not provide medical assistance for all poor persons. Even under the broadest provisions of the federal statute, Medicaid does not provide healthcare services even for very poor persons unless they are in one of the designated groups. Of these designations, low income is only one test for Medicaid eligibility for those within these groups; their resources also are tested against threshold levels as determined by each state within federal guidelines. States generally have broad discretion in determining which groups their Medicaid programs will cover and the financial criteria for Medicaid eligibility.[9]

Coverage under the Medicaid program

The Medicaid program allows considerable flexibility. However, some federal requirements are mandatory if federal matching funds are to be received. A state's Medicaid program must offer medical assistance for certain basic services to most categorically needy populations. Within broad federal guidelines and certain limitations, states determine the amount and duration of services offered under their Medicaid programs. States may limit, for example, the number of days of hospital care or the number of physician visits covered. Two restrictions apply: (1) limits must result in a sufficient level of services to reasonably achieve the purpose of the benefits, and (2) limits on benefits may not discriminate among beneficiaries based on medical diagnosis or condition. With some exceptions, a state's Medicaid Plan must allow recipients to have some informed choices among participating providers of health care, and to receive quality care that is appropriate and timely.[9]

Payment for Medicaid services

Medicaid recipients are required to pay relatively small average expenditures each year. The program provides coverage for almost 17 million children, who otherwise would usually receive little or no medical care. The data for 2000 indicates that Medicaid payments for services for these children (who constitute more than 46 percent of all Medicaid recipients) averaged only a little more than $1,000 per child.[9] There are, however, certain other specific groups for whom Medicaid is at least as essential: those comprising far fewer persons, but ones who have much larger per-person expenditures. The Medicaid program pays for almost 45 percent of the total cost of care for persons using nursing home facilities or home health services in the United States.[1] The data for 2000 shows that Medicaid payments for nursing home facilities and home health care totaled $51.8 billion. The 2000 payments for healthcare services for over 35 million Medicaid recipients averaged $5,921 for healthcare expenditures.[1,6]

Medicaid managed care

A significant development in Medicaid is the growth in managed care as an alternative service delivery concept different from the traditional fee-for-service system. Under managed care systems, HMOs, prepaid health plans or comparable entities agree to provide a specific set of services to Medicaid enrollees, usually in return for a predetermined periodic payments per enrollee. Medicaid managed care programs are growing rapidly. The number of Medicaid beneficiaries who are now enrolled in some managed care program continues to increase, and may soon approach 50 percent of all Medicaid enrollees. Several states have converted their entire Medicaid programs into managed care.[9]

Overall cost of the Medicaid program

Medicaid paid for 14.7 percent of all health spending in 2000.[1] Slow spending growth rates over the past four years have led to stability in Medicaid's share of overall health spending. With anticipated impacts from the Balanced Budget Act of 1997, it is projected that total Medicaid outlays may be $250 billion in fiscal year 2003, with an additional $5.8 billion expected to be spent for the Children's Health Insurance Program.[1,9]

Managed care

With the passage of the 1973 Health Maintenance Organization (HMO) Act, healthcare delivery in the United States has experienced tremendous change. This act was the catalyst for the dramatic increase in the number of HMOs and the managed care revolution. Managed care grew out of the concern for increasing healthcare costs and now has a prominent role in health care. Managed care is defined as the provision of health care with a corresponding concern for the appropriate use of resources.[11] Under managed care, financing and delivery of health care is integrated. The assumption of responsibility and accountability for the health of a defined population and the subsequent acceptance of financial risk are the basis for the managed care movement. Managed care organizations are categorized according to the degree of control over cost and the provision of services where both physicians and members are

Figure 1 Consumer cost sharing

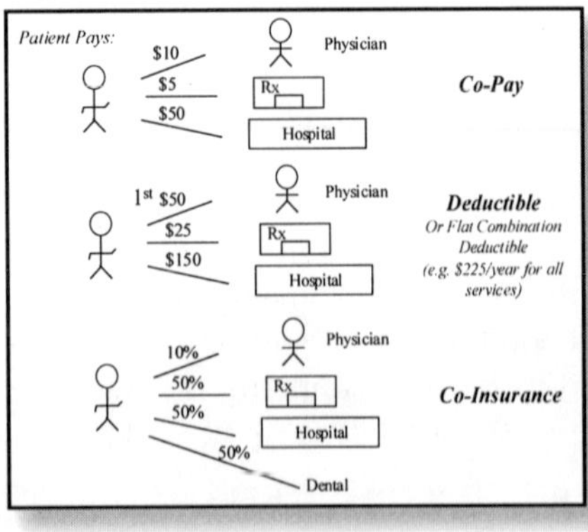

at financial risk.[12] Financial risk for the member results in cost sharing, which may be in the forms of copayments, deductibles or co-insurance (see Figure 1).

Types of Managed Care Organizations (MCOs)

The HMO is the most common MCO. There are various types of health maintenance organizations such as staff, group practice, network, independent/individual practice association (IPA), and direct contract models. These models are differentiated by how the HMO is linked to the providers and the subsequent delivery and access to healthcare services. There are also Preferred Provider Organizations (PPOs), which differ from HMOs by the provision of services (see table 3). For example, the PPO is a homogenous group of providers who collectively offer a single type of service; the HMO is a heterogeneous group of different providers who collectively offers comprehensive health care.[12]

Table 3 HMO models

HMO Models	Linkage of Providers*
Staff	Organizations employ the physicians who provide care to the members
Group	Organizations that contract with multi-specialty physician groups to provide physician services for enrolled members
Network	Organizations that contract with multiple group practice physician groups
Independent/Individual Practice Association (IPA)	Organizations contract with individual physicians to create healthcare delivery systems

*Only physicians are used as providers in the above table; however, providers can include other healthcare professionals such as dentists and pharmacists.

Another type of managed care organization is the Point-of-Service Health Maintenance Organization (POS HMO), which is a hybrid of PPOs and HMOs. In the POS plan, members can obtain care through an HMO provider network for the lowest out-of-pocket cost. If members wish to access the larger PPO network, they are required to pay higher out-of pocket costs. Other types of MCOs are the Exclusive Provider Organization (EPO), which is similar to PPOs but requires members to access only contracted providers, and the physician-hospital organizations (PHOs), which are healthcare delivery systems jointly owned by hospitals and the affiliated physicians. To complicate matters further, in practice, these are not discrete models but mixed models with organizations offering a combination of the above managed care options.[12]

Trends in managed care enrollment

Both the public and private sectors have adopted the managed care trend largely in part as a response to rising healthcare costs and the need to contain cost. MCO enrollment trends are presented in Chart 6. Medicare and Medicaid managed care programs were discussed in previous sections of the chapter. Employees covered by managed care accounted for 89 percent of all insured workers in 1998, up from 53 percent in 1993. When offered a choice of managed care plans, employees are moving away from health maintenance organizations (HMOs) to less restrictive plans such as point-of-service (POS) plans and preferred provider organizations (PPOs). Enrollment in PPO plans rose from 27 percent of total employer-based enrollment plans in 1993 to 43 percent in 1999.[13]

Chart 6 Managed care enrollment

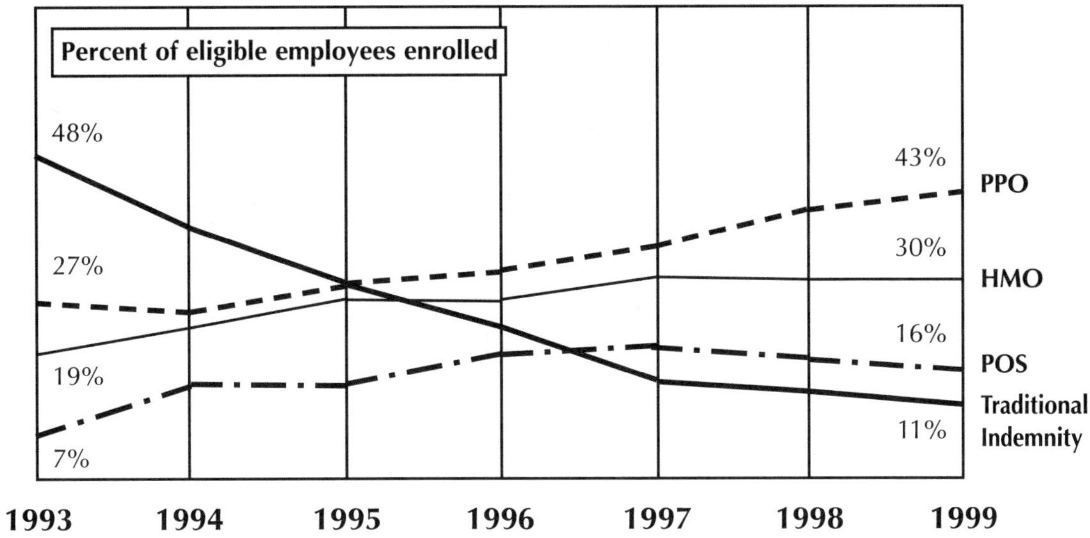

Source: 1999 National Survey of Employer-sponsored Health Plans, Mercer/Foster Higgins

Accreditation

Healthcare payors and providers are increasingly being held accountable for the delivery of quality health care. As a result, healthcare entities must undergo accreditation, which entails documented evaluation that measures whether healthcare institutions meet predefined standards of operation. The accreditation process is like a "seal of approval" indicating to purchasers of healthcare service that institutions meet a competitive standard of quality and value. There are several organizations that accredit healthcare institutions. They include the Joint Commission on Accreditation of Healthcare Organizations (JCAHO, pronounced "jay-co"), the National Committee on Quality Assurance (NCQA), and the American Accreditation Healthcare Commission. The Joint Commission is the oldest and largest accrediting body and is best known for accrediting hospitals and home health agencies. In order to receive Medicaid and Medicare reimbursement, healthcare institutions must meet Joint Commission standards. The government does not require MCOs to be accredited; however, there is a strong incentive for an MCO to demonstrate the quality of the care it provides. NCQA is the most prominent accrediting body for MCOs which use the Health Plan Employer Data and Information Set (HEDIS) system to measure performance of managed care organizations.[12]

Conclusion

Health care in the United States is a complex system that is financed by both private and public funds. Important factors that have influenced and will continue to influence the shape of health care include population characteristics, disease patterns, information technology and medical technology. With advances in pharmaceutical technology, the use and delivery of prescription and nonprescription medications will have a significant impact on health and healthcare delivery in the future. As a result, pharmacy technicians will be utilized in ways that maximizes the use of their knowledge and skills. Therefore, pharmacy technicians must develop a knowledge base consistent with the practice setting and enhance that knowledge though participation in continuing education programs and practice experience.

References

1. National Health Expenditure Projections 1998-2008, www.hcfa.gov/stats/, January 10, 2000.
2. 2000 Annual Reports of the Board of Trustees of the Federal Hospital Insurance and Supplementary Medical Insurance Trust Funds, www.hcfa.gov, April 20, 2000.
3. HCFA Actuarial Data, Health Care Financing Administration, Office of the Actuary, 1998.
4. Bruce Stuart, et. al., "Prescription Drug Costs for Medicare Beneficiaries: Coverage and Health Status Matter," The Commonwealth Fund, January 2000.
5. United States Census Bureau, Current Population Survey, www.uscensus.gov, March 1999.
6. Personal correspondence, Office of the Actuary, Health Care Financing Administration, May 19, 2000.
7. Bennefield, R.L., Dynamics Of Economic Well-Being: Health Insurance, 1993 to 1995 Who Loses Coverage And For How Long? Current Population Report, United States Department of Commerce, June 22, 1998.
8. Blakely, S., Severing The Link Between Health Insurance and Employment: What Happens If Employers Stop Offering Health Benefits?, *EBRI Notes,* Washington, D.C., Vol. 20, No. 3, August 1999, pp. 136-159.
9. Waid, M.C., Brief summaries of Medicare & Medicaid Title XVIII and Title XIX of the Social Security Act, Health Care Financing Administration, Department of Health and Human Services, June 25, 1998.
10. Medicare and You 2000, Health Care Financing Administration, Publication No. HCFA-10118, March 2000.
11. Ito, S.M., Blackburn, S., Pharmacist's Guide to Principles and Practices of Managed Care Pharmacy, Alexandria, VA, 1995, pp. 1-14.
12. Navarro, R.P., Managed Care Pharmacy Practice, Gaithersburg, MD, 1999, pp. 285-301.
13. National Survey of Employer-sponsored Health Plans, Mercer/Foster Higgins, 1999.

About the author

Stephanie D. Taylor received her master's of science degree and doctorate of psychology in Pharmaceutical Administration from Ohio State University and her bachelor's degree in pharmacy from Auburn University, Auburn, Alabama. She completed an administrative hospital pharmacy residency with Riverside Methodist Hospitals in Columbus, Ohio. Dr. Taylor is a faculty associate of the University of Michigan Center on Medication Use, Policy and Economics and an assistant professor of social and administrative sciences at the University of Michigan College of Pharmacy in Ann Arbor, Michigan. Prior to working at the University of Michigan, she was a pharmacy consultant for Assisted Care Partners in Columbus, Ohio, and a critical care pharmacist with Riverside Methodist Hospitals in Columbus, Ohio.

Self-assessment questions

1. It is estimated that _____ million Americans lack healthcare coverage.
   a. 5
   b. 12
   c. 44
   d. 50

2. Approximately what percent of the nation's heathcare dollar is paid out-of-pocket by the patient?
   a. 38 percent
   b. 45 percent
   c. 17 percent
   d. 7 percent

3. The federal health insurance provided to people over the age of 65 is typically covered under which healthcare program?
   a. Medicaid
   b. Medicare
   c. Blue Cross and Blue Shield
   d. Managed care

4. The federal-state health insurance that provides for the basic healthcare services of needy persons is covered under which health care program?
   a. Medicaid
   b. Medicare
   c. Blue Cross and Blue Shield
   d. Managed care

5. Which of the following is ***not*** an example of a managed healthcare organization?
   a. HMO
   b. PPO
   c. POS
   d. FDA

6. Which of the following is true about Medicare?
   a. Dental care is covered.
   b. Cost sharing is required.
   c. It is administered by the Food and Drug Administration.
   d. It only covers persons age 65 and older.

7. Medicare Part C is also referred to as:
   a. Medicare Managed Care.
   b. BBA.
   c. Managed Care for Medicare (MCM).
   d. Medicare Plus Choice/Medicare+Choice.

8. Which of the following is ***not*** true about Medicaid?
   a. Each state establishes its own Medicaid eligibility standards.
   b. Medicaid provides coverage for nearly 17 million children.
   c. Medicaid accounted for 14.7 percent of the nation's healthcare dollar in the year 2000.
   d. Medicaid provides medical assistance for all poor persons.

9. Managed care organizations are primarily accredited by what accrediting entity?
   a. MCO
   b. JCAHO
   c. NCQA
   d. HCFA

10. Accreditation measures were developed for health care organizations to assure that:
    a. healthcare programs receive appropriate reimbursement.
    b. high quality services are provided in healthcare.
    c. licenses are granted to healthcare providers.
    d. healthcare costs are contained.

CHAPTER
2

TRAINING, EDUCATION AND CERTIFICATION FOR PHARMACY TECHNICIANS

Dianne E. Miller, R.Ph., and Jennifer L. Pakkala, B.A.

Learning objectives

Upon completion of this chapter, the technician should be able to do the following:

- ♦ List the skills and knowledge that should be obtained before performing the functions of a certified pharmacy technician.
- ♦ List the different methods of obtaining educational training to become a pharmacy technician and describe the advantages of each method.
- ♦ Explain the difference between certification and licensure.
- ♦ Describe the role of PTCB.

Introduction

The increasing involvement of pharmacists with patient care activities has increased the need for fully trained and qualified pharmacy technicians who are able to assume the more technical roles in pharmacies to relieve the pharmacist of these functions.

Employment opportunities for pharmacy technicians have been greatly expanded over the last several years and the trend is expected to continue. Substantial growth in the technician work force will be needed to meet these demands; therefore, the outlook for pharmacy technicians is very promising.

Certain skills and knowledge are needed to be a pharmacy technician. The following section provides a list briefly describing skills that, according to several pharmacy educators and state and national pharmacy organizations, are deemed necessary to have in order to perform the duties of a pharmacy technician.

Controlling inventory

Pharmacy technicians need to know how to account for medications, equipment, devices, and supplies within the pharmacy practice. Inventory control involves much more than counting the number of items on a shelf or tablets in a bottle.

With respect to inventory control, pharmacy technicians need to know how to:

- Follow established policies and procedures of inventory control.
- Handle the receipt, storage, and removal of items.
- Document their activities when receiving, storing, and removing items.
- Identify items that need to be ordered when supply is low or a demand is anticipated.
- Locate a needed item when it is not readily available at the pharmacy.
- Communicate problems and concerns regarding inventory to the pharmacist in charge.
- Maintain a secure inventory to prevent and deter theft both by patients and staff.

Receiving prescriptions or medication orders

When receiving a prescription from a patient/patient's representative, prescriber, or other healthcare professional, the pharmacy technician must know how to read the prescription correctly to avoid errors such as an overdose or dispensing the wrong medication.

A technician must:

- Know the procedures for receiving and ordering prescriptions or medication orders.
- Assess the prescription or medication order for completeness with respect to such items as patient, physician, medication information, and dosing instructions.
- Assess the prescription or medication order for accuracy, authenticity, legality, and reimbursement eligibility.
- At the direction of a pharmacist, add missing information to the prescription or medication order when appropriate or alert a pharmacist when an incomplete prescription has been received.
- Communicate effectively when receiving a prescription or medication order.

Processing prescriptions or medication orders

The pharmacy technician plays an important role through filling prescriptions or medication orders. By completing the dispensing process, technicians allow pharmacists to spend more time providing patient-focused care.

When filling a prescription or medication order, the technician is responsible for:

- Understanding his or her role and the role of the pharmacist in the drug distribution process.
- Knowing the proper procedures for retrieving drugs from inventory and preparing medications.
- Following safety and quality assurance procedures to ensure the integrity of the medications and the workplace.
- Being proficient in calculating and measuring medications.
- Labeling drug products accurately, adding auxiliary labels when necessary.
- Practicing correct methods of handling hazardous wastes, sharps, and infectious materials.
- Recording the prescription or medication order in the patient's profile.
- Abiding by the laws, regulations, and standards that govern the preparation of medications for dispensing.

Compounding

Before there were pharmaceutical manufacturers, pharmacists made medications through combining the chemical ingredients—compounding. Even though the overwhelming majority of drugs are already prepared, this method of preparing medications by hand is still alive and well in community pharmacies, since some patients require special or unique doses, forms, or flavors of medicines that are not commercially available. In the institutional setting, compounding also involves the preparation of intravenous solutions, parenteral nutrition, and chemotherapy solutions.

Today, many pharmacy technicians are relied upon to perform this specialized task. The certified pharmacy technician should be proficient in all types of compounding, which includes the preparation of sterile, non-sterile, cytotoxic, and hazardous drug products.

Compounding requires that a pharmacy technician:

- Calculate the appropriate amount of each ingredient using correct and appropriate techniques.
- Accurately measure the appropriate ingredients as permitted by state laws.
- Know the compatibility, stability, and storage requirements for chemicals within a compounded medication.
- Apply quality assurance procedures described in the Good Manufacturing Practices as defined in the United States Pharmacopeia National Formulary (USP-NF). (See Chapter 28 on Operations and Medication Control.)

- Work in accordance with laws, regulations, and standards that govern the preparation of compounded products.

Maintaining pharmacy records

Included in the process of drug distribution is careful record keeping for the purposes of controlling inventory levels and maintaining patient profiles. The pharmacy technician is largely responsible for creating and maintaining such records.

To maintain accurate drug distribution records, the pharmacy technician must:
- Be proficient in using the pharmacy's computer database to enter, retrieve, and maintain information.
- Know the methods for distributing medications and recording their distribution in various practice settings.
- Follow the laws, regulations, and standards as they pertain to entering, retrieving and maintaining patient profiles.

Supporting pharmaceutical care

With the implementation of pharmaceutical care, pharmacy technicians will be called upon to assume greater roles in the pharmacy so pharmacists can spend more time interacting with patients.

Pharmacy technicians can assist a pharmaceutical care practice in a variety of ways. Technicians can:
- Understand the importance of pharmacist-patient consultations.
- Know the legal requirements (such as OBRA '90) for pharmacist-patient consultations.
- Complete pharmacy tasks within the scope of a pharmacy technician's practice that allow a pharmacist to spend time providing patient-focused care.
- Help the pharmacist identify patients who desire or require counseling on medication use, equipment, and/or devices.
- Develop techniques to effectively ask patients if they desire or need to be counseled by a pharmacist.

Billing third party insurers

A patient paying for a prescription with cash is a rarity; most patients' medications are covered by insurance companies, and it is the insurance company (a third party payor) that then reimburses the pharmacy. Each insurance company has different requirements for billing and receiving reimbursement, which may be continually revised.

To effectively bill and receive reimbursement for pharmacy services, a technician must:
- Determine how patients intend to pay for the pharmacy goods or services they will receive.
- Verify a patient is covered by an insurance company.
- Know the methods of payment and operating techniques of third party payors.
- Be familiar with the products and services covered by insurance companies.
- Correctly bill and collect payment for pharmacy goods and services.
- Know which items are taxable and which are not.

Monitoring patients

Increasingly, pharmacy professionals are playing a role in monitoring a patient's progress during their drug therapy.

Advancing patient care through drug therapy monitoring means pharmacy technicians will need to:
- Understand the purpose of a monitoring program.
- Assist the pharmacist's monitoring of a patient's drug therapy by learning to perform specific monitoring activities.
- Know how to use the computer database to aid in patient monitoring.
- Follow the laws, regulations, and standards governing the confidentiality of patient information.

Using pharmacy equipment

Proper use and maintenance of equipment and devices used in the pharmacy will help keep these mechanisms working properly and ensure safety for patients and pharmacy staff members.

Properly using pharmacy equipment means that the pharmacy technician should:

- Know how to maintain, troubleshoot, and repair pharmacy equipment and devices.
- Be able to clean a laminar airflow cabinet and a vertical flow hood (chemotherapy hood).
- Know how to calibrate commonly used equipment and devices.

Storing medications

Pharmacy professionals constantly relay the importance of proper drug storage to their patients to preserve the properties of the medications.

This holds true for the pharmacy as well, both for medications that are already on the market and investigational drugs. This means the pharmacy technician must:

- Learn the storage requirements of all medications carried in the pharmacy, including repackaged medications and investigational drugs.
- Know the legal storage requirements for controlled substances.
- Understand how pharmacy practice settings contribute to the development of new drug products.
- Know the policies and procedures involved when filling an order for an investigational drug product.
- Assist the pharmacist in the preparation, storage, and distribution of investigational drugs.
- Complete the required paperwork to record the preparation and distribution of investigational drug products.

Educational opportunities

Individuals who are interested in becoming pharmacy technicians should appropriately evaluate all available opportunities that support their interest to become a qualified pharmacy technician. The following will briefly describe various options that prepare individuals to serve in the role of a pharmacy technician.

Individuals who desire to become pharmacy technicians should exhibit excellent mathematical abilities, communication skills, and problem-solving techniques. Foreign language skills may be beneficial when the pharmacy has a large population of patients who don't speak the common language of the area. These characteristics will serve as a strong foundation to build upon when pursuing specialized education developed for technicians. A variety of educational programs are available and should be chosen based upon commitment to advancing a career as a pharmacy professional and devotion to obtaining an education.

College

Most states have community colleges that offer one- to two-year pharmacy technician educational programs. The one- and two-year programs usually consist of two and four, 15-week semesters, respectively. Most programs not only include a didactic (instructional) portion, but also offer practical experience.

Didactic pharmacy courses may include topics such as: pharmacy operations, institutional pharmacy, ambulatory pharmacy, pharmacology, introduction to pharmaceutical concepts, drug distribution systems and procedures, administration of medications, law and ethics, pharmacy calculations, inventory controls, and field experience.

Required supportive courses might include biology, microbiology, general and organic chemistry, interpersonal relations, communications, economics, composition, medical terminology, computer literacy, algebra, and trigonometry. Course topics and program requirements will vary between educational institutions and length of the educational program.

The practical or field experience ranges from 10 to 30 weeks of internship and involves 12 to 15 educational contact hours per week. At the minimum, the practical experience involves performing functional tasks in a laboratory simulation, but can be as elaborate as actually working at a pharmacy practice site under faculty supervision. Obviously, two-year programs not only have a more intensive didactic course outline, but also offer a more in-depth practical experience.

Several advantages exist for those pursuing a college-developed, technician training program. Individuals who complete one-year programs usually receive a certificate, while two-year programs usually result in an associate's degree. In addition, some course credits from two-year programs can be transferred to apply toward a pharmacy degree for those who later choose to become a pharmacist.

Military training

Pharmacy technician educational opportunities exist within the United States armed forces. Military technician training programs have similar curriculum content and contact hours to civilian programs; however, practical experiences tend to be more innovative than the average practice setting.

The curriculum outline might include topics such as: pharmacy administration, pharmaceutical calculations, pharmacy compounding, pharmacology, computers and typing, dispensing, supply services, sterile products, and a clinical rotation. Average contact hours range between 600-800 hours, including didactic courses and field experience.

Advantages to military training may include worldwide travel and pharmacy experiences not normally available at traditional practice sites. Due to the nature of government armed services, military personnel are commonly exposed to cutting-edge technology. Depending on the branch of service, an individual in the military would obtain a variety of life skills in addition to technician training.

Vocational schools

Another avenue to obtain educational training is through vocational schools or adult education programs. Vocational institutions are usually privately owned and may or may not be bound by state educational requirements. The primary goal of a vocational school is to train an individual to perform a job and be employable upon completion of the program. Due to the wide variety of educational programs taught at vocational schools, the programs offered usually have a limited curriculum, focusing on fundamental skills that prepare students for employment.

Vocational education offers many advantages. The educational programs tend to be based on a more practical level, highlighting the functional skills that must be acquired to perform the duties of a pharmacy technician. Individuals who are beginning their careers or re-engineering an old one as a result of job displacement find vocational schools to be an efficient and effective method to obtain new job skills and enhance their employment marketability. Many high schools have even developed programs that allow students to begin their vocational training during the school year.

Adult education programs usually focus on subject matters rather than complete educational programs. They can serve as introductory courses or provide supplemental knowledge to strengthen an area of weakness. Adult education provides an opportunity to meet the needs of nontraditional students who cannot afford to make full-time commitments to their education. Another advantage to adult education is that it is usually very economical.

Independent study

Some individuals have elected to complete independent study courses to enhance their knowledge base of the responsibilities of a pharmacy technician. These reference materials, Internet-based programs, or video courses can be used to supplement on-the-job training opportunities in preparation for the national certification examination. Independent study would be very challenging for individuals who have not had prior pharmacy experience.

Independent study materials can be obtained through many pharmacy-related organizations. These references have been found to be very beneficial when utilized as a study guide to prepare for the certification exam. Another advantage to independent studies is the freedom from time constraints because they can be completed at one's convenience.

While many educational opportunities exist for individuals interested in pursuing a career as a pharmacy technician, the educational trend has been moving toward formalized education. This trend is expected to continue and become more necessary as the responsibilities of the pharmacy technician increase with the pharmacist's involvement in patient care.

Certification

Various recognitions of a professional's knowledge, including credentialing, accrediting, certifying, licensing, or registering can be achieved upon completion of formalized educational or training programs. It is important to understand the definitions of these terms to make an informed decision when choosing a career path.

The American Society of Health-System Pharmacists' Task Force on Technical Personnel in Pharmacy has compiled definitions of these terms:

Credentialing: The general process of formally recognizing professional or technical competence.

Accreditation: The process of granting recognition or vouching for conformance with a standard (usually refers to recognition of an institution).

Certification: The process by which a non-governmental agency or association grants recognition to an individual who has met certain predetermined qualifications specified by that agency or association.

Licensure: The process by which an agency of government grants permission to an individual to engage in a given occupation upon finding that the applicant has attained the minimal degree of competency necessary to ensure that the public health, safety, and welfare will be reasonably well protected.

Registering: The process of making a list or being enrolled in an existing list. (In an occupational setting, it may or may not be illegal to carry out a particular function without being registered.)

While different states have different requirements, the national Pharmacy Technician Certification Board (PTCB) certification program is the only national certification program currently available and the most widely accepted recognition for pharmacy technicians within the United States. PTCB was founded in January 1995 by the American Pharmaceutical Association (APhA), the American Society of Health-System Pharmacists (ASHP), the Illinois Council of Health-System Pharmacists, and the Michigan Pharmacists Association. The goal of PTCB was to create a consolidated, voluntary, national certification program for pharmacy technicians that would promote consistency throughout the country.

While PTCB is responsible for the development and implementation of policies related to national certification for pharmacy technicians, the Professional Examination Service (PES), which specializes in the development and administration of national certification and licensure examinations, is the company that administers the PTCB certification examination. The examination contains 125 multiple-choice questions, each with four options but only one best answer. The questions randomly address different functional areas from all practice settings to test the technician's knowledge base. The functional areas addressed on the exam fall into three major categories: assisting the pharmacist in serving patients, maintaining medication and inventory control systems, and participating in the administration and management of pharmacy practice. The final exam score is based upon the number of correctly answered questions so testing candidates should attempt to choose an answer for each question.

As previously discussed, the preparation leading to national certification of a pharmacy technician can vary greatly, dependent upon the individual's experience with the profession of pharmacy. In all cases, candidates who elect to take the national certification examination must possess either a high school diploma or general equivalency diploma (GED) before an application can be submitted. PTCB Candidate Handbooks, which include applications for the exam, can be obtained directly from PTCB and many state professional pharmacy organizations. The Candidate Handbook provides complete information on the PTCB certification processes: eligibility requirements, application procedures, the examination, and recertification (maintaining certification or renewal).

Summary of PTCB recertification (renewal) process

- PTCB certification must be renewed every two years.
- Twenty (20) contact hours of technician-appropriate continuing education are required for recertification; one (1) must be in pharmacy law.
- All continuing education must be earned within the two-year certification period and may not be completed after the expiration date.
- Recertification materials will be sent to certified technicians approximately 60 days before the certification expiration date.
- Appropriate recertification fees must be paid.
- Audits are conducted randomly by PTCB. If audited, provide a list of all continuing education hours on the application and send copies of the continuing education certificates as proof of completion.

Individuals who meet all eligibility requirements and successfully pass the examination are awarded the privilege of using the title of "CPhT" following their name, which represents the designation of "Certified Pharmacy Technician." Once certification is achieved, recertification (renewal) is required every two years. A total of 20 contact hours of technician-appropriate continuing education in pharmacy-related topics is required within the two-year period. At least one contact hour must be in the area of pharmacy law each renewal period.

Acceptable pharmacy technician continuing education can be obtained through a variety of methods. Acceptable continuing education certificates for certified pharmacy technicians include the American Council on Pharmaceutical Education (ACPE) certificate of Continuing Pharmaceutical Education Participation; the American Association of Pharmacy Technicians (AAPT) certificate of Continuing Education Service Participation; the PTCB Universal Continuing Education Form; and certificates of participation generated by other national, state and local pharmacy professional organizations, state boards of pharmacy, or educational organizations.

Individuals who are interested in becoming certified pharmacy technicians or who would like additional information should contact any of the following organizations:

American Association of Pharmacy Technicians
P.O. Box 1447
Greensboro, NC 27402
(336) 275-1700; FAX (336) 275-7222
www.pharmacytechnician.com

American Pharmaceutical Association
2215 Constitution Avenue NW
Washington, DC 20037-2985
(800) 237-APhA; (202) 628-4410; FAX (202) 783-2351
www.aphanet.org

American Society of Health-System Pharmacists
7272 Wisconsin Avenue
Bethesda, MD 20814
(301) 657-3000; FAX (301) 657-8817
www.ashp.com

Illinois Council of Health-System Pharmacists
4430 Manchester Drive
Suite G2
Rockford, IL 61109
(815) 227-9292; FAX (815) 227-9294
www.ichpnet.org

Michigan Pharmacists Association
815 N. Washington Avenue
Lansing, MI 48906-5198
(517) 484-1466; FAX (517) 484-4893
www.mipharm.com

National Pharmacy Technician Association
3920 FM 1960 W, Suite 240
Houston, TX 77068
(281) 866-7900; FAX (281) 895-7320
www.pharmacytechnician.org

Pharmacy Technician Certification Board
2215 Constitution Avenue NW
Washington, DC 20037-2985
(202) 429-7576; FAX (202) 429-7596
www.ptcb.org

Pharmacy Technician Educators Council
1426 Prince Street
Alexandria, VA 22314
(703) 739-2330; (605) 394-4034, extension 308; FAX (703) 836-8982
www.mbnet.mb.ca/ptec

Conclusion

As pharmacists' roles shift toward patient care activities, knowledgeable pharmacy technicians will be instrumental in executing the more technical functions that were once only performed by pharmacists. In Chapters 6 and 7, the direction of pharmacy will be more fully discussed, which will help you to understand why technicians with the proper education and training, as well as Certified Pharmacy Technicians, will be essential in the pharmacy.

References

1. American Society of Health-System Pharmacists Task Force, Model Curriculum for Pharmacy Technician Training, American Society of Health-System Pharmacists, Bethesda, MD, 1996.
2. Communication from Ronald Lukasiewicz, McAuley Pharmacy Inc., to the author. May 2, 1997.

3. American Pharmaceutical Association, American Society of Health-System Pharmacists, "White Paper on Pharmacy Technicians," Journal of the American Pharmaceutical Association, Washington, DC, Vol NS36, No. 8, pp. 515-120, August 1996.

4. Pharmacy Technician Certification Board, 2000 Candidate Handbook-National Pharmacy Technician Certification Examination, Pharmacy Technician Certification Board, Washington, DC, 2000.

5. Flanagan, M., "Voluntary Technician Certification Program Reflects Changes in Practice," American Pharmacy, Washington, DC, Vol. NS35, No. 5, pp. 18-23, May 1995.

About the authors

Dianne E. Miller received her bachelor's degrees in pharmacy and applied biology in 1987 from Ferris State University in Big Rapids, Michigan. She has completed a variety of certificate courses and post-graduate training, including the University of Pittsburgh's Smoking Cessation Specialist Certification Program, the National Institute for Pharmacists Outcomes Osteoporosis Care Certificate Program, University of Tennessee's Asthma Patient Management Certificate Program, American Pharmaceutical Association's Pharmacy-Based Immunization Delivery Certificate Course, and Central Michigan University master's level courses in administration. Miller is the Associate Executive Director at the Michigan Pharmacists Association in Lansing, Michigan. Prior to joining the staff at the association, she was a staff pharmacist for Ingham Regional Medical Center in Lansing, Michigan, where she continues to work as a relief pharmacist.

Jennifer L. Pakkala is the Director of Marketing & Communications for the Michigan Pharmacists Association in Lansing, Michigan, where she is responsible for expressing the association's positions to pharmacy professionals, healthcare professionals and the general public. She received her bachelor's degree in journalism from Michigan State University in 1993.

Self-assessment questions

1. Which functions would be ***not*** appropriate for a pharmacy technician to complete?
   a. Compound an ointment
   b. Prepare an intravenous solution
   c. Obtain a patient's insurance information
   d. Counsel a patient about their prescription

2. Certification can be defined as a:
   a. process of granting recognition or vouching for conformance with a standard.
   b. process of formally recognizing professional or technical competence.
   c. process by which a non-governmental agency or association grants recognition to an individual who has met certain predetermined qualifications.
   d. process of making a list or being enrolled in an existing list.

3. Vocational schools offer all of the following advantages except:
   a. highlighting functional skills.
   b. providing students with associate's degrees.
   c. serving as a tool for re-engineering.
   d. improving employment opportunities.

4. How many continuing education credits are required for recertification (renewal)?
   a. 5
   b. 10
   c. 20
   d. 30

5. Recertification (renewal) for certified pharmacy technicians (CPhTs) occurs every______years.
   a. one
   b. two
   c. three
   d. five

CHAPTER 3

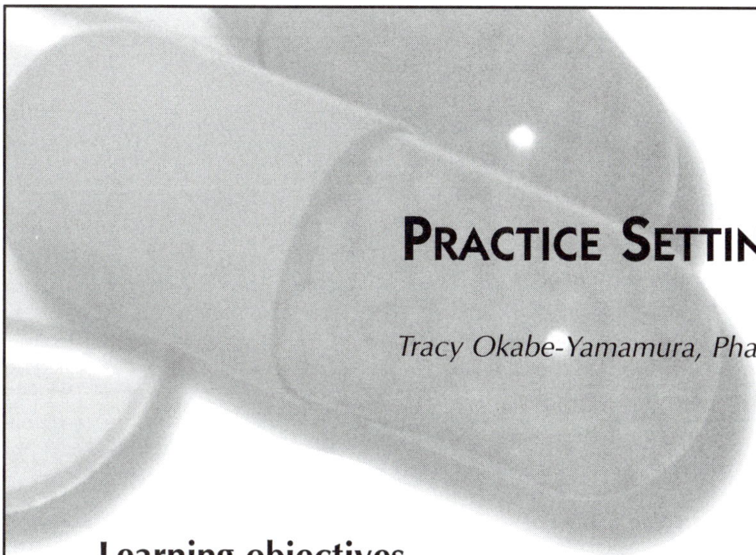

PRACTICE SETTINGS

Tracy Okabe-Yamamura, Pharm.D.

Learning objectives

Upon completion of this chapter, the technician should be able to do the following:

- Understand the different practice sites for a pharmacist or pharmacy technician.
- Know the difference between institutional and ambulatory practice for a pharmacist or pharmacy technician.
- Name the four criteria for classifying hospitals or institutions.
- Understand Internet pharmacy and the role of the pharmacist and pharmacy technician.

Introduction

Pharmacy technicians work in a variety of practice settings that are of two general types: ambulatory (community, outpatient, retail) settings and institutional (hospital, extended care facility, nursing home) settings.[1] There are also some practice settings that overlap ambulatory and institutional practice. Each type of practice setting allows for areas of specialization. In all practice settings, pharmacy personnel share the same professional objectives. These objectives include the preparation and provision of properly packaged and labeled medications according to federal and state laws for the care of the sick or injured. In all areas, a pharmacist provides patient counseling to ensure that the customers/patients are well informed about their medication(s). This information includes the indication for use, the dosing regimen, and potential side effects.

Pharmacy technicians are vital pharmacy personnel members. Well-trained pharmacy technicians have a working knowledge and understanding of pharmaceutical and medical terms along with the general chemical and physical properties of drugs. Technicians can be involved with the essential functions related to drug purchasing and inventory control, repackaging and labeling of drug products, aseptic compounding, parenteral admixture operations, and contemporary drug distribution systems.[2] In addition, technicians may work in a variety of different practice settings that are outside the traditional pharmacy setting such as in managed care, Internet pharmacy, or with industry (pharmaceutical companies). Because of their skilled training, pharmacists rely on pharmacy technicians to help them with multiple tasks associated with pharmacy operations. Pharmacy technicians must be able to work efficiently and accurately, follow written policies and procedures (see Chapter 29), and work with minimal supervision by a pharmacist. Technicians, however, do not make independent professional judgments on matters that by law are the domain of the pharmacist. Also, they are not responsible for communicating drug information to patients.[1]

Following is a brief introduction to the ambulatory and institutional practice settings; a complete description of each setting will be found in Chapters 4 and 5, respectively.

Ambulatory pharmacy practice

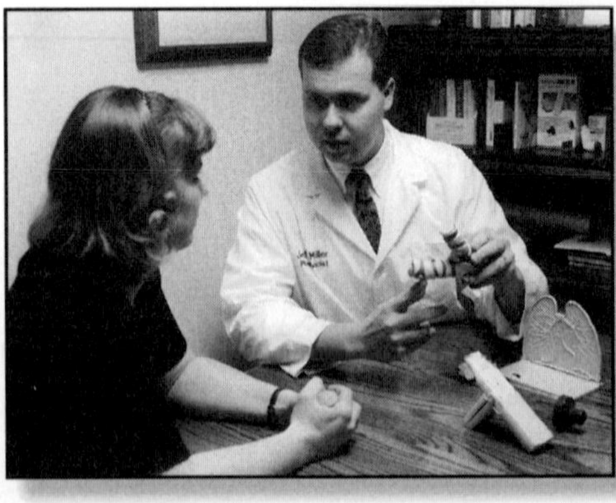

Ambulatory pharmacy practice includes the non-acute settings of community pharmacies, clinics, managed care settings, and mail order pharmacy services. Community pharmacies include privately owned pharmacies, chain pharmacies (corporate), and clinic pharmacies. They are readily accessible to the public and are in an excellent position to establish a professional and positive rapport with their patients and community. Some community pharmacies provide special services such as home delivery or individual charge accounts that are not available in other locations. Additional clinical services include blood pressure checks and immunizations. In ambulatory clinic settings, pharmacists can be involved in a variety of activities such as monitoring a patient's blood thinning medications and cholesterol, teaching patients about asthma and diabetes, and analyzing patients for risk of developing bone loss. Pharmacy technicians in these settings provide a variety of professional and clerical duties.

Pharmacy technicians working in the managed care setting such as a Health Maintenance Organization (HMO) or Preferred Provider Organization (PPO) clinic pharmacy may serve a specialized group of ambulatory patients. Pharmacy technicians often work closely with clinical pharmacists in assuring appropriate utilization of drug therapy. Pharmacists are often responsible for reviewing and analyzing pharmacy data received from the HMO and providing feedback of pharmacy prescribing performance to physicians. Educational programs can be developed on a formal or informal basis related to specific prescribing issues such as the utilization of non-sedating antihistamines in the treatment of allergies or the use of outpatient antibiotics for upper respiratory conditions. Programs like these are designed to provide physicians with best practice guidelines to assist in the most appropriate prescribing practices. In addition, pharmacists may design programs involving self-injectable medications to ensure proper utilization. Refill clinics may be established and operated by a pharmacist to manage pharmacy utilization. Pharmacy technicians can be responsible for prior authorization. Prior authorization is a service that the health plan maintains as part of the pharmacy benefit. For certain medications, specific criteria for use may be developed. The prior authorization process is used to ensure that patients meet the established criteria before the medication is dispensed at the community pharmacy.[3]

Mail order pharmacies provide services to patients similar to a community, retail, or chain pharmacy. Technicians provide clerical or professional support to pharmacists from a main distribution center that services a large population of patients and health providers. Since medications are provided to patients via the mail, technicians in this setting interact mostly with other workers and do not have direct patient contact.

Institutional pharmacy services

Pharmacy support personnel who practice in an acute care setting, such as a hospital, have limited visibility to patients compared to their counterparts practicing in an ambulatory (or non-acute) setting. Acute care pharmacy services may differ in scope and complexity from those of ambulatory pharmacy. There is some overlap, however, between acute and non-acute pharmacy practice in the type of services provided, as well as the need to provide seamless health care for patients as they transition back and forth between ambulatory, home, or institutional care. In most regions, hospital lengths of stay are decreasing as patients are sent home or to other non-acute settings to complete their recovery process. The intensity of service for hospitalized patients has increased as less severe illnesses are treated on an outpatient basis. Therefore, the continuity of care for patients between acute and non-acute care is especially important.

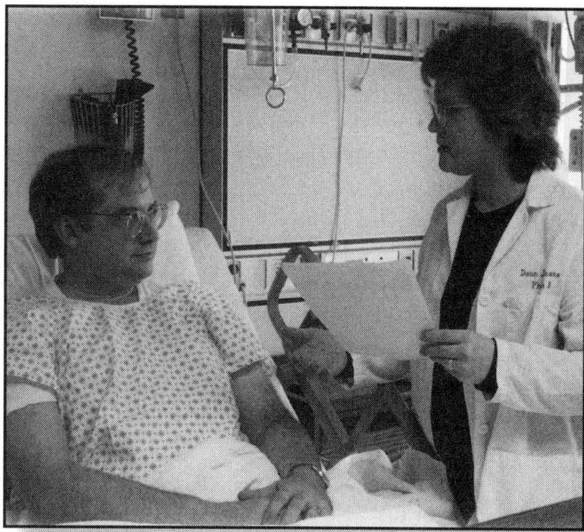

Healthcare institutions (hospitals) are classified by four criteria:[1]

- scope of service (general or specialty)
- length of patient stay (acute or chronic)
- ownership (government, private, corporations)
- bed capacity

Combinations of these criteria can influence the nature of the pharmacy within the institution and the type of services that the pharmacy provides. Government ownership may be at any level (federal, state, county, or municipal). Non-governmental ownership may be by church, fraternal organizations, or community. The type of ownership of a hospital can affect the type of medical and pharmacy services provided because they are dependent upon the policies or finances of the owning group.

Most institutional pharmacies provide a broad range of services including parenteral (non-oral) admixtures, unit-dose distribution, and patient drug dosing and therapy monitoring. Pharmacy technicians play a key role in many activities of an inpatient pharmacy. Technicians are usually responsible for preparation of IV piggybacks, syringes, or large volume parenterals, as well as chemotherapy doses. Technicians who fill patient cassettes with the appropriate medications accomplish unit-dose distribution. In addition, technicians may be responsible for the maintenance of automated dispensing units (such as a Pyxis or SureMed device). There may be opportunities for pharmacy technicians to be a part of a patient, drug therapy-monitoring care team working on a specific nursing unit. There have been reports of institutions that have developed clinical duties for technicians such as calculating creatinine clearances or reviewing certain lab values as a way to streamline pharmacist activities.

Long-term care facilities[1]

A long-term care (LTC) facility may be a nursing home or skilled nursing facility (SNF). Generally, patients may remain in these facilities for extended periods of time, and the complexity of medication regimens and the frequency of medication change is less compared to a hospital. The LTC facility provides nursing and other health- or social-related services to the chronically ill or elderly. Technicians help with drug preparation and distribution, and may assist the pharmacist with some aspects of clinical monitoring of patient drug therapy.

Home care[4]

Home care pharmacies provide pharmaceutical products and clinical monitoring services to patients of all ages in their homes, including home infusion therapy, oral medications, home hospice pharmaceutical services, and parenteral and enteral nutrition. Pharmacists practicing in home care pharmacies provide a specialized form of pharmaceutical care to the patients they serve. Infusion services may be based in hospitals, long-term care pharmacies, or community pharmacies or operated by independent or multi-site organizations and are an integral part of the overall continuity of patient care. A variety of medical conditions are treated at home following a short hospitalization or while avoiding hospitalization altogether. Pharmacy technicians practicing in a home infusion pharmacy may compound medications in a variety of delivery systems such as intravenous bags, syringes and portable pump devices.

Other pharmacy practice settings

There are other classifications of pharmacy practice settings that cannot be neatly included with either the ambulatory or institutional pharmacy categories. These settings, which tend to be highly specialized, are discussed below.

Nuclear pharmacy[5]

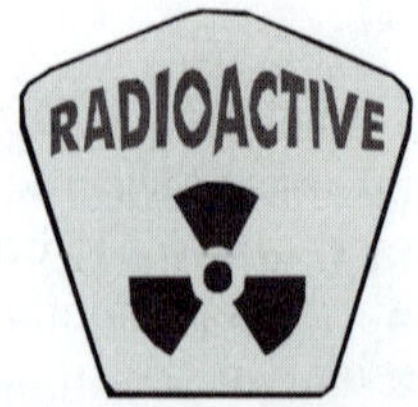

Nuclear pharmacy is a practice setting that incorporates the safe and effective use of radioactive pharmaceuticals for diagnosis and treatment. Radioactive pharmaceuticals contain small amounts of unstable, or radioactive, elements. With proper handling, the use of radioactive elements is very safe and can be used in a variety of diagnostic imaging tests and therapeutic treatment regimens for certain disease states. A nuclear pharmacist is a licensed pharmacist who has received specialized training in the practice of nuclear pharmacy. In this setting, pharmacy technicians compound special doses and control the inventory and storage of these agents.

Internet pharmacy[7]

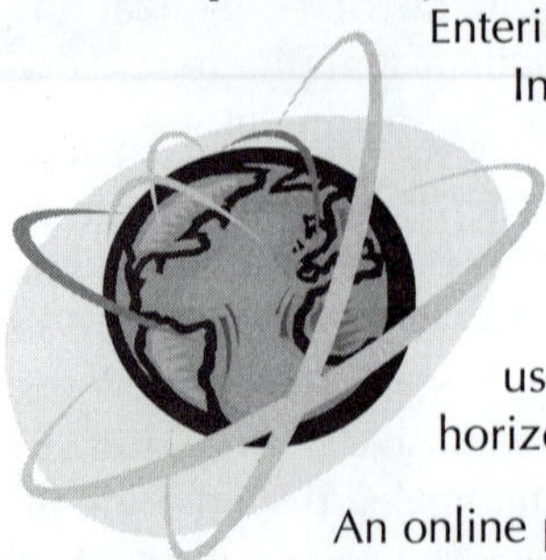

Entering the 21st century, there is an exciting trend in the development of Internet pharmacy. The principal advantage of Internet pharmacies is the convenience of shopping for prescription and nonprescription items from the comfort and privacy of home. Easy access to health information is also an extremely important feature. As consumers become more actively involved in the maintenance of their health and more savvy with the use of personal computers, a greater number of opportunities are on the horizon for both pharmacists and pharmacy technicians.

An online pharmacy must meet the specified requirements for every state to which it intends to dispense medications. It *cannot* and *should not* dispense medications without receiving a valid prescription.

The federal government, in cooperation with the National Association of Boards of Pharmacy (NABP) and professional pharmacy associations, will determine how to provide oversight to online pharmacies. One way to determine if an online pharmacy is operating legitimately and has met all the rules and regulations required to legally dispense medications is to look for the Verified Internet Pharmacy Practice Site (VIPPS) symbol awarded by the NABP. Information about this credential can be reviewed at the NABP website (*http://vipps.nabp.net/verify.asp*). As of January 1, 2001, 15 online pharmacies had been awarded the prestigious VIPPS credential.

Opportunities for pharmacists in Internet pharmacy include dispensing medications, participating in the technical aspects of website development, providing drug information to consumers, and developing informational content, including disease management guidelines. Pharmacy technicians are also vital for the efficient functioning of an Internet pharmacy, including assisting with the dispensing process and becoming involved with technical projects in website development.

Internet pharmacies have only scratched the surface of opportunities that will become available in cyberspace. Analysts estimate that by the year 2004, consumers will be spending an estimated $10 billion for health-related items purchased over the Internet. As personal computing becomes a more integrated part of society over the coming years, the need for pharmacists and pharmacy technicians in cyberspace will certainly increase.

Industry

The pharmaceutical industry is another area of pharmacy practice where pharmacy technicians are utilized. Because of their knowledge of medications, pharmacy technicians may find employment opportunities as a research assistant or a sales representative for a pharmaceutical company or a wholesaler. Pharmacists in this setting may practice as clinical liaisons and can be involved with pharmacoeconomic studies, outcomes research, and disease state management. Technicians can assist physicians, pharmacists, and other healthcare providers with tools to improve patient care and outcomes.

Pharmacy support companies[6]

Pharmacy technicians may work for organizations whose products support pharmacy practice. An example would be a company that provides automated distribution systems for pharmacy or materials management. Technicians in this role can be intimately involved with driving product development, an ongoing process from inception to release of the product to market. Product development can be a complex process involving both project planning and development. By interacting with customers, sales and field operations, and evaluating the competitive development in the marketplace, technicians may help develop new software features, software feature enhancements, new hardware, or a whole new product. The pharmacy technician can aid in facilitating project development, completing quality assurance activities, and managing the testing of the software or product.

Academia

As pharmacy technician training becomes more formalized, there is an increased need for experienced pharmacy technicians to teach tomorrow's technicians. Many community colleges that offer associate's degrees for successful completion of pharmacy technician training programs are utilizing technicians as instructors.

Conclusion

The practice of pharmacy was once merely thought of as the "corner drugstore," but changes in the way health care is delivered have expanded the practice site choices for pharmacists and technicians alike. Pharmacy professionals are creating new roles in ambulatory, institutional, and all other classifications of pharmacy practice. The rapid changes in health care will dictate a constant expansion of the profession of pharmacy, and these changes will provide many opportunities for those individuals who choose to enter the profession.

References

1. Pharmacy Certified Technician Training Manual, Michigan Pharmacists Association, Lansing, MI, 1997, p. 35.
2. Practice Standards of ASHP 1995-96, American Society of Health-System Pharmacists, Bethesda, MD.
3. Personal communication, Marilyn Stebbins, Pharm.D., Clinical Pharmacy Manager, CHW Medical Foundation/Medical Clinic, 2000.
4. Minimum Standards for Home Care Pharmacies, American Society of Health-System Pharmacists, 1999.
5. University of Arkansas for Medical Sciences, College of Pharmacy at Little Rock, Arkansas, website, http://nuclearpharmacy.uams.edu/.
6. Personal communication, Jennifer Cartright, Product Development Manager Omnicell.com, 2000.
7. Personal communication, M. Evelyn Rose, Pharm.D., Assistant Director of Clinical Pharmacy, Drug Information, PlanetRx.com, Inc.

Bibliography

Pharmacy Certified Technician Training Manual, 7th Edition, Michigan Pharmacists Association, Lansing, MI, 1997, pp. 35-37.

About the author

Tracey Okabe-Yamamura, Pharm.D., is a clinical pharmacy specialist at Mercy San Juan Medical Center in Carmichael, California. The medical center is a part of a multi-facility region of hospitals in the greater Sacramento area and includes services for oncology, trauma, cardiology, and other acute care specialties. Her current responsibilities include pharmacy support for a regional oncology service line, clinical staff development, continuous quality improvement, and preceptorship for pharmacy students and residents. Dr. Okabe-Yamamura is a graduate of the University of California, San Francisco, School of Pharmacy and completed a clinical pharmacy residency at the University of California Irvine. Her past positions include clinical coordinator at Pacific Hospital of Long Beach and Clinical Pharmacist for FHP, Inc.

Self-assessment questions

1. Which of the following pharmacy practice sites does ***not*** utilize pharmacy technicians?
   a. Long-term care pharmacy
   b. Mail order pharmacy
   c. Pharmaceutical industry
   d. All of the above utilize pharmacy technicians

2. Which of the following is ***not*** considered an ambulatory pharmacy practice site?
   a. Community pharmacy
   b. HMO clinic pharmacy
   c. Long-term care pharmacy
   d. Internet pharmacy

3 Which of the following is a true statement regarding a long-term care facility?
   a. It may be a nursing home or skilled nursing facility.
   b. Generally, patients are young and acutely ill.
   c. Patients are usually prescribed complex, frequently changing medication regimens.
   d. Patients do not remain in these facilities for long periods of time.

4. In what type of pharmacy practice setting would a technician most likely prepare intravenous solutions?
   a. Community pharmacy
   b. HMO clinic pharmacy
   c. Institutional pharmacy
   d. Internet pharmacy

5. Which of the following statements is false regarding Internet pharmacies?
   a. Internet pharmacies offer the convenience of shopping from one's home.
   b. All Internet pharmacies have received Verified Internet Pharmacy Practice Site (VIPPS) symbol awarded by the NABP.
   c. Pharmacy technicians assist with the dispensing process and sometimes become involved with technical projects in website development.
   d. The need for pharmacists and pharmacy technicians employed by Internet pharmacies is expected to increase.

Chapter 4

Ambulatory Care Pharmacy

Jennifer A. James, Pharm.D., and Matthew C. Osterhaus, R.Ph.

Learning objectives

Upon completion of this chapter, the technician should be able to do the following:

- Define the terms *prescription* and *over-the-counter* drugs.
- List the parts of a written prescription order.
- List the technician functions when receiving a written prescription order.
- Understand the purposes of the patient medication profile.
- List the information that must appear on the prescription label.
- Differentiate between the two types of third party drug programs.
- List five inventory-related functions that may be performed by a technician.
- Explain the reasons for growth in home health care.

Introduction

The technician practicing in ambulatory or community pharmacy serves the non-institutionalized, "walk-in" patient. Ambulatory pharmacies can be categorized by the type of setting they are located in or by the management structure employed. Settings may include retail drug stores, grocery stores, large discount stores, community medical clinics, or outpatient hospital clinics. Management or ownership structure may be independent, franchise, or corporate – commonly referred to as "chain." Mail order or Internet pharmacies provide similar services to ambulatory patients, but the patients communicate with the pharmacy in writing or by telephone rather than being able to walk in.

The number of prescriptions dispensed to ambulatory patients in recent years has been increasing dramatically. Among the factors responsible for this growth is earlier discharge from hospitals, a lengthening of life span and the availability of truly innovative pharmaceutical drugs for use by the ambulatory patient. The various types of ambulatory pharmacies have not shared equally in the increasing number of prescriptions dispensed. Chain pharmacies have significantly expanded prescription volumes and have increased the number of pharmacy sites, while the market share of independent pharmacies has declined. The type of pharmacy site will influence the tasks assumed by the technicians, as well as the policies of the individual employer and the pharmacy regulations in the specific state. However, the one characteristic common to nearly all ambulatory settings is frequent patient contact.

Types of medications

Medications are known by both a brand or trade name and by a generic name. The same medication may be made by a number of different manufacturers. Every medication goes through a strict approval process with the FDA before it is released for general use.

Medications are classified as nonprescription over-the-counter (OTC) or prescription. OTC medications can be purchased without a prescription order and are labeled and packaged for a lay person's safe and effective self-use. A medication is classified as prescription if it is habit-forming or not safe for unsupervised use. Prescription medications have traditionally displayed a statement on the manufacturer's container called the Federal Legend that states "Caution: Federal law prohibits dispensing without a prescription." However, a recent regulation allows this statement to be replaced with the words "Rx Only." Prescription medications are further classified by federal and state law into schedules depending on their degree of physical and psychological dependence. (Chapter 30 discusses the federal schedules.)

Federal law requires prescription medications to be prescribed by a licensed medical practitioner, and each state has laws regarding prescriptive authority. A prescription is an order for a medication issued by a licensed medical practitioner such as a physician, dentist, veterinarian, nurse practitioner, podiatrist, or physician's assistant. Each practitioner is able to prescribe medications for their patients within the scope of their practice. In some situations, pharmacists can prescribe or manage a limited number of prescription medications within specific protocols. Occasionally, a prescriber may issue a prescription for an OTC drug. The prescriber may not be aware of the OTC status or the patient may need to follow specific instructions different from those indicated on the OTC label. When such a prescription is received, the technician should consult the pharmacist to determine how this order must be processed.

Figure 1 Prescription order

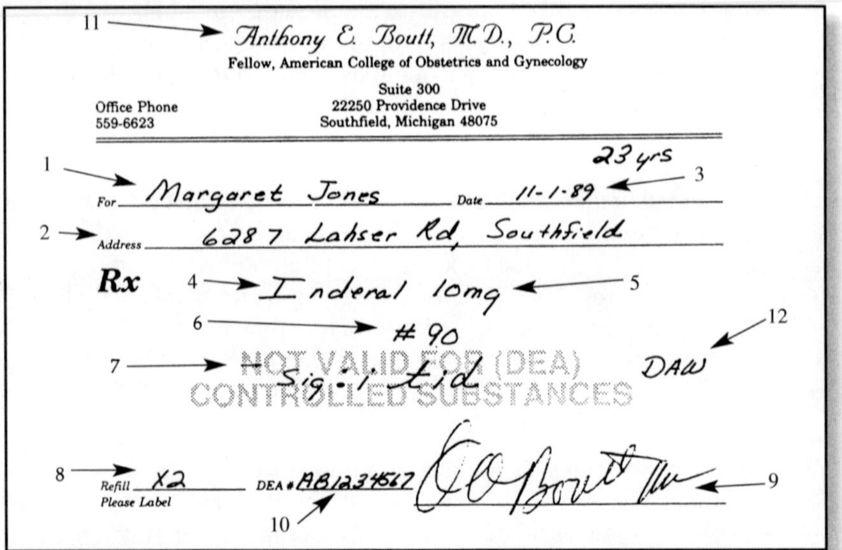

Prescription order

A prescription serves as a clear, written communication from the prescriber to the pharmacist containing the information required to accurately dispense medication to the patient. In practice, prescription orders may not contain all of the required information or may be illegible due to poor handwriting. The pharmacist, intern, or technician must then obtain the needed data from the patient or prescriber before processing the prescription. If a prescription is difficult to interpret or appears fraudulent, the technician should refer the concern to the pharmacist for his or her professional judgment. The key to the numbers on the sample prescription order (see Figure 1) are as follows:

1. Patient name
2. Patient address (required for controlled substances)
3. Date prescription was issued

4. Medication name
5. Medication strength
6. Quantity to be dispensed: number of tablets, milliliters of liquid, or grams of ointment
7. Directions for use, commonly abbreviated "Sig," which is Latin for "take thou"
8. Number of refills
9. Signature of prescriber or authorized representative
10. Prescriber DEA number (required for controlled substances)
11. Prescriber printed name, address, and telephone number usually preprinted
12. Some states may require indication of whether to substitute generic or formulary equivalent medication, such as "DAW" indicating "dispense as written."

Receiving the written prescription order

The prescriber usually writes the prescription order on a prescription blank, but may telephone an order directly to the pharmacy or send it by other electronic means when allowed by law. If the prescription is not received in writing, it must immediately be reduced to writing. State laws and a pharmacist's professional judgment determine whether this task can be delegated to the technician. When receiving a prescription order from a patient, the technician must initially review it for completeness. If information is omitted by the prescriber or is illegible, the proper information must be entered at the time the prescription is presented at the pharmacy.

The technician should also ask how the patient plans to pay for the medication; i.e., cash, insurance or charge. If a patient has insurance coverage, the specific insurance information, commonly provided to patients on a wallet-size card, should be obtained prior to processing the prescription. Most prescription benefits use real-time, online claims settlement. The technician must be knowledgeable with third party insurance programs with which the pharmacy participates. Technicians may also be responsible for running the cash register.

Patient medication profiles

A patient new to the pharmacy may be interviewed or asked to complete a written medication and medical history questionnaire. It is used to create a patient profile with all of the patient's personal information, as well as a record of all medications dispensed by a pharmacy to the individual patient or family. This record may also include OTC medications used, drug allergies, major medical conditions, and other relevant information. In today's ambulatory pharmacy, patient medication profiles are usually computerized; however, a few remaining ambulatory pharmacies maintain manual patient medication profiles. The technician may be responsible for initiating and updating these records. All information entered should be reviewed by the pharmacist.

By law, the pharmacist is responsible for completion of prospective drug therapy review each time a new medication is dispensed. This review includes verifying the prescription order is indicated for the patient, the dose is appropriate for the patient, and the medication will work well and not interfere with the other medications a patient is taking. Many computerized, prescription processing software systems include drug interaction software to alert the pharmacist when a problem may be present. When potential problems are flagged on the computer, the technician must alert the pharmacist. Pharmacists have a broad knowledge about drug therapy that they apply to patient care.

Prescription labeling

The technician is frequently responsible for preparing the prescription label. This task is usually performed with the aid of a computer, and familiarity with the prescription processing software is essential. If the instructions are difficult to understand, the technician consults the pharmacist for assistance

Figure 2 Sample prescription label

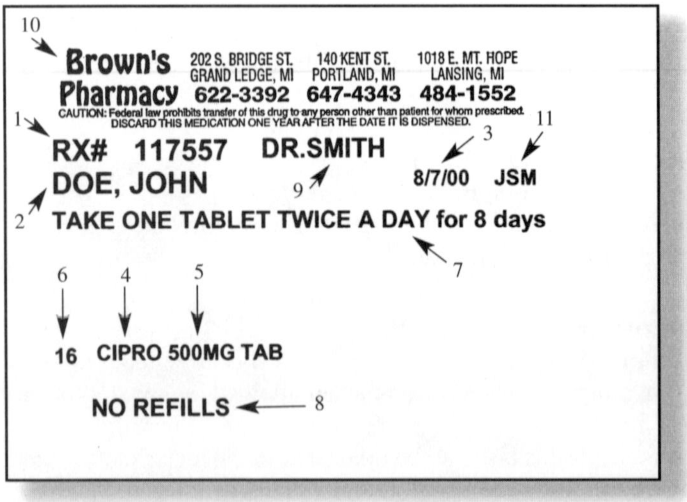

in clarifying the prescriber's intent. The label information must be accurate and easy for the patient to understand. The key to the numbers on the sample prescription label (see Figure 2) are as follows:

1. Prescription number
2. Patient name
3. Date prescription was filled by the pharmacy; some states also require the original date
4. Medication name; state regulations vary as to whether the brand name, generic name, or manufacturer are required
5. Medication strength
6. Quantity dispensed
7. Directions for use written out in full text, easy for the patient to understand
8. Number of refills remaining
9. Name of prescriber
10. Pharmacy name, address, and telephone number
11. Initials of pharmacist dispensing the prescription

The Poison Prevention Act of 1970 requires the use of safety caps for most oral prescription drugs. Requests by the patient or the prescriber for a non-child resistant container must be documented on the prescription order. The technician should determine if the patient will wait to have the prescription filled or when they will return for the medication. If the patient decides to wait, they should be given an estimate of the time required to fill the prescription.

Directions for use

The labeled directions for using the prescribed medication must be accurate and easy to understand. Abbreviations, which are commonly used by the physician to give the instructions to the pharmacist, should be avoided because they may be confusing to the patient. (Please refer to Chapter 8 on Terminology.) Use words to designate numbers for quantities and frequency. Instructions must be complete. "Take one capsule two times a day" is preferred to "One 2 times a day." For example, "Take one tablet every four hours as needed for headache" is preferred to "Take one tablet every four hours as needed." See chart for sample terms recommended for prescription labeling.

Type of medication	Word choice	Example
Oral	"Take," if adult	Take one tablet daily
	"Give," if child	Give two teaspoonfuls
External	"Apply"	Apply sparingly to arm two times
Suppositories	"Insert," specify place	Insert one suppository rectally
Drops, (eyes, ears, or nose)	"Place or instill," specify organ	Place one drop into right eye
Subcutaneous or intramuscular	"Inject"	Inject one unit subcutaneously
Oral drops	"Take by mouth"	Take five drops by mouth

Preparing the prescription

The technician may be involved in counting and pouring medications. In performing these tasks, the technician obtains the prescribed drug from the shelf. Each medication has a unique 11-digit identifier know as the National Drug Code (NDC), which is usually used to record the medication into the patient profile. The first five digits indicate the manufacturer of the drug; the next four digits indicate the drug and are unique for each drug, formulation, and strength; the final two digits indicate the package size or type. The NDC is used to ensure selection of the correct product for dispensing. The ordered quantity is counted or poured from the stock bottle, placed into a suitable prescription container and capped securely. The written prescription order, accurately prepared label, appropriate stock bottle and correctly filled prescription container are assembled for the pharmacist to validate. After the pharmacist verifies the prescription, the bottle is returned to the shelf.

Figure 3 Auxiliary labels

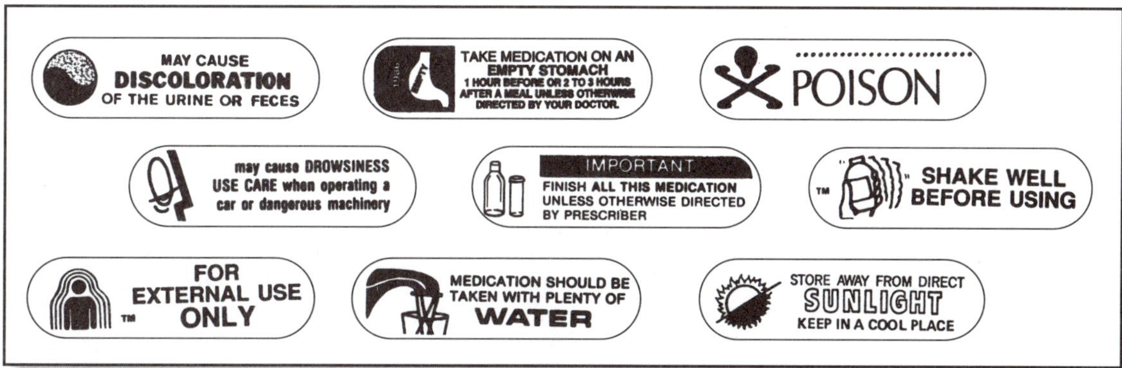

Patient information and counseling

Patient contact and communication are the core of ambulatory pharmacy practice. The required information on the prescription label provides the minimum necessary information for a patient to be capable of administering a medication. Frequently, the prescription label alone is inadequate for a complete understanding of proper medication usage. Auxiliary labels are small labels that bear additional information, reminders, or warnings about the medication. These labels are conspicuously attached to the prescription container so that they do not cover other label information. The pharmacist chooses these labels unless a protocol has been established for the technician to follow. (See Figure 3. Note that actual labels are available in color.)

Patient counseling is the responsibility of the pharmacist and cannot be delegated or assumed by the technician. A federal law commonly referred to as OBRA '90 and individual state pharmacy practice acts provide guidelines for the amount of information pharmacists are responsible for providing to patients. Counseling includes advising patients about both prescription and OTC medications. Topics covered by the pharmacist should include medication uses, instructions for administration, common side effects, precautions, what to do if a dose is missed, and storage requirements. It is best to provide this information verbally in person to allow the patient to ask questions of the pharmacist, as well as providing it in writing for the patient to refer to later. Most pharmacy computer systems generate written drug information for the patient specific to the medication ordered. The pharmacist must be available to the patient to ask questions; some states require the pharmacy to offer a toll-free telephone number for patients to use.

Many pharmacists are expanding their current pharmacy services to offer additional patient education, disease state management, or preventative health screening sessions. These are usually provided by appointment in a private, office-like area of the pharmacy department for an additional fee which is paid by the patient or billed to the patient's insurance company. Common conditions covered include asthma, diabetes, high cholesterol, hypertension, osteoporosis, weight management, and smoking cessation. Technicians are in the position to act as a receptionist, secretary, workflow coordinator, and billing agent to assist the pharmacist in the provision of expanded services. It is very important that technicians have a good understanding of these services and the benefits they provide to patients because technicians often receive the initial questions about these services from the patient.

Processing refills

Federal law limits the number of refills that can be authorized for controlled substances. For medications that can be given refills, some state laws allow the transfer of any remaining refills from one pharmacy to another. Some states do not allow the delegation of this authority to a technician. Customarily, the pharmacist or pharmacy intern at the receiving pharmacy telephones the originating pharmacist and receives a verbal copy. The verbal information is immediately reduced to writing to include the usual elements of a prescription, the original date written, date last dispensed, number of remaining refills, pharmacy and pharmacist it was transferred from, their prescription number, and their telephone number. The technician must be familiar with the pharmacy rules and regulations governing the transfer of prescriptions between pharmacies.

A request for a prescription refill may be made in person, by telephone, or by e-mail. When requested in person, the patient may present an empty labeled container, a prescription receipt, the prescription number, or the name or description of the medication. When receiving a request for a refill, the technician records the prescription number, the name of the medication, the patient's name and phone number, the pick-up time, and any special requests. The computerized prescription processing software will generate a refill transaction and automatically decrease the number of remaining refills. A manual medication profile system requires retrieval of the original prescription and the patient's profile to allow documentation of the refill on the prescription or profile. The technician is often responsible for verifying patient compliance with prescribed therapy by checking the days' supply per refill with the refill dates in the prescription profile. The label is typed and the medication counted, placed in the appropriate container, and labeled for the pharmacist to check. The pharmacist is not required to do the same extensive counseling, but should offer to review or answer any questions for the patient.

Third party insurance drug programs

Many patients have prescription benefits provided by private or government insurance programs. These programs are called third party insurance payors because, in addition to the pharmacist and patient, they are a "third party" involved in the financial transaction related to the prescription. Individual plans vary greatly from patient to patient and are often difficult for patients to understand. The third party copayment may be calculated as a percentage of the medication cost or a certain fee, depending on whether the medication is brand or generic. Third party payors typically impose restrictions on their covered services, such as limiting quantities dispensed, requiring use of generic drugs, or reimbursing at a maximum allowable cost (MAC) for selected medications. Computers can assist in tracking the insurer's restrictions, but it is imperative that the technician assess current restrictions. Many also limit the number of medications they will cover to certain medications they approve, which they refer to as "formulary medications."

The technician is frequently responsible for billing third party payors, reconciling payments received, and preparing claims for submission by patients who have "out-of-pocket" plans. (An out-of-pocket program requires that the patient pay the pharmacy the total prescription charge, then the patient submits a claim to the insurer and is reimbursed directly.) The computer simplifies these tasks by allowing real-time, online settlement of prescription claims. Third party insurers pay only for services provided to a subscriber or eligible dependents insured on the date of the service, thus coverage can be verified right at the time of the transaction. A specific amount, the copayment, is usually paid to the pharmacy by the patient at the time of service. The third party payor then pays the pharmacy the remainder of the allowable charge. Some small insurers are not equipped to receive automated claims, in which case the pharmacy technician manually completes claim forms.

Compounding medications

The profession of pharmacy is rooted in the compounding of medications. Today, some pharmacies offer specialty prescription compounding to meet the unique needs of their patients. Dermatologists, hospice providers, or veterinarians may use pharmacy compounding services more frequently than other prescribers. The dosage form may be capsules, creams, elixirs, lip balms, injectables, lollipops, liquids, ointments, solutions, suppositories, suspensions, tablets, or troches. The request may be to create a formulation that is no longer commercially available or to put together a certain combination of medications. Some ambulatory care pharmacies possess a laminar flow hood or vertical flow hood to compound intravenous solutions for home administration. Some states allow the pharmacy technician to be assigned compounding duties by written procedures under the direct supervision of the pharmacist.

Inventory procedures

Expenditures for inventory far exceed any other single cost of operating an ambulatory care pharmacy. Good inventory control reduces these costs while minimizing out-of-stock situations. Inventory control procedures used in ambulatory pharmacies vary from the basic "want book" system of writing items low in stock into an order book as you notice them, to a sophisticated, computer-assisted perpetual inventory. The technician is frequently assigned inventory tasks that may include:

- placing drug and device orders by telephone, electronic order device, computer, or in person with a representative
- checking in an order, verifying items listed on the invoice are received
- pricing drugs products, devices, and miscellaneous merchandise
- storing drug products and devices in the appropriate area (i.e., shelves, refrigerator, freezer)
- rotating shelved stock; placing earliest expiration date in front
- removing outdated or recalled items from inventory and returning them to the wholesaler or manufacturer
- preparing invoices for payment and maintaining filed invoices

Monetary policies and security

The technician must be familiar with the pharmacy's policies for payment of services and merchandise. Written policies and procedures should be coupled with thorough training. Technicians should be able to price prescription and OTC items and understand which items are taxable and non-taxable.

To be able to operate the cash register, technicians should know the computer system, check-cashing policy, and credit card authorization procedure. Some pharmacies continue to offer the additional service of private charge policies for their patients.

Ambulatory pharmacies possess items of value including cash, controlled substances, and general merchandise. Security procedures to safeguard these assets must be thoroughly understood by the technician. These policies and procedures may include specific actions about suspected shoplifting and how to respond to a robbery (or attempt). Most pharmacies employ an alarm system that may consist of both a panic alarm for use during hours of operation and an alarm activated only when the pharmacy is closed.

Long-term care

Patients residing in nursing homes or long-term care facilities must have access to pharmacy services. These services are sometimes provided by ambulatory care pharmacies, although in recent years an increasing number of patients are being served by specialized long-term care pharmacies that combine aspects of ambulatory care with hospital care into their professional practice. This trend has resulted from the increasing number of elderly and in part from changing needs of many of these patients who a few years ago were cared for only in the hospital. Pharmacy services may include unit-dose drug distribution, total parenteral or enteral nutrition, intravenous therapy, oxygen concentrators, and ventilator and respiratory unit care, along with all of the backup systems necessary. While providing these services, they must, in most cases, develop policies and procedures that ensure proper delivery of pharmacy services to patients located away from the pharmacy itself. Technicians practicing in pharmacies serving the long-term care patients assume a variety of duties that, in many instances, resemble hospital pharmacy more than ambulatory pharmacy.

Home health care

Over the past decade there has been a dramatic shift in healthcare delivery from the acute care hospital to the home. This shift, spurred by efforts to contain hospital costs, resulted in discharging patients "quicker and sicker." Other factors contributing to home healthcare growth include: patients' desire for more control over their own health care, an aging population with degenerative health conditions, and enhanced technology that allows people with chronic health conditions to live longer and more productively. This trend in home health care promises to continue escalating the need for medical equipment and supplies in the home.

Home health care may range from simple procedures such as dressing changes to complex ones involving intravenous fluids, nutrients, or medications. Pharmacies may provide a number of these services either independently or through consignment arrangements with a medical equipment company. In a consignment arrangement, the pharmacy does not own the medical equipment, but dispenses the item and shares in the revenue. With most home medical equipment, patients require instruction in proper use or a professional fitting. The pharmacy technician may gain the necessary knowledge and skills to render professional fittings or instruction. This training is available through the product's manufacturer, specific agencies, or professional associations (i.e., local ostomy association). In some instances the technician may complete certification as a fitter of mastectomy, ostomy, orthotics, or transelectrical neurostimulator (TENS) products.

Depending upon the equipment and insurance plan, the equipment may be rented or sold as predetermined with the carrier. The home medical equipment covered by an insurance plan must be prescribed by the patient's physician and often requires the pharmacy to have an original order with further documentation beyond the components of a standard prescription, such as the medical diagnosis. Home medical equipment is a fully or partially covered benefit under many insurance plans including Medicare Part B and Medicaid. This coverage is usually verified with the insurer before the professional transaction occurs. The verification process may be verbal by telephone or written by letter of prior approval stating that upon a review of the patient's diagnosis, a specific piece of equipment will be covered. The pharmacy may also have the patient pay the entire amount at the time of purchase, bill the insurance company, and have the payment sent directly to the patient.

Conclusion

Delegation of technical functions to technicians allows pharmacists to focus their time on the provision of high quality patient care. Attention to detail and prevention of medical errors is important for every member of the pharmacy staff. Teamwork is particularly important in an ambulatory care pharmacy setting because patients are often in the pharmacy waiting while technicians and pharmacists perform separate tasks to complete the patient order. Customer service focused on the philosophy that the patient comes first allows for ambulatory care pharmacies to succeed. Motivated technicians are a key component in the success of ambulatory care pharmacy.

Acknowledgment

The authors and publisher wish to acknowledge John Baughman, R.Ph., for his extensive contributions to this chapter in the previous edition of this manual.

Bibliography

Pharmacy Certified Technician Training Manual, 7th edition, Michigan Pharmacists Association, Lansing, MI, 1997, pp. 39-47.

About the authors

Jennifer A. James received her doctorate of pharmacy from Virginia Commonwealth University Medical College of Virginia School of Pharmacy in 1999. She is currently completing a one-year residency with the University of Iowa focused on the provision of pharmaceutical care in the community setting. Osterhaus Pharmacy in Maquoketa, Iowa, is her primary practice site. Upon completion of the residency, she will be an Assistant Clinical Professor at the University of Connecticut School of Pharmacy.

Matthew C. Osterhaus received his bachelor's degree in pharmacy from the University of Iowa College of Pharmacy in 1980. He is an adjunct faculty member of the University of Iowa College of Pharmacy serving as a preceptor for Community Care Pharmacy Practice residents and Doctor of Pharmacy students in Pharmaceutical Care. Osterhaus is a community and consultant pharmacist who owns and operates Osterhaus Pharmacy in Maquoketa, Iowa. He is a member of Outcomes™ Certified Pharmaceutical Care Network and has been instrumental in furthering community-based research in Iowa. He is an active member of his local, state, and national pharmacy associations, serving in a variety of leadership positions. He has been a member of the Iowa Board of Pharmacy Examiners for seven years and is currently serving as chairman.

Self-assessment questions

1. What is the definition of an over-the-counter medication?
   a. A medication labeled with the Federal Legend on the manufacturer's container.
   b. A medication that can be purchased without a prescription order that is labeled and packaged for a lay person's self-use.
   c. A medication that is habit forming and not safe for unsupervised use.
   d. A medication a patient requests from the pharmacy to be passed to them over the counter.
2. Who is not legally allowed to prescribe prescription medications?
   a. Veternarian
   b. Physician
   c. Medication aide
   d. Dentist
3. Which of the following elements is ***not*** a required component of a prescription order?
   a. Patient height, weight, and date of birth
   b. Prescriber name, address, telephone number, and signature
   c. Date prescription was issued by the prescriber
   d. Medication strength, quantity, and directions for use
4. Which of the following should be included on a patient's profile?
   a. OTC medications used
   b. Drug allergies or intolerances
   c. Major medical conditions
   d. All of the above
5. Which of the following elements is ***not*** a required component of a prescription label?
   a. Date prescription was dispensed by the pharmacy
   b. Prescriber DEA number, address, telephone number, and signature
   c. Medication strength, quantity, and directions for use
   d. Pharmacy name, address, telephone number, and pharmacist initials
6. The National Drug Code (NDC) identifies all of the following, except:
   a. the quality assurance agent who checked the medication.
   b. the manufacturer of the drug.
   c. the package size or type.
   d. the drug formulation and strength.
7. Prescription processing duties which are appropriate for pharmacists to delegate to technicians include all of the following, except:
   a. a final check of prescription.
   b. greeting and offering to help patients as they approach the pharmacy department.
   c. counting or pouring medications.
   d. preparing and submitting billing paperwork or electronic claims.
8. On what type of medication prescription must the prescriber's Drug Enforcement Administration (DEA) number appear?
   a. Legend medications
   b. Generic medications
   c. Controlled substances
   d. OTC medications
9. Which of the following inventory tasks are technicians ***not*** frequently responsible for?
   a. Placing drug and device orders
   b. Rotating shelved stock; placing earliest expiration date in front
   c. Removing outdated or recalled items from inventory
   d. Independently destroying controlled substances
10. What is the reason for growth in home health care?
   a. Patient's lack of desire for control over their own health care
   b. Decrease in technological advances in health care
   c. A growing elderly population living longer due to advances in health care
   d. Increase in the number of hospitals

Chapter 5

Institutional Pharmacy

Patricia A. Camazzola, Pharm.D.

Learning objectives

Upon completion of this chapter, the technician should be able to do the following:

- ♦ Describe the pharmacy responsibilities within an institutional pharmacy practice setting.
- ♦ Describe advantages of a unit-dose drug system versus floor stock or individual prescription systems.
- ♦ Explain the technician's role in creating patient profiles.
- ♦ Give examples of medications that may not be unit-dose packaged in a unit-dose system.
- ♦ Describe the process by which a drug formulary is developed and maintained.
- ♦ Explain the difference between therapeutic and generic equivalence.
- ♦ List the necessary components of a medication order.
- ♦ Discuss reasons why a pharmacist reviews a patient's medication profile.

Institutional pharmacy

Institutional pharmacy may be defined as the practice of pharmacy in a hospital setting or intermediate-care facility (such as extended care facilities and nursing homes). Pharmacy services are usually coordinated via a pharmacy department that procures, stores, prepares, and distributes medications to patients. Additional responsibilities of an institutional pharmacy include ensuring that medications are used safely and appropriately. Pharmacists are involved in determining that medications are appropriately selected, monitored, and dosed. This has also been referred to as clinical pharmacy, patient-oriented care, or patient-focused care.

Medication orders

A physician (or appropriate prescriber) must prescribe a drug prior to dispensing or administering it to a patient. Medication orders are written in a specific section of the patient's medical record. The medication order usually includes the:

- ■ patient's name, location, hospital identification number/Social Security Number/administration number, and birth date/age
- ■ name of the medication
- ■ dosage
- ■ frequency of administration
- ■ route of administration
- ■ signature of the prescriber
- ■ date and hour the order was written.

Figure 1 Patient medication profile

HP1.1.1 — ACTIVE DRUG PROFILE—ORDER ENTRY —

PATIENT: xxxxxxx xxxxxxx 2997837 LOCATION: MAT 120-B
ADMISSION DATE: 10/19/89 AGE: 25 SEX F WEIGHT: 70.91 (KG)
SERVICE: OB # OF ACTIVE ORDERS: 11 HEIGHT: 157.48 (CM)
DIAGNOSIS: TERM PREGNANCY/
ALLERGIES: NO PATIENT ALLERGIES/

* ACTIVE DRUG PROFILE *

	DRUG NAME	FORM	DOSE	RT	FREQUENCY	STATUS
1.	LACTATED RINGERS	IVLV	1000ML	IV	Q8	ACTIVE
2.	ACETAMINOPHEN 300MG/ CODEINE 30	TAB	1 TAB	PO	Q3–4PRN	ACTIVE
3.	IBUPROFEN	TAB	400MG	PO	Q4PRN	ACTIVE
4.	ERGONOVINE MALEATE	TAB	0.200MG	PO	Q6PRN	ACTIVE
5.	MASSE BREAST CREAM	CRM	1 APPL	TP	PRN	BULK
6.	PCA MORPHINE SULFATE 2MG/ML	IVPB	120MG	IV	TITRATE	ACTIVE
7.	MORPHINE SULFATE	INJ	5MG	IM	Q3PRN	ACTIVE
8.	NALOXONE HCL	INJ	0.400MG	IM	PRN	ACTIVE
9.	SIMETHICONE	TAB	80MG	PO	HSPRN	ACTIVE
10.	SECOBARBITAL SODIUM	CAP	100MG	PO	HSPRN	ACTIVE
11.	DOCUSATE SODIUM	CAP	200MG	PO	HSPRN	ACTIVE

With the exception of emergency situations, the pharmacist must receive a direct copy of the medication order. Direct copies may be obtained by self copying, non-carbon record (NCR) order forms, electromechanical (copy machine or fax machine), or with computer systems.

Technician utilization in patient medication profiles

A pharmacy technician may be responsible for retrieving all medication orders from multiple sources. The technician should review each medication order and ensure that it contains the patient's name, location, and prescriber's signature. The technician may also be responsible for entering the medication order into the pharmacy's computer system or a manual, patient profiling system. These technician-processed medication orders are commonly referred to as "unverified." By law, a pharmacist must review and interpret every medication order. The pharmacist may utilize supplemental information within the computer system or reference books to determine that the medication selected is dosed appropriately, based on the patient's age, weight, height, and clinical parameters. The pharmacist also reviews the patient's complete drug regimen or profile and determines if drug interactions, allergies, drug duplications, overlapping therapies, or contraindications for other reasons exist. Any problems or uncertainties must be discussed and resolved with the physician or prescriber prior to proceeding. Once all concerns are resolved, the pharmacist must check or verify that all information has been entered into the computerized or manual system accurately. The information becomes part of the patient's medication profile. (See Figure 1.) Other information that should be part of the profile includes:

- patient's full name, date hospitalized, age, sex, weight, hospital identification number, and diagnosis/reason for admission

- clinical test results
- sensitivities, allergies, or contraindications
- medications dispensed, dates of original orders, strengths, dosage forms, quantities, frequencies, and stop dates
- pharmacist's initials

Medication distribution systems

Within hospital environments there are various types of distribution systems. These include individual-prescription, floor-stock, and unit-dose systems. Many hospitals utilize a combination of floor-stock and unit-dose systems to meet the needs of patients comprehensively.

Technician utilization in an individual prescription system

In an individual prescription system, physician orders are filled with a sufficient supply of medication for several days. The manufactured dose nearest to the prescribed dose is dispensed to the nursing unit. For example, a physician orders ampicillin 350mg by intravenous piggyback (IVPB). The pharmacy dispenses ampicillin 500mg vials to the nursing unit. The nurse is then required to utilize 350mg from each 500mg vial to prepare the IVPB. The nurses need more time to prepare the dose for administration, and there is an increased risk for dosage errors. There is additional time spent by pharmacy personnel to process returns of medication when the patient is discharged or the drug is discontinued.

Technician utilization in a floor-stock system

In a floor-stock system, the nursing unit uses a bulk supply of medication and dispenses doses for the patient from a container holding multiple doses or from an automated dispensing machine. The container is subsequently replenished by the technician and checked by a pharmacist when a written request is received from the nursing unit. The nursing unit must also process the patient charges for doses used in this system. This method, although convenient for the nursing staff, has a number of disadvantages, including increased potential for errors and decreased inventory control.

Technician utilization in unit-dose drug distribution

The unit-dose system of medication distribution is a pharmacy-coordinated method of dispensing and controlling medications in healthcare institutions. The unit-dose system may differ in form depending on the specific needs of the institution. However, certain elements are basic to all unit-dose systems. Medications are contained in single-unit packages. They are dispensed in as ready-to-administer a form as possible, and usually not more than a 24-hour supply of doses is delivered to the patient care area at any time. The unit-dose system of drug distribution was developed to:

1. reduce medication errors
2. increase drug use control within institutions
3. minimize drug waste and pilferage
4. reduce nursing preparation time
5. provide a mechanism for accurate and efficient billing
6. allow full utilization of the professional training and capabilities of all involved members of the healthcare team
7. enhance or improve the quality of patient care

A unit-dose system provides the opportunity for checks and balances that lessen chances of medication errors and missed doses and increase communication between nursing and pharmacy staffs. The system places a greater responsibility for the appropriate procurement of medications on pharmacists, creating a greater need for trained technical and supportive personnel.

Benefits of unit-dose drug distribution system

Benefits obtainable with a unit-dose system were identified based on the criteria presented above. An efficient drug distribution system should provide the following benefits:

- Nursing time spent ordering, picking up, preparing, and pouring medications is virtually eliminated, allowing more time for direct patient care activities.
- Charting of medications is more accurate and less time consuming. The need for medication tickets, trays, and pre- and post-charting is eliminated. Charting is done as medications are administered as the Medication Administration Record is kept right with the cart.
- Medication errors are dramatically reduced, decreasing the potential for patient harm and malpractice suits against the hospital and its staff.
- Control of drug use on the nursing units is improved. Since medications are provided as they are used, drug pilferage and illicit use of medications are reduced.
- Patient billing is more accurate as patients are charged only for those medications actually administered to them.
- The patient profile or the Medication Administration Record can serve as an ongoing charge document, thereby eliminating the need for drug credit forms and additional charge documents.
- The pharmacist's education and experience equip him or her to monitor drug stability and special storage requirements of particular drugs until they are delivered to the patient care units.
- The system's simplicity allows for smoother running operations, with fewer chances of error and easier orientation for new nurses.

Types of unit-dose systems

The type of unit-dose system utilized in a hospital is determined by the hospital's physical layout, equipment available, allocation of personnel, and procedures required for the efficient distribution of medications. There are three major types of unit-dose systems:

- Centralized systems
- Decentralized systems
- Combined systems that include both centralized and decentralized functions

Technician utilization in centralized unit-dose systems

Centralized drug delivery provides a system where orders are interpreted, drug doses chosen, and medication placed in the patient drawers of medication carts. This task is a major responsibility of pharmacy technicians trained in a central pharmacy. Larger hospitals may have two or more centralized pharmacies, each serving a defined number of patient beds. Utilizing a centralized system concentrates technician workload to the extent that large-scale production techniques can be applied. This is a great advantage in the preparation and packaging of those products not available in unit-dose forms.

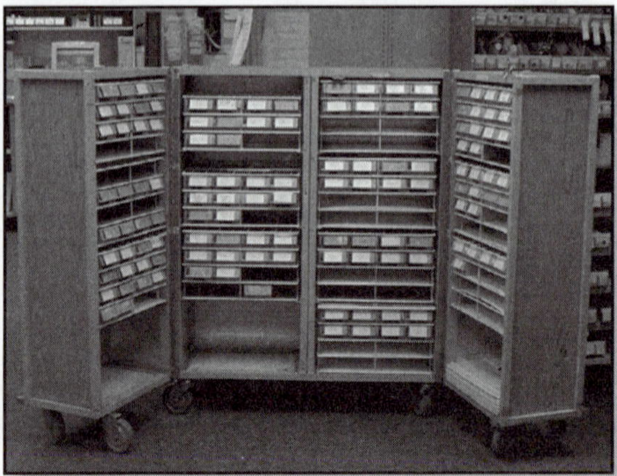

Patient drawers in a medication cart for delivery to nursing unit

The utilization of a centralized method of drug delivery is primarily determined by the physical characteristics and layout of the hospital. If adequate means for delivery of medications on time are not present (elevators, pneumatic tubes, personnel), the centralized system will be slow, inefficient, and ineffective.

Technician utilization in decentralized unit-dose systems

Decentralized drug delivery refers to systems in which one or more satellite pharmacies are assigned throughout the hospital and utilized to distribute medications. In this system, pharmacy technicians support the routine packaging of medications carried out centrally. The decentralized system provides an environment conducive to communication between physicians, nurses, pharmacists, technicians, and patients. Disadvantages to the initiation of decentralized services are primarily related to cost. Loss of economy is sustained in the need for multiple renovation of pharmacy sites, need for somewhat larger drug inventory to stock the satellites, and the need for more pharmacy personnel.

Systems combining centralized and decentralized functions

Combination unit-dose methods refer to those systems where certain distributive activities are performed in the patient care areas, while the rest are performed centrally. Combination systems provide advantages in that those activities benefiting from economics of scale, such as extemporaneous packaging and labeling and the physical function of filling the medication carts, can be done centrally by well-trained pharmacy technicians, while those activities that may improve patient care, such as interpretation of the physician's order, maintaining patient profiles, and communicating with physicians, nurses, and patients, can be decentralized.

Technician utilization in unit-dose packaging and labeling

Almost all medications are prepared by manufacturers in single, unit of use, or unit-dose packages. Those products not available in this form must be repackaged by the department of pharmacy to comply with the needs of the unit-dose system. Labeling unit-dose products must include the medication name(s) and dose strength, the manufacturer's or pharmacy's control number, and the drug expiration date. Packaging and labeling medications in accordance with the above recommendations will ensure that:

- each dose is identifiable up to the time it is administered.
- the drug is maintained in a sanitary form.
- liquids and injections are more accurately measured.
- injections are reconstituted with proper diluents and are ready for immediate use.
- drug waste is dramatically reduced. Waste due to discarding the unused portion of a three- to five-day supply of medication and waste due to using only a portion of a single-dose ampule can be all but eliminated under a unit-dose system.

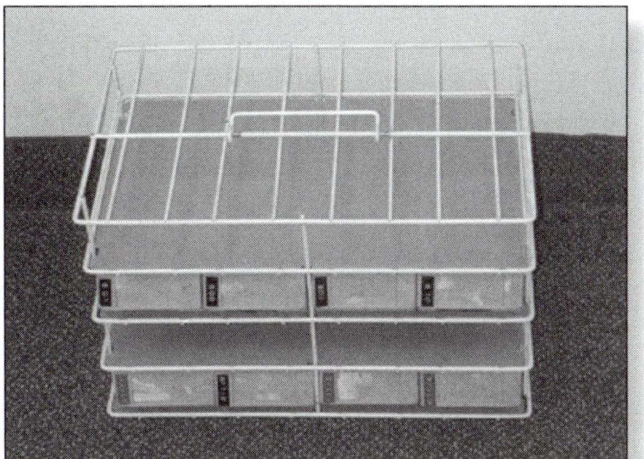

Patient drawers in a cassette

Technician utilization in unit-dose cassette exchange

Cassettes or unit-dose bins are exchanged, usually by pharmacy technicians at scheduled times unique to each institution. The cassettes most recently filled and updated are exchanged for those in use on patient care areas. Procedure for exchange follows a similar pattern. The filled medication cassettes are transported to the nursing unit at the exchange time. The medication cart is unlocked and the filled cassettes exchanged for those used during the previous medication time period. During this exchange, non-unit-dose medications are transferred to the replacement cassettes. Non-unit-dose medications may include preparations such as: ophthalmic preparations, oral liquids, ointments, and creams. The patient's name and location must be verified

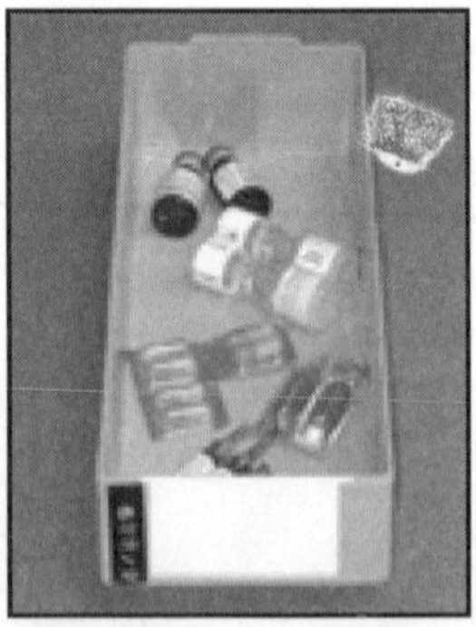

Patient medication drawer with a 24-hour supply of unit-dose medications

on all medications that are transferred between cassettes. At the completion of the exchange, the pharmacy technician locks the cart and the "used" cassettes are returned to the pharmacy for refilling.

Unit-dose exceptions

The philosophy of unit-dose drug distribution is to provide all medications in a ready-to-administer size and form. In practice this cannot always be accomplished for a number of reasons that include: stability, volume, manufacturer availability, and federal law regulations. Each pharmacy has special dispensing techniques that will apply to medications falling into these categories. Controlled substances are examples of medications falling into one of these categories. Controlled substances require special attention due to the record keeping requirements established by federal and state laws. (See Chapter 30 for these requirements.) Other medications are not unit-dose packaged because it is impractical and uneconomical. Examples of these are eye drops and ear drops, ointments, and irrigating solutions. Medications that are not dispensed in unit-dose form require special labeling. The label must contain the patient's name and room number, the date, and the name and strength of the drug.

Automated medication distribution systems

Pharmacists face high expectations for ensuring the accuracy of medication distribution, inventory management, and cost control. As a result, automated medication distribution systems have been developed that ensure reliability, accuracy, and security.

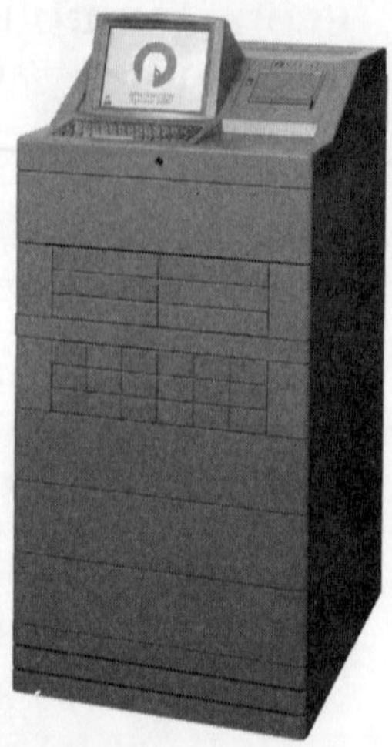

A Pyxis® automated medication distribution system

Automated medication distribution systems were originally designed to store and improve the accountability of narcotics control in the patient care area. Similar to the technology of an automated teller machine, these devices secure medications and require the healthcare professional to enter a password and specific patient information prior to opening a drawer or bin containing the desired medication. Following success with narcotic access and control, the system was expanded to STAT and "as needed" medications, and in some settings replaced the unit-dose cart system. In these settings, 90 percent to 95 percent of the patients' doses are dispensed through the automated distribution system. Subsequent to implementing the system, pharmacy administrators report significant reductions in missing dose reports and medication errors. The system also frees up pharmacists' time and allows their increased involvement in providing clinical pharmacy services versus distributive services.

A summary of benefits obtainable through implementation of an automated dispensing system include:

- dramatically decreased medication inventory
- reduction in labor costs
- reduced diversion of medications
- reduced medication errors
- increased productivity allowing increased pharmacist involvement in clinical services

Barcoding technology

Many disciplines of health care have looked at barcoding technology as a mechanism to improve accuracy, increase productivity, and control inventory. A barcode is a series of computerized lines or bars and numbers specific for a particular product, service, or patient.

Many healthcare computer information systems have incorporated barcode technology. In these systems, patients wear wristbands containing a patient-specific barcode. Medications are dispensed from the pharmacy department with barcode identifiers specific for each drug. The nurse administering the medication to the patient scans the barcode on a patient's wristband and scans the barcode on the medication label. This verifies that the correct medication is given to the correct patient. In addition, the medication administration is recorded in the medical record, and the medication is billed to the patient's account. This improves productivity through elimination of additional documentation procedures.

0 71709 18274 8

Barcoding technology has also been incorporated into inventory control procedures. Goods in/out, counting and picking stock can all be accomplished more effectively with barcoding. Tracking pharmaceutical inventory using barcodes has resulted in reduced paperwork, errors, duplication, and time.

Administration schedules

Medication administration schedules are important as they can affect the degree that a patient obtains benefit from a drug. Schedules are determined for each specific drug to provide the patient with maximal benefits and minimal side effects. Most institutions have standard administration times; therefore, it is important to be familiar with the institution's policies. An example of an administration schedule is included in Figure 2.

Technician utilization in automatic stop orders

The terminology *automatic stop orders* (ASO) refers to a procedure that automatically stops medication orders following a predesignated, specific duration of therapy. The medical and pharmacy staff decide which medications are to be included in such a policy. Criteria utilized in the formulation of these recommendations include evaluation of the medication, its intended use or indication, and the cost. Following the enactment of an ASO policy, the pharmacy personnel, including technicians, is responsible for stopping the order within a specified time. Examples of medications likely to be covered by such a policy include antibiotics, anticoagulants, controlled substances, and antineoplastic drugs.

Technician utilization in intravenous admixtures

A technician may assist the pharmacist in the preparation, labeling, and reconstitution of admixture intravenous (IV) solutions. The pharmacy technician needs a thorough understanding of aseptic technique and its application (see Chapter 27). Maintenance of special equipment such as laminar and vertical flow hoods, filters, and supplies used in the preparation of IV solutions may also be the responsibility of the well-trained technician. After a pharmacist has verified the preparation of the solution with the physician's order, a technician may store the IV until delivery to the nursing unit for administration to the patient. The compounding and admixture of large and small volume parenterals (injectable medications) must be undertaken by qualified trained personnel, usually technicians. Individuals who prepare these admixtures must have special training and follow written guidelines. In addition, the written procedures must be monitored to assure that all pharmacy requirements are met.

Pharmacy involvement in hospital committees

Since hospital structures are so large, it is necessary to utilize committee structures to gain appropriate input, address concerns, and develop and improve processes. The pharmacist must actively participate in a number of hospital committees. Among these committees are the Pharmacy and Therapeutics (P & T), Nursing/Pharmacy, Infection Control, Medication Use Review, Product Evaluation, Critical Care Committees, and others. The P & T Committee may be composed of physicians,

Figure 2 Example of an administration schedule

MEDICATION ADMINISTRATION SCHEDULES

(24-hour clock) Time / Frequency	0100	0200	0300	0400	0500	0600	0700	0800	0900	1000	1100	1200	1300	1400	1500	1600	1700	1800	1900	2000	2100	2200	2300	2400
DAILY										X														
BID										X								X						
TID										X				X				X						
TID P.C.										X				X				X						
TIC c MEALS or TID A. C.								X				X					X							
QID										X				X				X				X		
H.S.																						X		
(even hours) Q-2-H		X		X		X		X		X		X		X		X		X		X		X		X
Q-4-H		X				X				X				X				X				X		
Q-6-H						X						X						X						X
Q-8-H						X								X								X		
Q-12-H										X												X		
ORAL once daily ANTICOAGULANTS																		X						
HYPOGLYCEMICS " QD								(X)																
" BID								(X)									(X)							
" TID								(X)				(X)					(X)							
INJECTABLE ANTICOAGULANTS		X						X						X						X				

X = Scheduled time of administration

(X) = Hypoglycemics -
Administration times for hypoglycemics should coincide with patients' meal times. Refer to each nursing unit for meal time specifications.

pharmacists, nurses, administrators, continuous improvement coordinators and others as appropriate. The main objectives of the P & T Committee are:

- policy development that addresses the evaluation, selection, and therapeutic use of drugs and related devices
- education to meet the needs of professional staff related to medication use
- development of a list or formulary of drugs that are approved for use in the hospital and provide for its constant revision. The selection of medications to be included in the formulary should be based on therapeutic merits, safety and cost. The committee should minimize duplication of the same basic drug type, drug entity, or product.

Therapeutic and generic substitution

Therapeutic substitution or equivalents describes drugs that are *chemically different*; however, they can be expected to produce essentially the same therapeutic outcome and toxicity. The terms *generic substitution* or *equivalents* are defined as the substitution of drug products that contain the same active ingredient(s) and are chemically identical in strength, concentration, dosage form, and route of administration to the drug product prescribed. The P & T Committee is responsible for determining the drugs acceptable for therapeutic and generic substitution. Therapeutic and generic substitutions are identified to maintain or improve quality and provide cost containment through decreased duplication.

Conclusion

Within healthcare institutions, the pharmacy department plays a vital role in ensuring the proper use and administration of medications. Ensuring a patient's profile is as complete as possible is one job of the pharmacy technician. Because of the many different drug delivery systems, technicians working in the institutional pharmacy practice setting also need to know the benefits and limitations of each system. Pharmacy departments are also called upon to point out problems and suggest solutions that will improve the way health care is delivered in that institution.

About the author

Patricia A. Camazzola received her Doctor of Pharmacy degree from the University of Michigan College of Pharmacy and subsequently completed a pharmacy residency at Harper-Grace Hospitals in Detroit, Michigan. Dr. Camazzola is currently coordinating outcomes research and educational programs for Pfizer, Inc., as a clinical education consultant. She previously practiced in the Detroit Medical Center as a pharmacy director, assistant director, and drug information pharmacist. Dr. Camazzola is a past president of the Southeastern Michigan Society of Health-System Pharmacists and, at the time of the publication of this manual, is a member of the University of Michigan College of Pharmacy Board of Governors. In addition, she is an adjunct faculty member of the colleges of pharmacy at both the University of Michigan and Wayne State University.

Self-assessment questions

1. Within an institutional practice setting, the pharmacy department is responsible for all of the following, *except*:
   a. administering medications to patients.
   b. selecting proper medications.
   c. distributing medications to patients.
   d. procuring and storing medications.

2. Which is ***not*** a benefit of a unit-dose drug distribution system?
   a. Medication errors are reduced.
   b. Patient billing is more accurate.
   c. More time is spent charting medications.
   d. Control of medication use on the nursing units is improved.

3. All of the following must appear on a unit-dose product label, *except*:
   a. the medication name.
   b. the dose strength.
   c. the expiration date of the medication.
   d. the patient's name.

4. The hospital committee that is usually responsible for creating and maintaining the drug formulary is the:
   a. Nursing and Pharmacy Committee.
   b. Pharmacy and Therapeutics Committee.
   c. Product Evaluation Committee.
   d. Infection Control Committee.

5. Generically equivalent drugs are drugs that:
   a. are chemically identical in strength, concentration, dosage form, and route of administration.
   b. are chemically different, but expected to produce essentially the same therapeutic outcome and toxicity.
   c. are priced at exactly the same price.
   d. contain different active ingredients.

CHAPTER 6

PHARMACEUTICAL CARE

Kim D. Roberson, R.Ph.

Learning objectives

Upon completion of this chapter, the technician should be able to do the following:

- Define the concept of *pharmaceutical care.*
- List the five steps in the pharmaceutical care process.
- Describe the implications of drug-related problems for the U.S. healthcare system.
- Identify barriers to implementing pharmaceutical care.
- Discuss the skills required of pharmacy technicians when working with a team providing pharmaceutical care.

Introduction

During most of the 20th century, the standard of care for pharmacists was to assure "the right drug for the right patient at the right time." In the 1970s, studies began to provide valuable information about medication and the costs of medication misadventures. In 1995, a study by Jeffrey A. Johnson and J. Lyle Bootman[1] estimated the annual cost of medication related problems to be $76.6 billion, and it was clear that drug therapy problems pose a significant threat to society. Pharmacists began changing from "the right drug for the right patient at the right time" to asking themselves, "Did the drug work? Did the patient get better?"

The changing face of health care

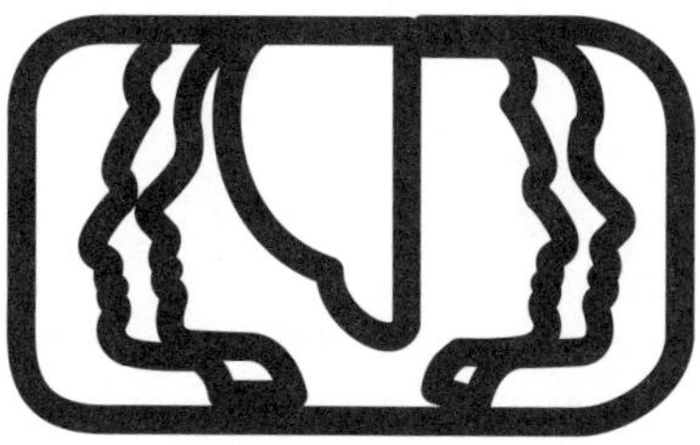

Over the past decade, the healthcare industry has begun to focus on standardizing care. One approach, called "disease management," uses a specified treatment plan or protocol for patients with a similar disease. The most economical and effective protocol can be selected by standardizing care and comparing treatment outcomes. During this same time, new and complex drug regimens were developed, and new information about these was more available in the medical and pharmacy literature. Recognizing the dangers with incorrect use of prescriptions, the federal government created new requirements for pharmacists as part of the Omnibus Budget Reconciliation Act (OBRA) in 1990. OBRA '90 required pharmacists to provide basic education when dispensing prescriptions so that patients would better understand how to use their medication and what to do in the event of a problem.

During the 1990s, two new tools—direct to consumer advertising (DTC) and the Internet—

allowed patients access to information that was previously restricted to pharmacists and physicians. Compared with previous generations, patients of the 1990s were more highly educated and capable of self-help care, including self-diagnosis, treatment selection and evaluating products and services. Patients began relying on pharmacists to help them select and manage their care, and the pharmacist's role had begun to shift. Pharmacists were recognized as the leading healthcare authority on medication and were easily accessible to patients daily, with many pharmacies open 24 hours per day. Pharmacists were a logical choice to evaluate patients' conditions and direct them toward appropriate care. As the decade came to a close, pharmacists collaborated more with physicians and patients and had begun to build a respected role in the management of drug therapy.

Pharmaceutical care

Drs. Charles Hepler and Linda Strand[2] define pharmaceutical care as "the responsible provision of drug therapy to achieve definite outcomes intended to improve the quality of a patient's life." From this definition, it is clear that the pharmacist's role to improve the quality of a patient's life encompasses more than simply dispensing prescriptions. According to Dr. Hepler, "pharmaceutical care involves classical problem solving applied to drug therapy" and "the pharmacist would follow a rational and consistent procedure."

In 1988, Dr. Strand published "Pharmacists Workup of Drug Therapy"[3] (PWDT), which served as the basis for the pharmaceutical care model. Three key components were identified:

1. Consistency, which allows outcomes comparisons
2. An emphasis on continual assessment and management to achieve those definite outcomes
3. A collaborative practice environment between pharmacists, physicians and other healthcare providers

In 1992, Strand, et al.,[4] described a nine-step process for pharmaceutical care. Others have described the process somewhat differently, combining some steps. In 1996, the American Pharmaceutical Association (APhA) released a multiple-day skills training program[5] that taught pharmacists a five-step pharmaceutical care process:

1. Gather appropriate information.
2. Evaluate the information to identify actual or potential drug therapy problems.
3. Develop a Pharmaceutical Care Plan (PCP) to address these problems.
4. Implement the plan.
5. Monitor and follow up to assure appropriate outcomes.

The pharmacist's role dramatically shifts from making sure the right drug product is dispensed to one focused on clinical assessment, therapeutic monitoring and patient education to assure the drug's effectiveness.

Many pharmacists have been providing elements of pharmaceutical care for years, but there has not been a consistent method of delivering these services, or the services were not well-documented. Pharmaceutical care addresses this problem, as pharmacists follow a documented process that results in more consistent outcomes.

In a pharmaceutical care model, pharmacists utilize their training in evaluating individual prescriptions to evaluate the patient's total drug therapy in a consistent method that is easily documented. In collaboration with the patient and physician, the pharmacist identifies actual or potential drug therapy problems. Drug therapy problems can be divided into seven categories:[6]

1. Unnecessary drug therapy
2. Wrong drug prescribed for the diagnosis
3. Dosage prescribed is too low
4. Drug will cause an adverse drug reaction

5. Dosage prescribed is too high
6. The patient cannot/will not comply with the prescribed dosage instructions
7. The patient needs other medications to optimize the treatment outcome

Once the drug therapy problem is identified, the pharmacist works with the patient and physician to develop a solution. This solution, or Pharmaceutical Care Plan (PCP), is documented, started and tracked. Often, it is adjusted as the patient progresses, or the PCP is continued until the treatment goal is reached or the patient is stabilized.

Barriers to the implementation of pharmaceutical care

So, what is keeping pharmacists from embracing this professional utopia? There are several barriers, which include:

- Pharmacist's reluctance to accept change
- Lack of confidence
- Lack of commitment
- Pessimism about pharmacy's future
- Lack of time
- Lack of current drug knowledge (perceived or real)
- Physical store layout
- High renovation or training costs
- Patient reluctance
- Lack of compensation
- Lack of technological support
- Lack of support help
- Potential increase in liability

Of all of these, one of the most critical assets to assuring a successful pharmaceutical care practice is the presence of enthusiastic, dedicated technicians. Without adequate support, pharmacists cannot focus their time on providing direct care services, as they must invest their time in dispensing prescriptions and processing claims with insurance companies.

The role of pharmacy technicians in pharmaceutical care

Pharmacy technicians are valuable assets in performing the technical dispensing functions traditionally done by pharmacists. When technicians are well trained and then given appropriate responsibilities, pharmacists can refocus their time and efforts to provide new patient care services. Pharmacy technicians work can be described in terms of three functions:[7]

1. Assisting the pharmacist in serving patients.
2. Maintaining medication and inventory control systems.
3. Participating in the management and administration of the pharmacy.

In many settings, pharmacists have delegated many functions in these categories to properly trained technicians. In 1999, a task analysis was completed that included the work performed by pharmacy technicians.[7] Table 1 lists primary functions of technicians within the three broad functions listed above.

The survey reported that the technicians devoted a majority of their work time to assisting pharmacists serve patients (community-based) 65 percent of their work time; hospital-based – 57 percent of their work time. Next, 25 percent of their time was devoted to maintaining medication and inventory control systems and 13 percent was dedicated to participating in the management and administration of the pharmacy.

Table 1 Technicians' primary areas of work

	Total[a] (%) (n = 281)	Community (%) (n = 115)	Hospital (%) (n = 113)	Other[b] (%) (n=53)
Assist in preparing outpatient prescriptions	58	90	27	55
Assisting in dispensing inpatient medications	42	11	82	21
Prepare IV admixtures	35	2	73	28
Purchasing/Inventory control	44	51	43	32
Billings	39	46	38	25
Non-sterile compounding	29	18	42	25
Prepackaging/repackaging	38	20	61	30
Educating/training other pharmacy technicians	15	16	15	11
Other	11	4	10	28

a. Percentages do not total 100 because multiple responses were permitted.

b. Includes home health care, long-term care, mail service facility, managed health care, educational/vocational training, military, and pharmaceutical industry

The predominant work areas for community-based pharmacy technicians were: (1) assisting in prescription dispensing (90%), (2) inventory control/purchasing (51%), and (3) billing (46%). Hospital-based pharmacy technicians predominant work areas were: (1) assisting in prescription dispensing (82%), (2) preparing intravenous solutions (73%), and (3) prepackaging/repackaging (61%).

In some instances, technicians may be limited in their activities due to state pharmacy rules or regulations, or by the degree of latitude that the supervising pharmacist authorizes. In most cases, the pharmacy technician performs critical support and quality assurance activities during the medication distribution process, bringing questions and problems to the attention of the pharmacist performing the final checks.

Recommended skills and training

Although highly variable and quite dependent on where technicians work or what pharmacist they work with, there are some universal requirements. Technicians should:

1. Be effective members of a team and support other team members. Have good "people skills."
2. Have a clear understanding of their role on the team, as well as understanding other members' roles.
3. Have a high degree of initiative, yet not overstep their limits, either legal or procedural.
4. Be an effective communicator, both verbal and written.
5. Have a basic understanding of prescription preparation including:
   - Pharmaceutical terminology and abbreviations
   - Pharmaceutical calculations
   - Basic medication classifications
   - Pharmacy computer system usage and procedures
   - Identification and appropriate response to problems that are personnel or system identified

6. Be able to keep patient information confidential. (See Chapter 30 for further discussion of patient confidentiality.)

These are elements common to any setting. Of course, each pharmacy or pharmacist may require other skills or specialized training, such as preparation of intravenous solutions or other prescription compounding.

Conclusion

Regardless of where a pharmacy technician works, it is certain that his or her role will be changing and evolving as the pharmacy profession evolves. What the future holds, no one knows, exactly. What it becomes will be determined by innovative pharmacists and technicians working together for the benefit of their patients.

References

1. Johnson, J.A., Bootman, J.L., "Drug-related morbidity and mortality, a cost-of-illness model," *Archives of Internal Medicine,* Vol. 155, pp. 1949-56, 1995.
2. Hepler, C.D., Strand, L.M., "Opportunities and responsibilities in pharmaceutical care," *American Journal of Hospital Pharmacy,* Vol. 47, pp 533-43, 1990.
3. Strand L.M., Cipolle R.J., Morley P.C., "Documenting the clinical pharmacist's activities: back to basics," *Drug Intell Clin Pharm.,* Vol. 22; pp. 63-67, 1988.
4. Strand L.M., Cipolle R.J., Morley P.C., "Pharmaceutical Care: an introduction," an article in *Current Concepts,* The Upjohn Company, Kalamazoo, MI, 1992, pp. 1-32.
5. "Positioning Your Practice for Pharmaceutical Care: An Individualized Blueprint for Change, Seminar 2: Finding & Solving Drug Therapy Problems," Modules 10-14, American Pharmaceutical Association, Washington, D.C., 1998.
6. "Positioning Your Practice for Pharmaceutical Care: An Individualized Blueprint for Change, Seminar 2: Finding & Solving Drug Therapy Problems," Module 9, American Pharmaceutical Association, Washington, D.C., 1998.
7. Muenzen, P.M., Greenberg, S., Murer, M.M.; "PTCB Task Analysis Identifies Role of Certified Pharmacy Technicians in Pharmaceutical Care," *Journal of the American Pharmaceutical Association,* Vol. 39, No. 6, pp. 857-859, November/December 1999.

About the author

Kim D. Roberson received his bachelor of science degree from the University of Arizona in 1976. He is currently the Senior Director for Professional Affairs at the Texas Pharmacy Association (TPA). Roberson joined TPA in 1996, and his responsibilities include providing or coordinating the education, training, research and marketing of pharmacists providing direct patient care services. His career in pharmacy includes experience as a nuclear pharmacist in Phoenix, Arizona, a hospital pharmacist and a community pharmacist with Smitty's Super Valu, Inc., a food/drug chain in Phoenix. Roberson held the position of pharmacy manager at Smitty's Super Valu until he was promoted to Senior Director – Pharmacy for the chain. Roberson was appointed to two consecutive terms with the Arizona State Board of Pharmacy and served until September 1992 when he became the Executive Director of the Arizona Pharmacy Association.

Self-assessment questions

1. What is the definition of pharmaceutical care according to Drs. Hepler and Strand?
   a. The responsible provision of drug therapy to achieve definite outcomes intended to improve the quality of a patient's life.
   b. Right drug, right patient, at the right time.
   c. Selection and dispensing of medication as ordered by the physician.
   d. The responsible provision of drug therapy to achieve the outcome as ordered by the physician.
2. The five steps of pharmaceutical care include all of the following, *except*:
   a. gather appropriate information.
   b. evaluate the information to identify actual or potential drug therapy problems.
   c. dispense the prescribed medication.
   d. monitor and follow up to assure appropriate outcomes.
3. Drug therapy problems are separated into ______ categories.
   a. three
   b. four
   c. five
   d. seven
4. Barriers to implementing pharmaceutical care include all of the following *except*:
   a. lack of finances to train staff.
   b. heavy pharmacy workload.
   c. legal restrictions.
   d. enthusiastic, dedicated technicians.
5. Responsibilities assigned to a pharmacy technician in a pharmaceutical care model include all of the following *except*:
   a. final check and dispensing of prepared prescriptions.
   b. settling claims and charges with insurance companies.
   c. ordering and checking in replacement inventory.
   d. repackaging bulk medications into "unit-of-use" quantities.
6. The Johnson and Bootman study showed that improper use of prescriptions costs the United States healthcare system:
   a. $26.6 million.
   b. $76.6 million.
   c. $26.1 billion.
   d. $76.6 billion.
7. The Task Analysis of the pharmacy technician's work categorized technicians' activities into three categories. These categories include all of the following *except*:
   a. assisting the pharmacist in serving patients.
   b. maintaining medication and inventory control systems.
   c. participating in the management and administration of the pharmacy.
   d. developing and implementing an effective Pharmaceutical Care Plan.
8. A pharmacy technician should have a basic understanding of all of the following *except*:
   a. pharmaceutical calculations.
   b. assessment and diagnosis of routine diseases, such as sore throats.
   c. pharmacy computer system usage and procedures.
   d. identification and appropriate response to problems that are personnel or system identified.
9. According to a 1999 study, pharmacy technicians spend the least amount of time in:
   a. billing.
   b. pharmacy administration.
   c. inventory control / purchasing.
   d. preparing IV solutions.
10. OBRA '90 requires pharmacists to:
    a. provide the patient with the medication name and strength, if authorized by the physician.
    b. provide prescriptions at the lowest price, but not below cost.
    c. provide patients with medication information so patients better understand their medication.
    d. provide Internet-based patient education.

Chapter 7

Current and Future Roles of Pharmacy Technicians

James B. Vander Linde, Pharm.D.

Learning objectives

Upon completion of this chapter, the technician should be able to do the following:

- ♦ List the skills a pharmacy technician should possess.
- ♦ Explain those factors that influence the role of the pharmacy technician.
- ♦ List the responsibilities of the pharmacy technician.
- ♦ Describe future opportunities for the pharmacy technician.

Introduction

Pharmacy technicians have an important role in the delivery of health care by assisting the pharmacist in the provision of pharmacy services. By definition, a pharmacy technician is a person who works under the supervision of a licensed pharmacist and is allowed to assist in pharmacy activities that do not require the professional judgment of a pharmacist. Pharmacy technicians were first utilized in the mid-1940s; the practice sites and duties that technicians were allowed to perform were initially limited. Today, pharmacy technicians can be found in nearly all institutional and ambulatory healthcare settings in which medications are dispensed. And, their responsibilities have broadened in scope, along with the skill required to fulfill those responsibilities in order to support the expansion of pharmacy practice. It is clear that pharmacy technicians continue to assume more responsibilities related to medication preparation, dispensing, and control as pharmacists increasingly depend on them to be an integral part of pharmacy practice.

Pharmacy technicians must practice under the supervision of a licensed pharmacist who assumes responsibility for their actions in the practice setting. Some state boards of pharmacy, however, have chosen to require that technicians in those states become registered or certified. Pharmacy technicians may also voluntarily choose to become certified through an examination process administered by the Pharmacy Technician Certification Board (PTCB). (See Appendix C for how to contact PTCB.) It is reasonable to expect that requirements for certification, registration, or licensure will increase as the professional role of pharmacy technicians continues to expand and becomes more consistently recognized from state to state.

The primary mission of pharmacy is to help people make the best use of their medications for the purpose of achieving outcomes that will improve their quality of life. This means that pharmacists and pharmacy technicians are involved with providing the medication, as well as providing the proper instruction and monitoring of therapy in order to assure those outcomes are met. This may involve providing medication and education for the purpose of assisting with the cure of a disease, preventing further disease progression, or controlling the manifestations of a disease so that the person can still maintain those day-to-day activities that provide quality and meaning to their life. The re-engineering of the practice of pharmacy to assume the responsibility for improving patient outcomes is what has been termed "pharmaceutical care." (Please refer to Chapter 6.) What has become increasingly apparent is that in order for the pharmacist to adopt a pharmaceutical care approach to practice, it is necessary that various responsibilities previously performed by the pharmacist be delegated to well-qualified, appropriately trained pharmacy technicians.

Pharmacy technicians have the opportunity to practice in several professional settings. These include ambulatory community pharmacy, hospital pharmacy, long-term care, home care, intravenous infusion services, pharmaceutical industry, academia, and mail order pharmacy. This list of practice opportunities is sure to expand as health care changes and pharmacy responds to the changes in order to keep pace with the opportunities in new practice environments.

There is some variation in the duties and functions that pharmacy technicians perform in the various practice settings. Some of this variation is due to a lack of consensus among pharmacists as to which duties should be delegated to pharmacy technicians and which should still be carried out by a pharmacist. Reasons for lack of consensus stem from differing beliefs and attitudes among pharmacists within the various practice settings, as well as individual state regulations that differ as to the functions that technicians are allowed to perform. However, there continues to be more collaboration in developing the role of pharmacy technicians, and there is agreement that technicians play a vital role in the delivery of pharmacy services. The role of pharmacy technicians is sure to expand as their competencies increase and as pharmacists respond to the demand for the provision of more cognitive services.

For any technician to perform his or her responsibilities optimally, he or she must be well-trained, appropriately supervised and work under clear policies and procedures that are based on ethical practice, patient safety, and continuous quality improvement. In addition, the technician should have an overall understanding of the healthcare industry and pharmacy's role in the healthcare system. To perform the duties and functions adequately, the technician should possess a working knowledge of pharmaceutical and medical terminology, medication names, abbreviations, and symbols used in prescribing, dispensing, administering, and charting medication. A general working knowledge of the chemical and physical properties of drugs handled in the manufacturing and packaging operations, along with knowledge of the usual medication strengths and dosages used in the delivery of pharmaceutical services, is required as well. Also, the pharmacy technician should have a thorough understanding of pharmacy law and state regulations governing the practice of pharmacy.

The profession of pharmacy should actively stimulate innovation in the use of pharmacy technicians in ways that will enhance the value of their contribution to health care within the pharmacy environment. The position of a pharmacy technician requires a person who can assume responsibility, is detail oriented and is accurate, for any mistake involving medications can have serious consequences on the health of the patient. A technician must be mindful that they represent pharmacy and that they share in the responsibility of shaping the image of the profession in the eyes of the public. Good communication and skill in dealing with all kinds of personality types is necessary, as well as an ability to anticipate the needs of pharmacists and patients. A successful pharmacy technician will exhibit a high degree of professionalism and will be adept at being discreet and keeping information confidential as often they will have knowledge of patients' personal health information. (See Chapter 30 on Legal Issues.)

Some of the specific duties and functions of pharmacy technicians have previously been discussed in the chapters covering those practice settings. PTCB commissioned an updated list of tasks that pharmacy technicians were currently responsible for in their areas of responsibility.[1] The analysis describes the work performed by technicians in terms of functions or broad areas of responsibility.

Specific responsibilities performed by technicians within each function, as well as the knowledge needed in order to perform those responsibilities, were also included in the report.

According to data from the February 1999 PTCB survey, about an equal number of technicians practice in community pharmacy (41 percent) and hospital pharmacy (40 percent). The other 19 percent practice in settings such as home-health, long-term care, managed care, and pharmacy mail service facilities. For those technicians practicing in community pharmacy, their primary responsibility was assisting in outpatient prescription dispensing. About one-half of community pharmacy technicians were also involved with purchasing functions, inventory management, billing, and processing of third-party prescription payments. Hospital-based pharmacy technicians spent the majority of their time assisting with the inpatient prescription dispensing, along with the preparation of intravenous (IV) fluids. The other major areas of technician work in the hospital environment involve the packaging and prepackaging of medications. In general, pharmacy technicians reported being involved with obtaining clinical information regarding the medical condition of patients, allergies, insurance coverage, and the initial evaluation of a prescription or medication order. Mathematical calculations were also important, as technicians reported that 30 percent of the work week involved performing tasks that required mathematical calculations.

In order for technicians to perform their tasks optimally, they must have adequate training. Technicians cited the most important areas of training focused on knowledge of drug names, classification of medication, and drug dosages. Also, mathematical calculations and conversions, aseptic technique and procedures for preparing intravenous products, pharmacy law and regulations, and customer relations and service were also deemed as necessary components of training for success as a pharmacy technician.

A pharmacy technician should have the basic knowledge and skills to be able to provide assistance to the pharmacist in three general categories of responsibility. These are: 1) assisting the pharmacist in serving patients, 2) maintaining medication and inventory control systems, and 3) participating in the administration and management of pharmacy practice. Specific duties in each of these categories include the following:

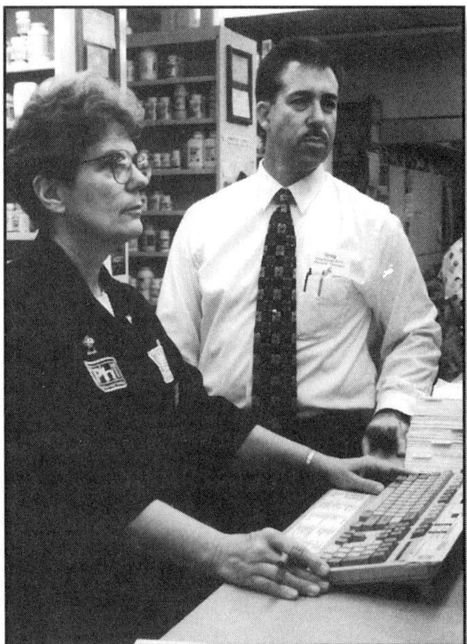

Assisting the pharmacist in serving patients

1. Receive a new or refill prescription or medication order. This may involve a telephone order or transmission via fax or computer. The technician should be skilled in knowing how to contact the prescriber if needed for clarification of the order.
2. Obtain from the patient or prescriber relevant patient information necessary for filling the prescription or medication order. This may include: diagnosis, medical history, medication use, allergies and adverse medication reactions, physical disabilities, and reimbursement information.
3. Collect data necessary for assisting the pharmacist in monitoring the clinical status of the patient. This may include data such as blood pressure and blood glucose.
4. Evaluate the prescription or medication order for completeness (all required information), accuracy, authenticity, legality, and reimbursement eligibility.

5. Update the patient's medical record or profile. This information may include medication history, allergies, medication duplication, and drug-disease, drug-drug, drug-laboratory, and drug-food interactions.
6. Process a prescription or medication order. This could include entering the prescription or medication order information into the patient profile; selecting the drug product; obtaining the medication from inventory; measuring, counting, or calculating the dosage forms for dispensing; recording the preparation of the prescription; packaging the dosage forms; applying prescription and auxiliary labels to the medication container; obtaining the appropriate patient education material; checking the accuracy of the preparation process; checking the prescription preparation of other technicians; and preparing the prescription or medication order for final check by the pharmacist.
7. Compound a prescription or medication order. Duties may include assembling the required equipment and supplies, calibrating the equipment used in the compounding process, performing calculations required to determine the dosage to be compounded, compounding medications according to formula, compounding bulk supplies of medication, preparing sterile products, preparing chemotherapy, and recording the preparation and/or the ingredients used in the compounding process.
8. Provide medication to the patient or the patient's representative. Duties may include properly storing the medication prior to dispensing, actually providing the medication to the patient or their representative, placing the medication in a dispensing system such as a unit-dose cart or a robotic dispensing system, delivering medication to patient care units, recording the distribution of non-controlled and controlled substances in the appropriate manner, and recording the distribution of investigational drugs.
9. Determine charges and obtain reimbursement for the pharmacy services provided.
10. Determine or verify coverage and obtain prior authorization from third party payors if necessary.
11. Provide supplemental information to the patient such as written teaching material and videos to increase the patient's understanding of the medication and appropriate administration and compliance.
12. Communicate with patients to determine if counseling by the pharmacist is desired.
13. Perform supervised drug administration functions.
14. Provide assistance to the pharmacist in monitoring patient laboratory data such as blood glucose, blood pressure, and cholesterol.

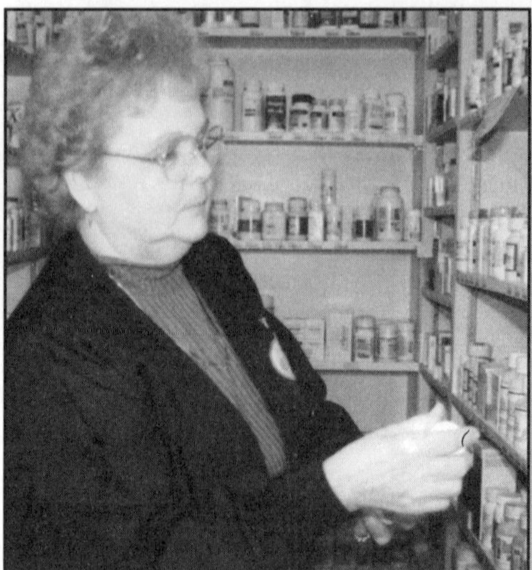

Maintain medication and inventory control systems

1. Identify the pharmaceuticals, durable medical equipment, devices, and supplies to be ordered.
2. Place the orders for pharmaceuticals, durable medical equipment, devices, and supplies in compliance with all applicable regulations.
3. Receive products and verify against the purchase order.
4. Place products into inventory, observing the proper storage conditions recommended for each product.
5. Perform non-patient-specific distribution of pharmaceuticals, durable medical equipment, devices, and supplies.
6. Remove from inventory those pharmaceuticals, equipment, and supplies that have been recalled,

have expired, have been discontinued, or whose use is so infrequent that it does not warrant maintaining them in the inventory.

7. Communicate the changes in product availability to patients and all appropriate healthcare professionals.
8. Be involved in implementing and monitoring policies and procedures designed to deter theft and/or drug diversion.
9. Maintain proper records for receiving, storing, and removing controlled substances from inventory.
10. Participate in performing inventories and the associated record keeping.
11. Maintain the necessary record-keeping systems for repackaging, compounding, recalls, and returns of pharmaceuticals and supplies.
12. Perform compounding of pharmaceuticals in bulk quantities.
13. Perform quality assurance tests on compounded pharmaceutical products.
14. Repackage pharmaceutical products.
15. Participate in quality assurance programs.
16. Communicate with representatives of pharmaceutical and equipment companies.

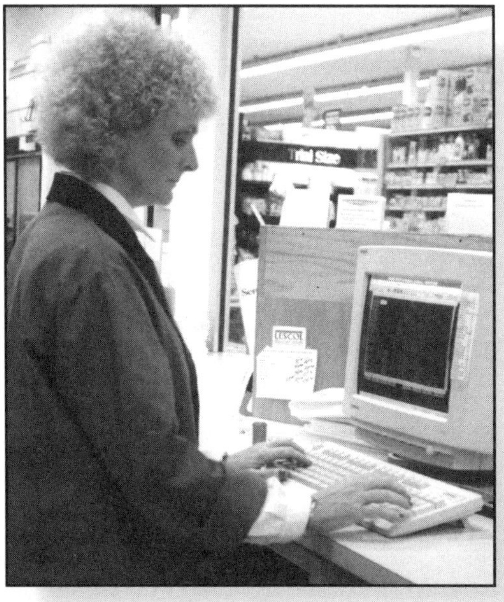

Participating in the administration and management of pharmacy practice

1. Coordinate and disseminate oral, written, and electronic communication throughout the practice setting.
2. Collect productivity information.
3. Participate in quality improvement activities and generate quality improvement reports.
4. Participate in assuring that the practice setting complies with federal, state, and local laws, regulations, and professional standards.
5. Participate in assuring that appropriate policies and procedures are in place, and that monitoring is performed regarding sanitation, management, and handling hazardous waste.
6. Participate in monitoring and recording routine sanitation, maintenance, and calibration of equipment.
7. Utilize manual or computer-based information systems to perform job-related activities.
8. Maintain software for automated dispensing technology.
9. Perform billing and accounting functions.
10. Communicate with third party payors to determine or verify coverage.
11. Conduct staff training.
12. Assist with establishing, implementing, and monitoring policies and procedures.

Future roles of pharmacy technicians

Predicting future roles of pharmacy technicians must take into consideration the history of the practice of pharmacy, as well as the historical progress of the role of the pharmacy technician. This must be coupled with observation and analysis of current trends that are anticipated to have a significant effect on the practice of pharmacy and role of the pharmacy technician. It must also be understood that predictions are only estimates based on information and influences that exist at the present time. Present and future influences such as healthcare reform, regulatory and legislative changes, reimbursement factors, changes in healthcare delivery systems, technological advances, changing population demographics, medical advances, the perception of the profession by society, and society's expectation regarding health care will continue to shape the profession of pharmacy and the role of the pharmacy technician. Therefore, future roles can only be discussed in the context that pharmacy, as a part of the changing pattern of health care, is a dynamic profession.

Conclusion

The profession of pharmacy is undergoing fundamental changes while health care and how it is delivered is being redefined. Along with these changes, the pharmacy profession is moving very rapidly toward an increasingly important role where information and technology to a large extent shape the profession. Advances in technology will drive automation along with the boom in information that will influence the role of the pharmacy technician. It can be expected that pharmacy technicians will be involved with the management of information and technology as it pertains to pharmacy services and pharmaceutical care. As the role of the pharmacist transitions into direct patient care services, technicians will be more involved with the day-to-day operations of the pharmacy. Technicians will become more multi-skilled practice extenders, supporting a variety of patient-focused services.

Some dispensing functions will continue with human labor, but the majority of repetitive tasks will be automated. In this area, the pharmacy technician will monitor, manage, and assure the quality and effectiveness of this technology. Pharmacy technicians can be expected to provide an essential component of pharmacy care or patient-centered care. The functions of the pharmacy technician will include many of the current duties, but will expand to include a variety of other tasks and services designed to continually improve the quality of health care provided by pharmacy.

Reference

1. Muenzen, P.M., Greenberg, S., Murer, M.M.; "PTCB Task Analysis Identifies Role of Certified Pharmacy Technicians in Pharmaceutical Care," *Journal of the American Pharmaceutical Association*, Washington, D.C., Vol. 39, No. 6, pp. 857-864, November/December 1999.

About the author

James B. Vander Linde received his bachelor's degree in pharmacy from Ferris State University College of Pharmacy in Big Rapids, Michigan, in 1979 and his Doctor of Pharmacy degree from Wayne State University College of Pharmacy & Allied Health Professions in Detroit, Michigan, in 1982. He completed a pharmacy practice residency at St. Lawrence Hospital in Lansing, Michigan. Dr. Vander Linde is currently the pharmacy manager at McPherson Hospital, St. Joseph Mercy Health-System in Howell, Michigan. He is a member of the American Society of Health-System Pharmacists and the Michigan Pharmacists Association.

Self-assessment questions

1. Which of the following statements regarding a pharmacy technician is true?
    a. The responsibilities of pharmacy technicians have not increased since the time when technicians were first utilized.
    b. A pharmacy technician must have a license to practice.
    c. Regulations governing the duties of a pharmacy technician are the same in every state.
    d. A pharmacy technician may assist in pharmacy activities that do not require the professional judgment of a pharmacist.
2. Which of the following statements best characterizes the role of the pharmacy technician?
    a. Pharmacy technicians have the same responsibilities in every pharmacy practice setting.
    b. A pharmacy technician is limited to practice in either a hospital or retail pharmacy setting.
    c. Pharmacy technicians must work under the supervision of a licensed pharmacist.
    d. There is consensus among all pharmacists regarding the duties of a pharmacy technician.
3. Which of the following is ***not*** a function of a pharmacy technician?
    a. Evaluating a prescription for accuracy
    b. Obtaining relevant patient information necessary for filling the prescription
    c. Updating a patient medical profile
    d. Dispensing a medication
4. When processing a prescription, what tasks would a pharmacy technician perform?
    a. Obtain the medication from inventory
    b. Collect productivity information
    c. Assure that appropriate policies and procedures are in place
    d. Assist the pharmacist in quality assurance
5. The term given to helping people make the best use of their medications for the purpose of achieving outcomes that will improve that person's quality of life is:
    a. Continuous Quality Improvement
    b. Pharmaceutical Care
    c. Pharmaceutical Plan
    d. Pharmaceutical Outcome
6. Medication inventory control responsibilities would include:
    a. receiving pharmacy-related products and verifying against the purchase order.
    b. assisting the pharmacist with patient clinical monitoring.
    c. performing billing functions.
    d. counting out the prescribed quantity of medication.
7. Responsibilities related to the management of pharmacy practice would include which of the following?
    a. Ordering durable medical equipment
    b. Assuring that the practice site complies with regulations and professional standards
    c. Repackaging pharmaceutical products
    d. Obtaining reimbursement information
8. Assisting the pharmacist in serving patients would include which of the following?
    a. Maintaining controlled substance inventory records
    b. Communicating with representatives of pharmaceutical and equipment companies
    c. Providing medication to the patient or the patient's representative
    d. Disseminating information via electronic means
9. Which of the following will most likely have a major influence on the future roles of pharmacy technicians?
    a. Pre-packaged medication
    b. New clinical monitoring devices
    c. Changes in healthcare delivery systems
    d. More effective medications
10. Which of the following statements is true regarding the future roles of pharmacy technicians based on current trends?
    a. The primary role of pharmacy technicians will be to count medication for filling prescriptions.
    b. The role of the pharmacy technician will not expand much beyond current practice.
    c. Pharmacy technicians will assume all direct patient care responsibilities.
    d. Pharmacy technicians will become more involved with the management of information and technology.

Part II: Operational Skills

CHAPTER

8

TERMINOLOGY

Wynefred Halpin Schumann, M.S.

Learning objectives

Upon completion of this chapter, the technician should be able to do the following:

- Define the listed medical and pharmacy terminology.
- Explain the routes of medication administration.
- Describe the types of pharmaceutical dosage forms.
- Name the chemical compounds as represented by their elemental symbols and molecular formulas.
- Define the meaning of symbols and abbreviations used in pharmacy.

Introduction

The following lists contain terminology, medication routes of administration, and pharmaceutical dosage forms. The prefixes, suffixes, symbols, and abbreviations are commonly used in the practice of pharmacy technology, pharmacy, medicine, and other health professions. These lists are not intended to be complete or exhaustive. Mastery of these terms provides the pharmacy technician with a solid core of information that may prove valuable in practice and as they continue studies as life-long learners. However, do note that each pharmacy practice will have an approved list of symbols and abbreviations, and pharmacy technicians should take care to learn and utilize those symbols and abbreviations that are approved in their workplace.

Basic principles of creation of pharmacy and medical terminology

To understand terminology and medical words, there are four important word parts that will help dissect and describe common words used frequently in pharmacy practice by pharmacy technicians. The four parts of words that are used are word roots, suffixes, prefixes, and a combination of vowels (a, e, i, o, u). These parts are further described as follows:

A word **root** is defined as the core of a word. Notably, each medical term may contain one or more word roots because it is the fundamental meaning of a complex word.

Examples:	*cardi/o*	meaning *heart*
	hepat/o	meaning *liver*

The **suffix** is a word part placed at the **end** of a word **root** to modify its meaning. Each medical term may contain a word **root** and may be modified or clarified by adding a **suffix** to the end of the word. Therefore, *-itis,* meaning *inflammation*, is added to the **root** word *cardi/o* or *hepat/o* to create the following words:

Examples:	*card-itis*	meaning *inflammation* of the *heart*
	hepat-itis	meaning *inflammation* of the *liver*

A **prefix** is the word part placed at the **beginning** of a word **root** to modify its meaning. Medical terms may contain a word **root** plus a **prefix** to modify or clarify the word. When the **prefix** *hyper* (excessive, more than normal) is added to the **root** word *kinetic* (motion) or the **prefix** *hypo* (deficient, less than normal) is added to the **root** word *tensive* (blood pressure), the following words are created.

Examples: *hyper-kinetic* meaning *increased activity* or motion
hypo-tensive meaning *decreased blood pressure*

Adding vowels between two word roots or between a word root and suffix helps with the pronunciation and often utilizes the letter "o." Adding the vowel "o" allows the **root** word *vas* (blood vessels) to combine with the **suffix** *–constrictor* and with the **suffix** *-dilator* to create these words:

Examples: *vaso-constrictor* meaning *narrowing* of the *blood vessels*
vaso-dilator meaning *widening* of the *blood vessels*

The following table provides several forms of each word for a comprehensive review.

Prefixes and suffixes	**Definition**
a-, an-	absence of, lacking, no
-algia	painful condition
ant-, anti-	inhibiting, opposing, relieving
ante-	before; forward
arter-, arteri-, arterio-	artery
arthr-, arthro-	joint
-ase	an enzyme
audi-, audio-	hearing, sound
aut-, auto-	self, self-regulating
bio-	life, living organisms
brady-	slow
cardi-, cardio-	heart
cervic-, cervico-	neck
-cidal, -cide	killing, killer
col-, coli-, colo-	colon
contra-	against, in opposition
cyst-, cysto-	bladder, sac
derm-, derma-, dermat-, dermato- dermo-, -derm	skin
dys-	abnormal, difficult, impaired
ect-, ecto-	outside, eternal
-ectomy	surgical removal
-emia	condition of the blood
end-, endo-	inside, within
enter-, entero-	intestine
-facient	causing, making
gastri-, gastro-	stomach

Prefixes and suffixes	Definition
-genic	producing, formed from
gluc-, gluco-	glucose
hem-, hema-, hemat-, hemato-, hemo	blood
hepat-	liver
hyper-	excessive, more than normal; above, over
hypo-	deficient, less than normal; below, under
inter-	between
intra-	inside, within
-itis	inflammation
macr-, macro-	large, long
mal-	abnormal, inadequate
micr-, micro-	small, minute; one millionth part
my-, myo-	muscle
nephr-, nephro-	kidney
-oma	tumor
ophthalm-, ophthalmo-	eye
-osis	any condition; abnormal or diseased condition
oste-, osteo-	bone
ot-, oto-	ear
path-, patho-, -pathy	disease
-penia	deficiency
peri-	around, enclosing
phag-, phago-	eating
phleb-, phlebo-	vein
pneum-, pneumo-	air, gas; lung
poly-	many, excessive
post-	after; behind
pre-	before; anterior
proct-, procto-	anus, rectum
psych-, psycho-	mind, mental
pulmo-	lung
rhine-, rhino-	nose
-stomy, -ostomy	surgical opening
sub-	below, underlying; slightly, inadequately
tachy-	fast
ther-, thermo-	heat, temperature
tox-, toxi-, toxic-, toxico-, toxo-,	poisonous
uria-	condition of urine or urination
vas-	blood vessels

General information

Following are definitions, abbreviations, and acronyms for a variety of classifications within health care. An alphabetical list of definitions is followed by an alphabetical table of abbreviations and acronyms for each classification.

The contents of these lists do not imply that these symbols and abbreviations are official, unambiguous or universally recognized. In fact, though commonly used, several of these abbreviations may be misinterpreted, or may be associated with different practice settings. Please note that the phrase *may be confusing* is added when the same abbreviation has two or more popular meanings. In some instances, it is valuable to interpret the abbreviation in the context in which is it used.

Examples:	*PT*	meaning the allied health specialty of *Physical Therapy*
	PT	meaning *Prothrombin Time*

Administration route

These abbreviations define the multiple methods of administering medications. The abbreviations are commonly based on Latin interpretations. Other abbreviations are from commonly defined acronyms using the first initial of each word.

Examples:	*PO*	per os	meaning *by mouth*
	IM	intramuscular	meaning *into the muscle*

Buccal: administering medication by placing it between the cheek and gum (the buccal pouch) where it will dissolve or disintegrate slowly.

Hyperalimentation: the administration of nutrients intravenously.

Infusion: the slow injection of a solution or emulsion into a vein or subcutaneous tissue.

Inhalation: the administration of a drug into the lungs or the respiratory tract by air pathway.

Intracardiac: the administration of a drug by injection into the heart.

Intradermal: the administration of a drug by injection into the skin.

Intramuscular: the administration of a drug by injection into the muscle.

Intrathecal: the administration of a drug by injection into the subarachnoid space surrounding the brain and spinal cord.

Intravenous: the administration of a drug by injection into a vein.

Nasogastric: the administration of a drug through a tube passed through the nose into the stomach.

Ophthalmic: the administration of a drug to the eye.

Parenteral #1: the administration by routes other than orally, but not intestinal.

Parenteral #2: the administration by injection; the most common injectable routes are intradermal, intramuscular, intravenous, and subcutaneous.

Rectal: the administration of a drug into the rectum or lower intestine.

Subcutaneous: the administration of a drug by injection beneath the skin.

Sublingual: the administration of a drug underneath the tongue.

Topical: the administration of drugs or medicine to the skin of the body.

Vaginal: the administration of a drug into the vagina.

Abbreviation	Meaning
a. d.	right ear
a. s.	left ear
a. u.	each ear
H	hypodermic
IC	intracardiac
ID	intradermal
IM	intramuscular
IV	intravenous
IVP	IV push; intravenous pyelogram *(may be confusing)*
IVPB	intravenous piggyback
l.	left
MDI	metered dose inhaler
NG	nasogastric
NPO	nothing by mouth
o. d.	right eye
o. s.	left eye
o. u.	both eyes
PICC	peripherally inserted central catheter
PO, per os	by mouth; orally
PR	per rectum
r.	right
Rec, rect	rectal, per rectum
s. l.	sublingual
SC, s.q., Sub-q	subcutaneous
Subling.	sublingual
Vag.	vaginal

Administration time

These abbreviations define the multiple times and series of times that drugs are administered. The abbreviations are commonly based on Latin interpretations. Other abbreviations are from commonly defined acronyms using the first initial of each word.

Examples:	*PRN*	pro ra nada	meaning *as needed*
	ASAP	as soon as possible	meaning *do not delay*

Abbreviation	Meaning
a. c.	before meals
a. m.	before noon; morning
Ad lib	at pleasure; as desired
ASAP	as soon as possible
b. i. d.	twice daily
D.A.W.	dispense as written; do not substitute with generic form of drug
DC	discontinue
h. s.	at bedtime
Hr.	hour
KVO	keep vein open
MR	may repeat
Non Rep, NR	do not repeat, no renewals
p. c.	after meals
p. m.	afternoon; evening
post	after
post op	after surgery
post partum	after delivery
Pre op	before surgery
PRN	as needed
Q	each, every
q. d.	daily, every day
q. h.	every hour
q. h. s.	every bedtime
q. i. d.	four times daily
q. o. d.	every other day
q. s.	a sufficient quantity
q. wk.	every week
STAT	at once, now
t. i. d.	three times daily
Ut. Dict	as directed
w., wk	week

Diseases

The following are examples of definitions, abbreviations, and acronyms of diseases that are commonly found in pharmacy practice.

Allergy: a condition of unusual or exaggerated specific sensitivity to a substance that is harmless in similar amounts to an average person.
Anemia: a blood deficiency of the hemoglobin that transports oxygen.
Arthritis: an inflammation of the joints.
Carcinogen: a substance that causes cancer.
Cystitis: an inflammation of the urinary bladder.
Decubitis ulcer: a sore caused by prolonged pressure on a patient's skin when confined to bed for a long period of time; also called a pressure sore or bedsore.
Fungus: a plant-like organism that lacks the green pigment chlorophyll.
Hepatitis: an inflammation of the liver.
Herpes simplex: an acute viral disease marked by groups of watery blisters on the skin and mucous membranes; also called *cold sores* when around the mouth area.
Hypertension: high blood pressure.
Jaundice: yellow appearance of skin, eyes and other tissues resulting from deposition of bile pigment.
Leukemia: diseases characterized by extremely high leukocyte counts.
Malignant: a condition tending to become progressively worse if untreated.
Metastasis: the spreading of disease from one organ or part of the body to another.
Nephritis: an inflammation of the kidney.
Pathogen: any disease-producing microorganism.
Pathology: the study of diseases, their causes, and the structural and functional changes they cause in tissues and organs of the body.
Phlebitis: an inflammation of the veins.
Pruritis: itching
Shock: a condition of acute peripheral circulatory failure due to interruption of circulatory control or loss of circulating fluid; characterized by clamminess of the skin, decreased blood pressure, feeble rapid pulse, decreased respiration, etc.
Symptom: a specific functional evidence of disease observed by the patient.
Syndrome: a set of symptoms occurring together and characterizing a particular abnormality.
Virus: a submicroscopic agent capable of growth and replication only within living cells; viruses cause many human diseases.

Abbreviation	Meaning
AIDS	acquired immune deficiency syndrome
CA	carcinoma
GERD	gastro esophageal reflux disease
HIV	human immunodeficiency virus
N & V	nausea and vomiting
PMS	premenstrual syndrome
URI	upper respiratory infection
UTI	urinary tract infection
HA	headache, hyperalimentation *(may be confusing)*

Dosage forms

This terminology defines the dosage forms commercially and professional prepared and includes more than 15 definitions of tablets in addition to the various types of drug dosage forms to maximize therapeutic and pharmacological effects.

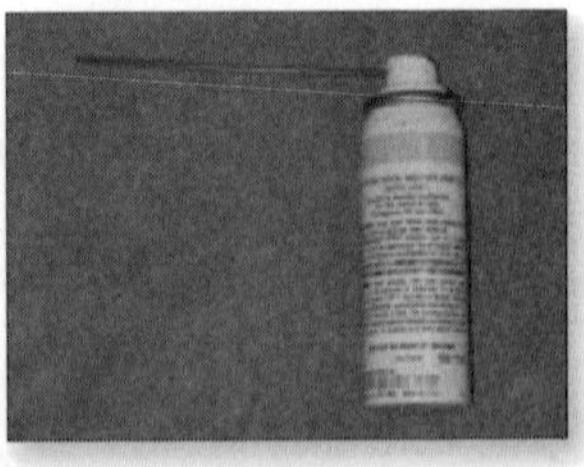

Aerosols: sprayable products employing propellants (liquefied gases) and valve systems to deliver medication. They are used for topical application to the skin, inhalation into the lungs, and local application in the nose and mouth. The medicinal agent may be a liquid or a finely divided powder. When used for inhalation therapy, a standard amount of drug must be delivered with each activation of the system. Metered-dose inhalers are used for this purpose.

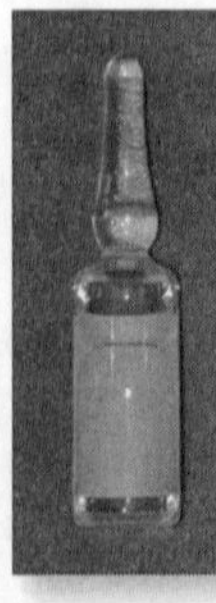

Ampule: a sterile glass or plastic container with single dose of parenteral solution.

Buccal: tablets that are placed in the buccal pouch (between the cheek and gum) where they dissolve or disintegrate slowly. The active ingredient is absorbed directly without passing through gastrointestinal tract.

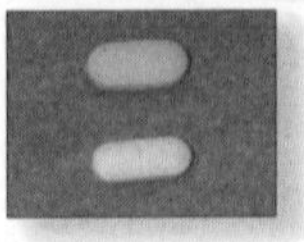

Caplet: tablets that are shaped like capsules.

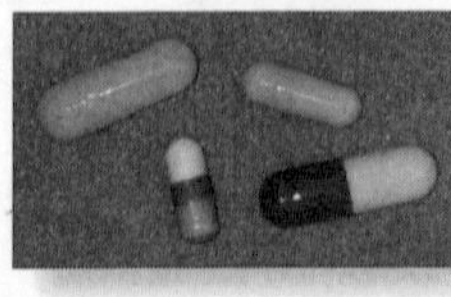

Capsules: a solid dosage form with the drug enclosed in a soluble shell of either hard or soft gelatin. Capsules can mask the unpleasant taste and odor of a drug by enclosing them in the almost tasteless shell. Capsule sizes range from the smallest (No. 5) to the largest (No. 000). Hard gelatin capsules typically contain powders or granules; soft gelatin capsules typically contain liquids. Capsules usually dissolve and release their contents in the stomach within 10 to 15 minutes. Extended- or timed-release capsules are formulated to release the drug over a prolonged period of time, usually between eight and 24 hours.

Chewable: tablets that are pleasant tasting and intended to be chewed or dissolved in the mouth and then swallowed.

Colloidal suspensions: see *gels*.

Creams: viscous liquid or semi solid emulsion of oil and water; generally applied topically to the skin, into the vagina, or into the rectum.

Effervescent: a tablet that contains a mixture of acid and sodium bicarbonate in addition to the active ingredient(s). These tablets release carbon dioxide and dissolve rapidly when placed in water.

Elixir: clear, sweetened liquid dosage forms whose primary solvents are water and alcohol. They may contain flavoring substances; medicated elixirs contain active medicinal agents.

Emulsions: semi-liquid or solid preparations containing fats and oils suspended with the aid of an agent that promotes and stabilizes the formation of the preparation.

Enemas: rectal preparations used for the evacuation of the bowel (evacuation enemas), for a system's absorption of drugs (retention enema), or for local effect on the lower intestine.

Enteric coated: tablets that have a special coating to prevent dissolution in the stomach; they dissolve in the intestine instead.

Essences: see *spirits.*

Extended-release: tablets that are formulated to release the drug over a prolonged period of time; referred to as controlled-release, sustained-action or timed-release tablets.

Eye insert: small, wafer-like pads designed for insertion under the eyelid where medication is released for an extended period of time.

Fluid extracts: liquid preparations of vegetable drugs containing alcohol as a solvent or preservative; manufactured with each milliliter containing the therapeutic constituents of one gram of the standard drug that is represented in concentration of 100% weight/volume.

Gels: semisolid suspensions of very small particles, usually in water; may be referred to as colloidal suspension.

Liniments: mixture of various substances in oil, alcohol solutions of soap, or emulsions intended for external application. They are often used for their rubefacient, or heat-producing, effects.

Lotions: fluid emulsions or suspensions intended for external application to the body.

Lozenges: tablets held in the mouth for slow dissolution; the medication stays in contact with mouth and throat for an extended period of time; also known as troches.

Matrix: tablets that contain the active drug in a wax matrix, formulated to provide a controlled-release of the drug to minimize high concentrations in the gastrointestinal tract.

Ointments: semisolid preparations intended for external application to the skin or mucous membranes.

Pellets (implanted tablets): tablets that are intended for surgical implantation in the subcutaneous tissue. These highly purified products release the drug over a long period of time.

Powders: finely divided solid materials intended for use internally or externally.

Solutions: liquid preparations containing one or more soluble chemical substances, usually dissolved in water.

Spirits: alcoholic or hydroalcoholic solutions of volatile substances that contain a high percentage of alcohol and require storage in tight containers to prevent loss through evaporation; sometimes referred to as essences.

Sublingual: tablets that are placed under the tongue. Sublingual tablets dissolve rapidly when the active ingredient is absorbed directly without passing through the gastrointestinal tract.

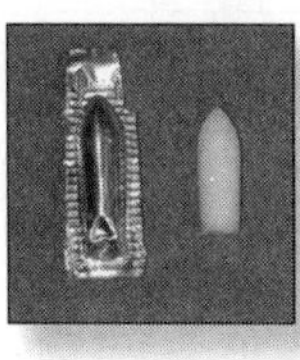

Suppositories: solid dosage forms that are usually manufactured in cylindrical, egg, or pear shapes for insertion into the rectum, vagina or urethra.

Suspensions: preparation of finely divided, undissolved drugs dispersed in a liquid. Suspensions are often supplied as powder intended for suspension in a suitable liquid vehicle prior to use. Suspension must be well-shaken before use.

Syrups: concentrated solutions of sugar (e.g., sucrose) in water or other aqueous liquid.

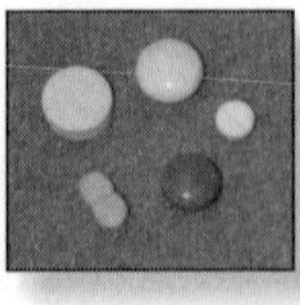

Tablets: compressed tablets are the most common dosage forms used in the United States. Most are swallowed whole with water and later disintegrate in the gastrointestinal tract. These solid dosage forms vary greatly in shape, size, weight, and other properties. Most tablets are made by compression in a large-scale facility. The granular medicinal substances are mixed with fillers, binders, and other agents. This granular mixture is subjected to high pressure utilizing dies and punches to form compressed tablets.

Tinctures: alcoholic or hydroalcoholic solutions prepared from vegetable drugs or from chemical substances. Tinctures usually contain 10% to 20% (w/v) of the drug.

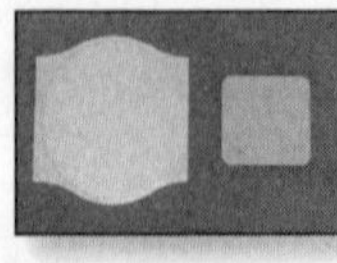

Transdermal: flat, topical systems (patches) intended to provide continuous, controlled-release of a drug through a semi-permeable membrane; applied to intact skin.

Vaginal: tablets, creams or ointments that deliver medication to the vagina; may be inserted into the vagina with the fingers or a delivery device.

Abbreviation	Meaning
Amp	ampule
Cap	capsules
Conc.	concentration
EC	enteric coated
El., elix	elixir
Ext.	extract
Fl.	fluid
Oint	ointment
oph., ophth.	ophthalmic
Pulv	powder
SOS	may repeat if necessary
supp, suppos	suppository
susp.	suspension
Syr	syrup
Tr., tinct.	tincture
ung, ugt	ointment

Elemental chemical symbols and molecular formulae

Elemental chemical symbols and the subsequent molecular formulae using those symbols are universally recognized and should not be ambiguous. Refer to any current chemistry text for additional formulae.

Chemical symbol	Chemical
C	carbon, elemental
Ca	calcium
Cl	chlorine
Cl^-	chloride
Cr	chromium
Cu	copper
Fe	iron, elemental
H	hydrogen
I	iodine, elemental
K	potassium, elemental
Mg	magnesium, elemental
Mn	manganese, elemental
Na	sodium, elemental
O	oxygen, elemental
O_2	oxygen
P	phosphorous, elemental
S	sulfur, elemental
Zn	zinc, elemental

Medicine, allied health and medical specialty

The table defines some common terms found in pharmacy and medical practice, and includes some professionals in health care who have frequent interaction with pharmacy technicians and pharmacists.

Examples: *CRNA* Certified Registered Nurse Anesthetists
Appendix A small pouch, with no known function, attached to the cecum

Aneurysm: a sac filled with blood and formed by a weakness in the walls of an artery or a vein.

Angina pectoris: an attack of chest pain caused by insufficient supply of oxygen to the heart.

Aorta: the largest artery in the body.

Appendix: a small pouch, with no known function, attached to the cecum.

Arrhythmia: any irregular heart rate.

Arteriosclerosis: any condition marked by thickening, hardening and loss of elasticity of the arteries.

Artery: blood vessels that carry oxygen away from the heart to the body cells.

Bacteria: unicellular microorganisms that have various forms and often cause disease.

Benign: a condition that does not threaten health.

Biopsy: the removal of a small piece of tissue for examination.

Congestive Heart Failure (CHF): the failure or diminished ability of the heart to supply blood to the tissues and organs of the body.
Electrocardiogram (ECG): a graphic record of the heart's electrical activity; sometimes called an EKG.
Electroencephalogram (EEG): a graphic record of the brain's electrical activity.
Erythrocyte: a red blood cell.
Excretion: a process by which material is eliminated from the body.
Fibrillation: a rapid, ineffective heart beat.
Gastric: pertaining to the stomach.
Hematocrit: the percent of the total blood volume composed of erythrocytes; also known as packed blood (or cell) volume.
Hyperkinetic: an abnormally increased motor function or activity.
Infection: the invasion of the body by pathogenic organisms.
Inflammation: a reaction of tissue to injuries; characterized by pain, heat, redness, and swelling.
Leukocyte: a white blood cell.
Mastectomy: the surgical removal of the breast.
Nosocomial: acquired at, or originating from, a hospital (e.g., nosocomial infection).
Ophthalmic: relating to the eye; route of administration to the eye.
Oral: pertaining to the mouth.
Otic: relating to the ear; route of administration in the ear.
Phobia: a fear of something.
Renal: pertaining to the kidneys.
Syncope: a temporary suspension of consciousness due to cerebral anemia; a faint.
Systemic: pertaining to or affecting the body as a whole.
Tracheotomy: an incision into the trachea thorough the skin and muscles of the neck to relieve obstruction to breathing.
Vertigo: dizziness.

Abbreviation	**Meaning**
Abd	abdomen, abdominal
ABG	arterial blood gases
Anes	anesthesia
Angi-, angio-	blood or lymph vessel
APTT	activated partial thromboplastin time
BM	bowel movement
BP	blood pressure
BS	blood sugar
BUN	blood urea nitrogen
Cath	catheter
CBC	complete blood count
CCU	coronary care unit
CHF	congestive heart failure
CHO	cholesterol
CPR	cardiopulmonary resuscitation
CRNA	Certified Registered Nurse Anesthetist

Abbreviation	Meaning
CVA	cerebral vascular accident
Diag, DX	diagnosis
EPO	erythropoietin, epoetin alpha
FBS	fasting blood sugar
G-CSF	granulocyte colony stimulating factor, filgrastim
GI	gastrointestinal
GU	genitourinary
Gyn	gynecological
H. pylori	*Helicobacter pylori*
HCT	hematocrit
HDL	high density lipoprotein
Hgb	hemoglobin
HR	heart rate
HRT	hormone replacement therapy
INR	international normalized ratio
LDL	low density lipoprotein
LPN	licensed practical nurse
LS	lumbo-sacral
MI	myocardial infarction
MRI	magnetic resonance imaging
N & V	nausea and vomiting
OB	obstetrics
Ortho	orthopedics
OT	occupational therapy
Oto	otology
Ped	pediatric
PET Scan	positron emission tomography
PT	prothrombin time; physical therapy *(may be confusing)*
pt	patient, pint *(may be confusing)*
RBC	red blood cells
SCr	serum creatinine
surg.	surgery
T	temperature
TC	total serum cholesterol
TCT	total clotting time
TIA	transient ischemic attack
TSH	thyroid stimulating hormone
UV	ultraviolet
VS	vital signs
w.; wk	week
WBC	white blood cell

Pharmacology: study of drugs and their effects on the body

Within pharmacy and medicine there is pharmacological terminology to describe a drug's action on the body. These terms may also describe classes of drugs.

Examples: *tetracycline* These broad-spectrum agents are effective against certain bacterial strains that resist other antibiotics.[1]

Absorption: the process by which substances (including drugs) are taken up and are transported to the bloodstream.

ACE Inhibitor: angiotensin converting enzyme inhibitors; used as an antihypertensive drug (e.g., lininopril).

Acidosis: an acid-base imbalance in which the pH of the blood becomes excessively low due to an inability of the body to maintain its proper alkali reserve.

Addiction: a pattern of compulsive drug use characterized by overwhelming involvement with the drug, securing its supply, and a high tendency to relapse after withdrawal.

Additive: a drug added to a solution intended for intravenous use (e.g., potassium chloride).

Additive response: when the effect of two or more combined drugs is equal to the sum of their individual effects.

Adverse Drug Effects (ADE): effects occurring other than the desired ones. Adverse effects may be divided into two groups, side effects and toxicities.

Alkalosis: an acid-base imbalance in which the pH of the blood becomes excessively high due to an inability of the body to maintain its proper acid reserve.

Allergen: a substance that stimulates an altered cellular response in the body and produces the symptoms of allergy (e.g., pollen).

Amebicide: a drug that destroys amoebas (one-celled organisms) or inhibits their growth (e.g., chloroquine phosphate).

Analeptic: a drug that stimulates the central nervous system (e.g., caffeine).

Analgesic: a drug that relieves pain (e.g., aspirin).

Anaphylaxis: a hypersensitivity reaction resulting from contact with a causative agent after prior sensitization to this agent. The mediating agent is histamine that may be released locally or systemically. Anaphylactic shock is a rare condition, but is often life-threatening.

Anesthetic: a drug used to eliminate sensation; may be administered to a specific body site to provide a local effect (e.g., lidocaine) or systemically to provide a general effect.

Anorectic: a drug that depresses appetite (e.g., diethylpropion).

Antacid: a drug or dietary supplement that counteracts or neutralizes stomach acidity (e.g., calcium carbonate).

Antagonist: a drug that opposes the action of another drug (e.g., amphetamines are antagonists to barbiturates).

Anthelmintic: a drug that destroys or paralyzes parasitic worms (e.g., piperazine); compare with vermicide.

Antibacterial: a drug that destroys bacteria or inhibits their growth or reproduction; compare with bactericidal, bacteriostatic.

Antibiotic: a substance produced by a living microorganism capable of killing or inhibiting the growth of another microorganism (e.g., penicillin).

Anticoagulant: an agent that prevents or delays the clotting of blood (e.g., warfarin sodium).

Anticonvulsant: a drug used to prevent or reduce the severity of convulsive seizures (e.g., phenytoin).

Antidepressant: a drug used to prevent or relieve depression (e.g., venlafaxine).

Antiemetic: a drug or agent used to prevent or reduce nausea and vomiting (e.g., prochlorperazine).

Antihistamine: a drug that antagonizes one of the effects of histamine (e.g., chlorpheniramine maleate).

Anti-inflammatory: a drug that counteracts or suppresses inflammation (e.g., ibuprofen).

Antineoplastic: a drug that destroys or inhibits tumor cells; a drug used in cancer chemotherapy (e.g., cisplatin).

Antipruritic: a drug that relieves itching (e.g., diphenhydramine HCl).

Antipyretic: a drug that reduces fever (e.g., aspirin).

Antiseptic: an agent that destroys or inhibits the growth of microorganisms and may be applied safely to living tissue (e.g., povidone iodine).

Antispasmodic: a drug that relieves or prevents spasms (e.g., atropine sulfate).

Antitoxin: an antibody capable of neutralizing the specific toxin that stimulated its production (e.g., tetanus antitoxin); compare with toxin.

Antitussive: a drug that relieves coughing (e.g., dextromethorphan).

Antiviral: a drug that inhibits the replication of viruses (e.g., ganciclovir).

Bactericidal: capable of killing bacteria; compare with antibacterial and bacteriostatic.

Bacteriostatic: capable of inhibiting the growth or reproduction of bacteria; compare with antibacterial and bactericidal.

Bioavailability: measures the rate and extent of systemic absorption of a therapeutically active drug.

Biotransformation: see metabolism.

Cathartic: a drug used to stimulate evacuation of the bowels (e.g., bisacodyl); compare with laxative.

Caustic: an agent that causes burning and destruction of tissue upon contact.

Chemotherapy: the prevention or treatment of a disease by administering chemical agents.

Contraindication: an aspect of a patient's condition that makes it unwise to pursue a specific treatment.

Cumulative effects: toxic effects resulting from repeatedly administering a drug faster than the body can metabolize or eliminate it.

Decongestant: a drug that relieves congestion and opens blocked air passages in the nose and bronchi (e.g., pseudoephedrine HCl).

Dependence: an altered state produced by habitual drug use; continued administration of the drug is necessary to prevent physical withdrawal symptoms or to maintain a psychological state of well-being.

Depressant: a drug that decreases the activity of a body process or functioning of a body organ (e.g., phenobarbital).

Disinfectant: an agent that destroys microorganisms on inanimate objects.

Distribution: the process that moves a drug from the bloodstream to the area where it will exert its pharmacological effect.

Diuretic: a drug that increases urine production (e.g., furosemide).

Emetic: a drug that causes vomiting (e.g., Syrup of Ipecac).

Expectorant: an agent that increases respiratory tract fluid and reduces the viscosity of mucous secretions (e.g., guaifenesin).

Fungicide: an agent that kills fungi (e.g., nystatin).

Hormone: a substance formed by one organ that is transported through the blood stream to a distant site where it affects the function of another organ (e.g., estrogen).

Hypersensitive: tending to exhibit an abnormally increased response to a drug or other agent.

Hypoglycemic: a drug that decreases the amount of glucose circulating in the blood (e.g., glipizide).

Idiosyncrasy: an abnormal or peculiar response to a certain drug in a particular individual (e.g., morphine producing excitement rather than depression).

Immunity: the ability to resist and overcome infection.

Laxative: a drug used to stimulate evacuation of the bowels or to promote softer, bulkier stools (e.g., docusate sodium); compare with cathartic.

Metabolism: a biochemical alteration of substances (including drugs) within the body.

Narcotic: a drug that induces insensibility and relieves pain but is also addicting, causing dependence and tolerance (e.g., morphine sulfate).

Pharmacodynamics: the relation of drug concentration and its pharmacological response.

Pharmacokinetics: the study of the rates at which drugs and their metabolites are absorbed into, distributed throughout, and eliminated from the body.

Respiration: the process by which an organism exchanges gases with its environment. It includes oxygen uptake and carbon dioxide release by breathing through lungs, diffusion through body surfaces, and diffusion through gills.

Sedative: a drug that exerts a quieting effect on mental processes or nervous irritability (e.g., secobarbital).

Side effect: an undesirable pharmacological effect of a drug produced when therapeutic doses of the drug are administered.

Teratogenic effect: the induction of a defect in an unborn child (fetus) produced by a drug administered to the mother.

Tolerance: a condition where a drug has a less than normal effect on the body; may develop when the drug is used repeatedly over a long period of time. When tolerance develops, the dose of the drug is usually increased to maintain a desired therapeutic effect.

Tranquilizer: a drug that relieves anxiety and tension (e.g., diazepam), producing a calming effect.

Vaccine: an agent administered to establish resistance to an infectious disease (e.g., polio vaccine).

Vasoconstrictor: a drug that causes a narrowing of the blood vessels (e.g., phenylephrine HCl).

Vasodilator: a drug that causes widening of the blood vessels (e.g., nitroglycerin).

Vermicide: a drug that destroys parasitic worms (e.g., thiabendazole); compare with anthelmintic.

Abbreviation	Meaning
ACTH	adrenocorticotropic hormone
ADR	adverse drug reaction
Alb	albumin
ANS	autonomic nervous system
APAP	acetaminophen
ASA	acetylsalicylic acid; aspirin
B & O	belladonna and opium
BC, BCP	birth control pills
BE	barium enema
Carb	carbohydrate
CNS	central nervous system
D5W	dextrose 5% in water intravenous fluid
DS	double strength
EtOH	ethanol, alcohol
HC	hydrocortisone
INH	isoniazid
IPPB	intermittent positive pressure breathing
LCD	liquor carbonis detergens; coal tar solution
LOC	laxative of choice
MOM	milk of magnesia
MS	morphine sulfate
MVI	multiple vitamin infusion
NS	normal saline, 0.9% sodium chloride
NSAID	nonsteroidal anti-inflammatory drug
NTG	nitroglycerine
OJ	orange juice
PCN	penicillin
PEFR	peak expiratory flow rate; peak flow
PPD	purified protein derivative
sat	saturated
SSKI	saturated solution potassium iodide
SSRI	selective serotonin reuptake inhibitors
SWI; SWFI	sterile water; sterile water for injection
TCN	tetracycline
tPA	tissue plasminogen activator
TPN	total parenteral nutrition

Pharmacy

The terminology in the practice of pharmacy describes terms used in pharmacy law, administrative rules, management and scope of pharmacy practice.

Examples:	*aa*	of each
	Ambulatory Pharmacy Service	Health care provided by pharmacy professional to the walk-in (ambulatory) patient.

Ambulatory Pharmacy Service: health care provided by pharmacy professional to the walk-in (ambulatory) patient.

Auxiliary labels: small labels printed with additional information, reminders, or warnings to the patient about drug use. Used to supplement direct patient counseling and the prescription label.

Brand name: the name assigned to a drug by its manufacturer; often called the proprietary or trade name of a drug.

Chemical name: usually the full, systematic name for the drug substances.

Generic name: a convenient and concise name in the public domain for medicines with the same ingredients that are available under different brand names from a variety of companies; often referred to as the nonproprietary name.

Nonprescription: medication that does not require a prescription; sometimes called OTC (over-the-counter).

Patient Medication Profile: a record of all medication prescribed for an individual patient. A profile may identify patient characteristics including age, height, sex, diagnoses, previous adverse drug effects, and allergies.

Prescription: a written or verbal order for a patient's medication or device issued by an appropriately licensed healthcare professional.

Sterilize: to render objects, wounds, etc., free of microorganisms, usually by destroying those present with heat or by other means.

Synergistic response: when the effect of two or more combined drugs is greater than the sum of their individual effects.

Toxicity: a harmful or poisonous effect on the human body.

Toxin: a poison produced by a living organism, often by a bacterium; compare with antitoxin.

Abbreviation	Meaning
aa	of each
Alk	alkaline
Aq dist	distilled water
Aq, aqua	water
AWP	average wholesale price
C	with
Cpd., cmpd	compound
CQI	continuous quality improvement
DEA	Drug Enforcement Administration
Disp.	dispense

Abbreviation	Meaning
DNA	deoxyribonucleic acid
DRG	diagnosis related group
DTD	dispense of such dose
DUE	drug utilization evaluation; see also drug utilization review
DUR	drug utilization review; see also drug utilization evaluation.
HMO	health maintenance organization
HX	history, as in medical history
ICU	intensive care unit
LAS	label as such
LR	lactated ringers
M	mix
m. ft.	mix and make
MAC	maximum allowable cost
Mixt	mixture
OBRA	Omnibus Budget Reconciliation Act
OP	outpatient
OTC	nonprescription (over-the-counter)
PPI	patient package insert
PPO	preferred provider organization
Rx	prescription; take
S	without
Sig.	label, let it be labeled
sol., soln.	solution
Ss	one-half
Tx	treatment
USP	United States Pharmacopeia
VO	verbal order

Weights and measures

The terminology found in pharmaceutical weights and measures for liquids and solids is based on the metric system. There is limited reference to the apothecary system, which is seldom used in current pharmacy practice. Further definitions are found in the Calculations chapter (Chapter 32).

Examples:	*mg*	milligram	meaning one-one thousandth of a gram
	ml	milliliter	meaning one-one thousandth of a liter

Abbreviation	Weight/Measure	Abbreviation	Weight/Measure
cc	Cubic centimeter	mg	Milligram
cm	Centimeter	ml	Milliliter
G, gm.	Gram	mm	Millimeter
gr.	Grain	mmol	Millimole
Gtt.	Drop	oz.	Ounce
kg	Kilogram	Tbsp.	Tablespoon
lb.	Pound	tsp.	Teaspoon
mcg	Microgram	u.; un.	Unit
mEq	Milliequivalent		

Conclusion

Understanding commonly used terminology and abbreviations are extremely important in the practice of pharmacy. Pharmacy technicians in all practice settings will utilize this information on a daily basis when interpreting medication directions for computer entry, calculating appropriate amounts of additives for intravenous solutions, understanding a patient's therapy for a particular diagnosis, etc. In addition, pharmacy technicians increase their ability to function more efficiently in the pharmacy and provide greater support to pharmacists when they enhance their knowledge of the items discussed in this chapter.

Reference

1. Shargel, et al., Comprehensive Pharmacy Review, 3rd edition, Williams & Wilkins, 1997; p 720.

Bibliography

Brooks, Myrna LaFleur, Exploring Medical Language, A Student-Directed Approach, 4th edition, Mosby, 1998.

Chabner, Davi-Ellen, The Language of Medicine, 5th edition, W. B. Saunders Co., 1996.

Facts and Comparisons, J. B. Lippincott Company, St. Louis, MO, 1995.

Masters, Thomas and Masters, Rebecca, Terminology for Allied Health Professions with Medical Terminology, A Visual Guide, Delmar Publishers, 1997.

Pharmacy Certified Technician Training Manual, 7th edition, Michigan Pharmacists Association, Lansing, MI, 1997.

About the author

Wynefred Halpin Schumann received her bachelor's degree in pharmacy from Ferris State University College of Pharmacy in Big Rapids, Michigan, and her master's degree from Wayne State University College of Pharmacy & Allied Health Professions (WSU-CPAHP) in Detroit, Michigan. She is currently serving as the WSU-CPAHP Assistant Dean of Student Services. Her prior pharmacy experience includes serving as a pharmacy technician trainer and subsequently a supervisor at St. Joseph Mercy Hospital in Ann Arbor, Michigan, and as the pharmacy director for McPherson Hospital Pharmacy in Howell, Michigan. In 1981 Schumann was a charter member of the Pharmacy Certified Technician

Board of Examiners administered by the Michigan Pharmacists Association (MPA) and has been appointed to the Pharmacy Technician Certification Board's Certification Council for 2001-2003. She is a Technician Advisory Board member at Oakland Community College in Bloomfield Hills, Michigan, and Henry Ford Community College in Dearborn, Michigan. Schumann has received many awards, including the 1988 MPA Pharmacist of the Year, the 1997 Southeastern Michigan Society of Health-System Pharmacists Student Research Preceptor of the Year, and the 1997 Wayne County Pharmacists Association John H. Webster Award for Exemplary Service to the Profession. She is also a Fellow of the American Association of State Colleges and Universities.

Self-assessment questions

1. The abbreviation "a.s." means:
   a. before meals.
   b. right ear.
   c. before noon; morning.
   d. left ear.

2. The abbreviation "b.i.d." means:
   a. each ear.
   b. twice daily.
   c. at bedtime.
   d. both eyes.

3. The abbreviation "q.d." means:
   a. daily, every day.
   b. four times daily.
   c. every other day.
   d. three times daily.

4. The chemical symbol "Ca" represents:
   a. aluminum.
   b. calcium.
   c. iron.
   d. sodium.

5. The chemical symbol "K" represents:
   a. hydrogen peroxide.
   b. iodine.
   c. bicarbonate.
   d. potassium.

6. A solid dosage form with the drug enclosed in soluble shells of either hard or soft gelatin is a:
   a. tablet.
   b. capsule.
   c. lozenge.
   d. emulsion.

7. A "liniment" is:
   a. a sprayable product employing liquefied gasses and valve systems to deliver medication used for topical application to the skin, inhalation into the lungs, and local application in the nose and mouth.
   b. a clear, sweetened liquid dosage form whose primary solvents are water and alcohol.
   c. a semi-liquid or solid preparation containing fats and oils suspended with the aid of an emulsifying agent.
   d. a mixture of various substances in oil, alcohol solutions of soap, or emulsions intended for external application, often used for their heat-producing effects.

8. A preparation of finely divided, undissolved drugs dispersed in a liquid is a:
   a. suspension.
   b. solution.
   c. emulsion.
   d. tincture.

9. An "elixir" is:
   a. a viscous liquid or semi-solid emulsion of oil and water.
   b. a semisolid suspension of very small particles, usually in water.
   c. a clear, sweetened liquid dosage form whose primary solvents are water and alcohol.
   d. a concentrated solution of sugar in water or other aqueous liquid.

10. In pharmacy weights and measures, a "mEq" represents:
    a. millimole
    b. milliliter
    c. milligram
    d. milliequivalent

11. In pharmacy weights and measures, the abbreviation for "drop" is:
    a. dp.
    b. Gtt.
    c. mcg.
    d. oz.

12. A small, sterile glass or plastic container with a single dose of parenteral solution is a(n):
    a. vial.
    b. ampule.
    c. spirit.
    d. analgesic.

13. A "vasoconstrictor" is:
    a. a drug that causes widening of the blood vessels.
    b. an agent that prevents or delays the clotting of blood.
    c. a drug that causes a narrowing of the blood vessels.
    d. a drug that antagonizes one of the effects of histamine.

14. A drug that relieves coughing is an:
    a. antitussive.
    b. antacid.
    c. antipruritic.
    d. anticoagulant.

15. An "arrhythmia" is:
    a. a substance that causes cancer.
    b. a drug or dietary supplement that neutralizes stomach acid.
    c. a special coating on tablets to prevent dissolution in the stomach.
    d. any irregular heart rate.

Chapter 9

Computer Applications

Dennis M. Gates, R.Ph., M.S.

Learning objectives

Upon completion of this chapter, the technician should be able to do the following:

- Name the basic components of a computer system.
- Define the terms *software* and *hardware*.
- Describe the basic functions that computers perform.
- Explain how a modem works.
- Define the terms *Internet, intranet,* and *World Wide Web*.
- Explain the difference between a *main frame computer* and a *microcomputer.*
- Explain the terms *local-area network* (LAN) and *wide-area network* (WAN).
- List the roles technicians have with computers.
- Describe the computer's use in various pharmacy practice settings.
- Describe the functions of an intravenous (IV) pharmacy computer system.
- Describe the computer's use in purchasing medications through a wholesaler or prime vendor.
- Describe future methods of entering information on a computer.

Introduction

Pharmacy technicians work closely with computers in all practice settings. They use computers to enter medication orders, verify insurance information, order medications from the wholesaler, and print medication refill lists. Pharmacy technicians, therefore, must have a basic understanding of computer terminology and applications. By becoming familiar with the operation of computer equipment and programs, the chance of causing a computer problem can be reduced, which ultimately will make computing more enjoyable.

Basic functions of a computer

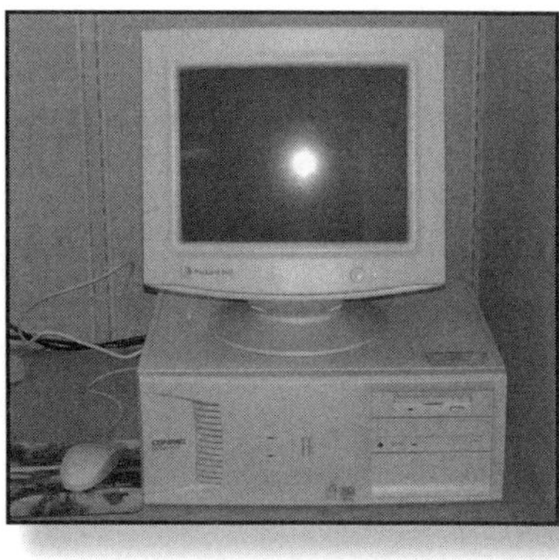

The computer does three basic functions: storing, processing, and communicating information. *Electronic data processing* is a phrase used to describe how computers work because electronic circuits accomplish each function. Inside the computer's tower case, critical components (e.g., *RAM* chip and *CPU,* which will be described later) are plugged into small sockets onto what is called the motherboard. Also, there are larger expansion sockets that can hold auxiliary circuit boards, otherwise known as cards (e.g., sound cards, network card). The term *hardware* describes all of the mechanical, electrical, and magnetic equipment that make up a computer system. The term *software* refers to programs written for the computer. Software programs provide instructions to the hardware to store, process, and communicate information.

Components of a computer

The basic computer includes a central processing unit (CPU) or processor, memory, storage, and input and output devices.

Processor

The CPU or processor serves as the computer "brain." The processor takes the information entered into the computer (*input*) and the instructions from the software to process the information. The speed of a computer refers to how fast the CPU can process or carry out an operation. The speed is measured in megahertz (MHz) or millions of cycles per second. In 2001, computer manufacturers are making processors that contain speeds of 1,000 MHz.

Memory

The memory is the computer's work space, similar to an individual's desk. This type of memory is called Random Access Memory (RAM). The RAM is not permanent, but only serves as the workspace for processing the input and the instructions from the software. Like desks of different sizes, computers are available with different size memory units. For example, in 2001, a common memory size is 128 megabytes (MB) of RAM, while in 1995, the 32 MB RAM computer was common.

Storage

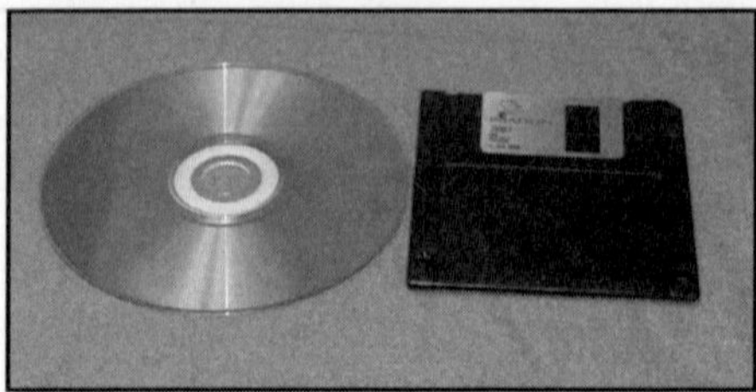

CD Rom **3.5″ disk**

Storage devices are similar to filing cabinets. When a computer is directed to retrieve information from a file, it "opens" the file, reads and writes information to it, and then "closes" the file. Large volumes of data are stored in files on magnetic disks, drums, tapes, or optical disks. Magnetic disks may be rigid plastic or hard disks that measure 3.5″. Plastic diskettes are used for storing smaller amounts of information and are used primarily with microcomputers. A 3.5″ disk can hold up to 1.44 MB of information, a *Zip* disk can hold up to 100 MB of information, and a Compact Disc (CD) can hold up to 650 MB of information. The hard disk drive is composed of microscopic components that mechanically work together to store large amounts of information. This information can either be retrieved or saved by the user. The hard disk drive is enclosed by a metal casing to protect the components from dust and installed directly in the central processing unit (CPU). An optical disk uses CD technology. An optical disk that contains data that cannot be changed is called a *CD-ROM* (compact disc, read-only memory). The term CD-ROM is actually misleading since these disks are used to store information and have nothing to do with memory.

Input and output

Computers process information using *input/output (I/O) devices*. These devices, also called peripheral devices, allow the computer to "read" and "write" information. The *keyboard* is the primary input device for the computer. The keyboard provides input directly into a terminal. Other examples of input devices are bar code technology, touch screen applications, and voice recognition systems. Two examples of *output* devices include the monitor screen and the printer. The screen is the television-like display module also called a *console* or cathode ray tube (CRT). The laser jet printer is a common type of printer.

Computers communicate with other computers through a modulator-demodulator (*modem*) to receive and send information over a telephone line. For example, a hospital pharmacist may use a modem to send intravenous solution preparation orders to an off-site compounding center or to order drugs from a wholesale company. In the year 2000, the industry standard modem transmits data at a rate of 57,000 bits per second (bps), or 57K. Previously, the most common modem transmitted data at 28,800 bps. Modems connect to computer bulletin boards, on-line computer services, and the *Internet.*

Types of computers

Two types of computers often used in pharmacies are main frame computers and microcomputers. Main frame computers are a large, complex group of machines that normally require multiple employees to maintain. A main frame computer may be used for hospital pharmacy computer systems. Microcomputers, or personal computers (a desktop, palm top, lap top, or notebook), are smaller and are normally maintained by the user.

There are three important points to remember when working with computers: (1) enter information accurately, (2) save and back up information consistently, and (3) handle floppy disks appropriately. The computer cannot correct information entered incorrectly. Entering faulty information is called "garbage-in" and this leads to faulty output or "garbage-out." The computer must follow accurate and detailed instructions to operate correctly. By organizing the information to be entered (e.g., patient medication orders), the potential for errors in data entry is greatly reduced.

Precautions with computer use

As people become comfortable working with computers, they often fail to back up information. Eventually, the user may inadvertently lose a diskette, or a *"virus"* may affect the operation of the computer. If these events happen, the user cannot retrieve the data. It is important that all information entered is duplicated on floppy diskettes or the hard disk. Remember to copy information every time the computer is used. Information is also lost when users inappropriately handle diskettes. Computer users should follow these recommendations for handling diskettes:

DO NOT

- touch the recording surface of a diskette.
- write on a disk label with a ballpoint pen or pencil. Use a felt-tip pen.
- bend the disk.
- spill any liquids (e.g., coffee) on the diskette or the computer.
- overheat the disk (e.g., leaving the diskette in the car on a warm day).
- expose the disk to magnetic fields like color television monitors, the telephone ringer, or magnet accessories on work desks.

Your computer should always be plugged into a surge protector. A surge protector will prevent your computer's motherboard and all internal electronics from damage in case of a high-voltage power irregularity. At any time, an abnormal electrical current or power surge can occur and cause significant damage to your computer hardware. A surge protector is used to prevent these abnormal electrical currents from damaging your systems. Abnormal electrical currents can occur from a bad thunderstorm with lightning or when electricians test the emergency power generator at your facility. An Uninterruptible Power Supply (UPS) contains not only a surge protector, but also includes a battery that will keep your computer operating and monitor working in case of a total blackout (i.e., total loss of power). If a blackout occurs, with a UPS, you will have approximately seven minutes to shut down your system.

Applications

People use word processing software to generate letters, memorandums, policies and procedures, and chapters in textbooks. Documents can be saved, then retrieved and updated at a later date. Features such as spelling and grammar checks, a thesaurus, and various font types and sizes are available with word processing software. These tools allow the user to be more efficient in creating high-quality documents. Pharmacy managers use word processing software to type memorandums and reports.

People also use software to create spreadsheets. A spreadsheet is a document that contains several rows and columns of information. Mathematical formulas within the spreadsheet software can automatically calculate the sum or product of numbers listed in a row or column. Pharmacy employees use spreadsheet software to maintain payroll records and workload statistics. For example, a manager of a chain drug store may use a spreadsheet that contains 12 columns of data where each column represents a month, while each row represents the number of prescriptions dispensed by an individual pharmacy. The manager can then use the spreadsheet software to automatically calculate the total number of prescriptions dispensed by all of the drug stores and the average number of prescriptions dispensed each month.

Database software is an application used to create and store large volumes of data. Each category of information is contained in a different field. For example, a pharmacy manager may wish to create a database of information of all employees working in the pharmacy. The different fields of information can include the employee's name, telephone number, birth date, address, hourly rate, license or certification number, etc. After all of the information is entered, the manager can sort the information and create a report, such as a list of all employee names and their phone numbers. This can be accomplished by printing only two fields of information, the name field and the telephone number field.

People use computers to communicate with each other through electronic mail (*e-mail*). E-mail allows people to communicate with each other at work or at home. Users can send attachments (e.g., computer files) along with e-mail messages. Overall, e-mail improves communication between people.

A *local area network* (LAN) involves different computers linked together by radio, cables, or lasers to share software, hardware, and information. A LAN is common in businesses such as hospitals. A *wide area network* (WAN) involves the same concept of linking computers, except the area is much larger compared to a LAN. Connections are made by telephone lines, microwaves, or satellites within a city or country.

Technician roles with computers

Technician roles with computers include entering information, printing reports and labels, reviewing patient profiles, and maintaining the equipment. Pharmacy managers are relying on technicians to complete this technical work so pharmacists can spend more time providing clinical pharmacy services to the patient. Information entered by technicians includes medication orders, workload statistics, purchasing and inventory data, and database information (e.g., entering insurance information).

Pharmacy applications

Computer use in pharmacy has increased greatly over the last 20 years. Computers are used in three primary areas of responsibility: (1) management, (2) drug distribution, and (3) clinical services. In management, pharmacy managers use computers to maintain inventory, payroll, and budget records. Pharmacy employees also use desktop publishing software to create department newsletters. In hospital pharmacies, a newsletter can announce the addition of new medications to the hospital's formulary and is distributed to pharmacy and nursing employees and to physicians. In drug distribution, pharmacists and technicians use computers for maintaining patient medication profiles. Pharmacy profiles provide patient information such as height, weight, and allergy information, and a list of all of the medications the patient is currently taking and medications discontinued. In clinical applications, computers are used for storing and retrieving drug information, monitoring drug interactions and therapeutic incompatibilities, drug use review, and calculating medication doses.

Computer applications in community (ambulatory or outpatient) pharmacies

Community pharmacy (also known as ambulatory or outpatient) computer systems maintain prescription order information such as a patient name, an address, medication names, directions for use, quantity, etc. Outpatient computer systems create a label, price the prescription, process insurance information, and detect drug interactions and possible drug allergies. These systems also generate management reports and inventory control information.

Computer applications in hospital pharmacies

Order processing

Accurate medication order entry is essential to operate a pharmacy department efficiently. The entry of medication orders is difficult because many fields of a medication order are needed. Some examples of the fields include patient name, location, medication name, dose, frequency, duration, the route of administration, and special information such as comments or directions for use.

Pharmacy computer systems use mnemonic codes to make order entry easier. Mnemonic codes can have predefined information containing the most common frequency, the route of administration, and special comments. Mnemonic codes can be numeric (e.g., 5646), *alphanumeric* (e.g., acet325) or drug names (e.g., acetaminophen).

Medication orders entered by pharmacy technicians are placed in a "hold" file until pharmacists validate the order. The pharmacist validates the medication order for accuracy and safety for the patient. Until this validation step occurs, the order is not activated and the dose is not filled. If the physician does the order entry at a nursing unit, the pharmacist usually validates the order before it is dispensed and administered.

After entering a medication order on the computer, the information is part of the patient's medication profile. A standardized time for medication administration is based on the order frequency (e.g., aspirin 325 mg by mouth every day). In some hospitals, the standard administration time assigned to a daily frequency is 9:00 a.m. or 0900 in military time. Computer systems often use military time, so it is essential that pharmacy technicians understand military time and regular time (Table 1). Pharmacy staff, however, can change the administration time if the patient is to receive the medication later in the day. It is important to maintain most medications on a standard administration time. The advantage of established administration times is that it reduces the chance for a medication error. Examples of standard medication administration times used in hospitals are listed in Table 2.

Table 1 Military time compared to standard time

Standard Time	Military Time	Standard Time	Military Time
1:00 a.m.	0100	1:00 p.m.	1300
2:00 a.m.	0200	2:00 p.m.	1400
3:00 a.m.	0300	3:00 p.m.	1500
4:00 a.m.	0400	4:00 p.m.	1600
5:00 a.m.	0500	5:00 p.m.	1700
6:00 a.m.	0600	6:00 p.m.	1800
7:00 a.m.	0700	7:00 p.m.	1900
8:00 a.m.	0800	8:00 p.m.	2000
9:00 a.m.	0900	9:00 p.m.	2100
10:00 a.m.	1000	10:00 p.m.	2200
11:00 a.m.	1100	11:00 p.m.	2300
Noon	**1200**	**Midnight**	**2400**

Table 2 Example of standardized administration times

Abbreviation	Translation	Sample Administration Time				
BID	twice a day	0900	1700			
TID	three times a day	0900	1300	1700		
QID	four times a day	0900	1300	1700	2100	
q 6 hr	every 6 hours	0600	1200	1800	2400	or
		0900	1500	2100	0300	
q 12 hr	every 12 hours	0500	1700	or		
		0100	1300			

Unit-dose medication systems

The dispensing of unit-dose medications is one method pharmacists use to provide medications to patients. They generate computerized cart fill lists each day, reporting the number of doses needed for a 24-hour period. Pharmacy technicians fill these doses in patient-specific medication bins. Pharmacists use the computer-generated cart fill lists to check the medication bins.

Intravenous medication systems

Computer systems provide intravenous medication order processing capabilities, either as a stand-alone system or part of an integrated pharmacy system. These systems provide diluent, additive, and compatibility information; chemotherapy dilutions; total parenteral nutrition (TPN) order processing; patient billing; and medication scheduling capabilities.

Pharmaceutical purchasing

Computer technology plays an important role in purchasing medications. Medications stocked in the pharmacy will contain a bar code label on the shelf and on the medication's package. This bar code label contains ordering information such as minimum and maximum quantity levels and pricing information. A pharmacy technician can use a bar code *scanner* to order medications. After entering the ordering information into a hand-held bar code device by scanning the bar code label, the information is downloaded and sent electronically over a modem to a pharmacy wholesaler. Prior to placing an electronic order, a pharmacy technician can determine whether a wholesaler stocks a particular medication by dialing into the wholesaler's computer inventory system to determine the medication's availability.

Internet, intranets and the World Wide Web (WWW)

The Internet allows users in locations around the world to communicate by using computers and modems. Similar to the Internet is an *intranet,* which uses Internet technology but relies on a single server and can only be accessed by employees working within a company. The server acts as a storage area for files that can be accessed through a *network* connection by users at other computer stations. The purpose of an intranet is to share information. Employees can continuously access and update information. For example, a multi-hospital health system can use their intranet to post quality improvement activities for all of the hospitals within the system.

The World Wide Web (WWW) is a system of Internet servers that support specially formatted documents. The documents are formatted in a language called *HTML* (hypertext markup language) that supports links to other documents including text, graphics, audio, and video files. People can use an application called a web *browser* to easily access the WWW. The two most popular web browsers include Netscape Navigator and Microsoft's Internet Explorer.

The glossary lists several definitions of terms associated with websites and the Internet.

Future applications of computers in pharmacy

Some hospital pharmacies now have physicians enter patient medication orders directly. This allows more time for pharmacy staff to provide patient-centered clinical pharmacy services. In the future, computers will be more powerful, contain more memory, and yet be available in smaller sizes. Input devices will occur through voice recognition or touch screen applications. The Internet will continue to play an important role in pharmacy practice. People will be able to refill their prescriptions by typing in their prescription number directly into any pharmacy's website. Computers also will have an important role with automation and robotics in drug distribution. Pharmacy technicians must maintain competencies with computers through training, practice, and reviewing pharmacy policies and procedures.

Glossary of computer terminology

Address bar: the navigation area within a web browser into which a website's *URL* or domain name can be entered.

Alphanumeric: a code consisting of letters and numbers used for easier order entry of medication orders.

Back up: to make a second copy of important files or data by saving a file with a different name or by copying files to a different disk or tape drive.

Browser: any program used to view material prepared for the Internet or an intranet. Browsers are able to interpret *URLs* and *HTML* language, as well as several Internet file transfer protocols.

CD-ROM: Compact-Disc, Read-Only Memory.

Console: a television-like display screen or monitor; also called a cathode ray tube (CRT).

CPU: central processing unit; the computer's "brain;" the unit that processes information received (input) and turns information into results (output).

Data: information entered into the computer.

Domain name: the common name for an Internet address that is mapped onto its formal numeric Internet (*IP*) address.

E-mail: electronic mail.

Firewall: a software program used to separate a local network from the outside world, thus preventing unauthorized access.

Hardware: the physical components of a computer system including the mechanical, electrical, and magnetic parts.

Home page: the introductory page for a *World Wide Web* site or intranet site.

HTML: hypertext markup language; a language used for creating pages on a website. HTML is simply a collection of tags used to mark blocks of text and assign them special meaning.

Input/Output (I/O) device: equipment used to transfer information to and from a computer.

Input: information entered into a computer to be processed.

Internet: a network allowing computers in government, education, and industry throughout the world to connect.

Internet Service Provider (ISP): companies that can facilitate access to the Internet for a cost of approximately $10 to $20 per month.

Intranet: an Internet belonging to an organization, usually a corporation, that only employees or others with authorization can access. An intranet's website looks and acts just like any other website, but the firewall surrounding an intranet prevents unauthorized access.

IP address: the numerical Internet protocol address of a computer on the Internet. Every computer on the Internet has a unique numerical address.

Keyboard: the device used to enter information into a computer.

Local area network (LAN): groups of microcomputers connected by radio, cables, or laser to communicate with each other.

Modem: modulator-demodulator; a device allowing a computer to connect to a telephone line. Modems can either be located inside the computer's case or outside the case and connected to a computer's serial port.

Mouse: a device used to control the movement of a cursor or an object on a display terminal.

Network: refers to two or more microcomputers connected so they can share hardware and software.

Output: the results of a computer processing information.

Parallel port: sends several bits of data across eight parallel wires simultaneously; usually used for printers.

RAM: Random Access Memory; the computer memory accepts instructions from software diskette.

ROM: Read Only Memory; refers to the instructions that are preset within your computer that are responsible for making the computer operate properly.

Scanner: a device, usually connected to the computer's parallel port, used to transfer text or photos (illustrations) to the computer.

Serial port: sends data one bit at a time over a single, one-way wire; slower than a parallel port.

Software: programs developed to provide directions to the hardware to process information.

TCP/IP: Transmission Control Protocol/Internet Protocol; the basic communication protocol that is the foundation of the Internet.

URL: Uniform Resource Locator; the scheme used to address Internet resources on the World Wide Web or intranet resources on private networks.

Virus: an infectious computer program, often having an incubation period, that is created to cause damage, such as destroying data or damaging a computer's boot drive.

Website: a group of pages (i.e., HTML files) linked to one another in some sort of logical fashion using one or more domains controlled by the same organization.

Wide area network (WAN): groups of microcomputers connected by telephone lines, microwaves, or satellites over a wide geographic area such as a city or country.

World Wide Web: a system of Internet servers that support specially formatted documents.

Zip disks: a disk used for storing data; can hold up to 100 MB of information. A special Zip disk drive is required for storing information on and retrieving files from such disks.

Conclusion

Since the computer was introduced, it has been progressively changing the way people work and live. The healthcare system is utilizing computerization to aid in the delivery of faster and improved care to patients. Pharmacy technicians who have a thorough understanding and working knowledge of computers and their applications are true assets to the healthcare team.

Bibliography

Andrews, J., Ph.D., A Guide to Managing and Maintaining Your PC, 2nd edition, Course Technology, Cambridge, MA, 1998.

Computer PC Manual, Michigan Pharmacists Association, Lansing, MI, 1993.

Frankenfeld F.M., "Basics of Computer Hardware and Software," *American Journal of Hospital Pharmacy*, Vol. 50, pp. 717-24, 1993.

Graham, I.S., HTML Source Book Second Edition: A Complete Guide to HTML 3.0, Wiley Company Publishing, 1996.

Sharp, R., "The Pharmacist Guide to Understanding the Internet and Finding Your Way Around It," *Michigan Pharmacist,* Lansing, Vol 37, No. 7, pp. 4-8, July/August 1999 .

White, R., How Computers Work, 4th edition, Que, a Division of Macmillan Computer Publishing, USA, Indianapolis, IN, 1998.

About the author

Dennis M. Gates received his bachelor's of science and master's of science in pharmacy from Wayne State University College of Pharmacy & Allied Health Professions in Detroit, Michigan. He completed a one-year general pharmacy residency and a one-year advanced administrative residency at Detroit Receiving Hospital and University Health Center. Gates currently works at St. Joseph Mercy Hospital in Ann Arbor, Michigan, and has worked in managerial positions at the University of Wisconsin Hospital and Clinic, Detroit Receiving Hospital and University Health Center, and St. Joseph Mercy Hospital.

Self-assessment questions

1. The term used to describe the speed of a computer is:
   a. RAM.
   b. ROM.
   c. MHz.
   d. MB.

2. Which storage disk will store the largest amount of information?
   a. 3.5″ floppy disk
   b. Zip disk
   c. CD-ROM
   d. I/O device

3. Voice recognition is:
   a. an output device.
   b. an input device.
   c. the most common method for entering information.
   d. obsolete.

4. Which software application is commonly used to create a department mail list?
   a. Word processing
   b. Spreadsheet
   c. Database
   d. Desktop publishing

5. Which software application is commonly used to develop memorandums?
   a. Word processing
   b. Spreadsheet
   c. Database
   d. Desktop publishing

6. A UPS is used to:
   a. access the Internet.
   b. print documents.
   c. protect computers from a power outage.
   d. send electronic messages.

7. Bar code labels on medication storage shelves are used to:
   a. purchase pharmaceuticals.
   b. enter medication orders to create patient profiles.
   c. validate insurance information.
   d. access the Internet.

8. The military time for 11:00 p.m. is:
   a. 1100.
   b. 0100.
   c. 0011.
   d. 2300.

9. The WWW stands for:
   a. World Wrestling Foundation.
   b. Women Working for Women.
   c. World Wide Web.
   d. World Wide Width bands.

10. Networked computers used to connect computers within a health system are called:
    a. WAN.
    b. IP address.
    c. HTML.
    d. LAN.

Part III: Introduction to Pharmacology

CHAPTER 10

INTRODUCTION TO DRUG ACTION

Tracey Okabe-Yamamura, Pharm.D.

Learning objectives

Upon completion of this chapter, the technician should be able to do the following:

- Understand drug definitions and categories.
- Explain the difference between a medication's generic name and brand (trade, proprietary) name.
- Explain the difference between pharmacodynamics and pharmacokinetics.
- Understand the processes of *absorption, distribution, metabolism,* and *elimination.*

Introduction

The practice of pharmacy is a dynamic, patient-oriented health service. It applies a scientific body of knowledge to improve and promote patient health by means of appropriate drug use and drug-related therapy.[1] Pharmacists are knowledgeable of prescription and nonprescription drugs including their pharmacology (how they act), indications (what they are used for), dosage, mechanisms of action, contraindications (when not to use them) and adverse effects. Pharmacists must also consider the effects that the patient's age, sex, other disease states, drug therapies, or diets have on the drug's activity or disposition (what the body does to the drug).

Drug definition

In the United States, a drug is any substance, other than a food or device, intended for use in the diagnosis, cure, relief, treatment, or prevention of disease or intended to affect the structure or function of the body. More simply, a drug is any chemical that affects the body and its processes.

Drugs are divided into two categories: prescription and nonprescription. Prescription drugs are those that are safe for use only under medical supervision. Drugs in this category are available only with a written prescription from an authorized prescriber. Prescription drugs include controlled substances that are regulated by federal, state, and local laws because of the potential for abuse or dependence. Nonprescription drugs are those that are safe for use without medical supervision. They are sold over-the-counter (OTC) without a prescription and are commonly called "OTC" drugs. The Food and Drug Administration (FDA) is the government agency that determines whether a drug is prescription or nonprescription.

Drug names are divided into three categories: chemical, generic (non-proprietary), and trade (brand, proprietary). The chemical name describes the atomic or molecular structure of the drug. Usually the chemical name of a drug is too complicated or technical for everyday use. Exceptions are simple compounds such as sodium bicarbonate.

The generic name is the established (official) United States Adopted Name (USAN) of a drug. It is a generic (nonproprietary) name, and it refers only to the drug entity and not to a specific product.[2]

The trade (brand) name is the specific product name and is the name registered to a manufacturer holding the trademark. Usually the trade name is short and easy to remember so that doctors will prescribe it and consumers will look for it by name.

An example of the three drug name categories is illustrated below:

Trade (Brand, Proprietary) Name:	Catapres®
Generic (Non-Proprietary) Name:	clonidine
Chemical Name:	2-(2,6-Dichloroanilino)-2 Imidazoline

Although the trade (or brand) name of a drug may vary among manufacturers, each drug has only one chemical and one generic name. The FDA requires that generic versions of drugs have the same active ingredients as the original product. The generic drug must also be absorbed into the body at the same rate. The FDA publishes the *Approved Drug Products with Therapeutic Equivalence Evaluations* (commonly known as the "Orange Book"), which cites the agency's evaluation about how each generic product's therapeutic effect compares to the therapeutic effect of the referenced brand name product. The pharmacist uses the information on therapeutic equivalence when selecting generic drug products in clinical practice.

Drugs are usually categorized by therapeutic class. The American Hospital Formulary Service (AHFS) has developed standard drug class categories that are identified by number.[3] Within each drug class categories, subclasses are also outlined. For example, the therapeutic class of anti-infectives is classified as 08:00. Subclasses, such as antibiotics, are listed as 08:12. Further classes of antibiotics like the aminoglycosides are listed as 08:12:02.

Principles of pharmacology[2,5]

Pharmacology is the study of drugs and their interactions with the human body. There are two main considerations that influence the selection of a particular drug: pharmacodynamics (what the drug does to the body) and pharmacokinetics (what the body does to the drug).

Pharmacodynamics describes not only *what* the drug does to the body but also *where* the drug works and *how* the drug works. In order for the drug to work, it has to get to the right place in the body where the problem is occurring, and that is why the pharmacokinetics of the drug is important. Pharmacokinetics refers to the *quantitative* aspects of elements of drug disposition: absorption, distribution, metabolism, and elimination. (See Figure 1.)

Absorption, distribution, metabolism, and elimination[2,5]

Absorption is the process that brings the drug from the administration site into the bloodstream. Most drugs are administered orally. Once the drug is dissolved in the gastrointestinal system, absorption occurs primarily in the small intestine. The drug then passes through the liver into the systemic circulation. This is called the first pass effect (through the intestine). Some non-oral routes of administration avoid this first pass effect. These routes include the lower rectum (suppository or enema), sublingual (under the tongue), nasal, buccal (between the cheek and teeth), transdermal (through the skin), inhalation (through the lungs), and by injection. The injectable routes of administration are intramuscular (between the muscle tissue), subcutaneous (under the skin), and intravenous (into the vein). The intravenous route does not usually include absorption since the drug is being placed directly into the bloodstream.

Bioavailability is the term used to describe the rate and extent in which a drug is absorbed into the bloodstream. There are several factors that can affect the bioavailability of a drug, including the way in which the drug is manufactured, its chemical and physical properties, and the physiology of the patient taking the drug. Drug products are designed to release the active drug at a desired rate once it is taken into the body (i.e., how a tablet or capsule dissolves in the stomach). Two drug products may have the same active drug compound, but they may contain different inactive ingredients that can affect the rate and extent of absorption. Drug products are considered "bioequivalent" when they not only contain the same active ingredient, but also produce virtually the same blood levels over time. Bioequivalence ensures that the products are therapeutically equivalent and thereby are interchangeable.

> Absorption, distribution, metabolism, and elimination can be affected by the patient's:
> - Age
> - Sex
> - Weight
> - Disease states
> - Genetic factors

Distribution is the process that moves the drug from the bloodstream to the area where it will exert its pharmacological effect. This process involves transporting the drug at a molecular level across biological (cell) membranes. Drugs do not distribute evenly throughout the body. Some drugs tend to stay within the watery tissues of the blood and muscle, while other drugs may concentrate in specific organs such as the liver or kidneys. Drugs will bind to plasma proteins (such as albumin) to different degrees; if the drug binds tightly, it will be released into the bloodstream slowly. Some drugs do not bind to plasma proteins as readily; their concentration in the bloodstream will be greater.

Metabolism prepares the drug for elimination. Although metabolism occurs in many body organs, the primary organ is the liver, followed by the lungs and kidneys. Enzyme systems (oxidation, reduction, and hydrolysis) break the drug down into smaller units called metabolites. Metabolites can be inactive or active. An active metabolite is one that has pharmacological effects following the metabolic process. Some drugs are prodrugs; they are administered in an inactive form and are metabolized to the active compound.

Elimination is the process that removes the drug and its metabolites from the body. Drugs are eliminated primarily through the urine, although they can be eliminated through the feces, lungs, or skin. If one elimination process is damaged or slowed, an accumulation of the drug and/or its metabolite may occur in the body. This can result in toxic levels. Therefore, for some drugs, changes in doses or frequency of administration must occur when an elimination process is slowed or damaged. This is seen frequently in the elderly where kidney function is often decreased.

Figure 1 Example of pharmacodynamics

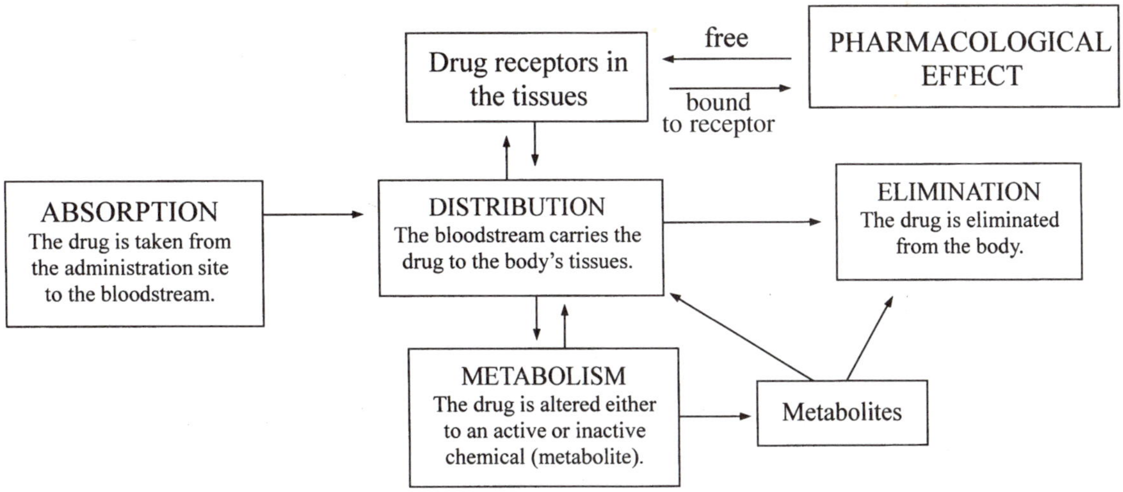

Absorption, distribution, metabolism, and elimination are dynamic processes and can be affected by many variables. Patient variables include: age, sex, weight, disease states, and genetic factors. These factors may all influence these processes and, therefore, how the body is affected by the drugs.

Figure 2 Drug at a receptor site

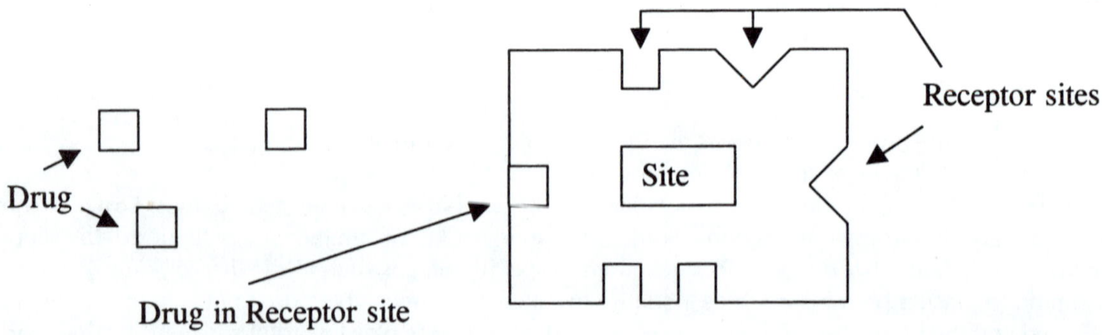

Adverse effects and toxicities[6]

Adverse effects can be described as an undesired effect that occurs when a drug is administered. These adverse effects can be divided into two groups: side effects and toxicities. Side effects are undesirable pharmacological effects of a drug seen at therapeutic doses. Side effects are an unavoidable part of the drug's action. Some examples of side effects include: drowsiness caused by antihistamines, constipation caused by narcotics, and dry mouth caused by anticholinergic agents. Toxicities, on the other hand, are harmful to the body. Toxicity can occur when the drug dose exceeds the recommended range, when therapy exceeds the recommended duration, or if a drug is not monitored properly. Most toxicities are avoidable when drugs are properly and carefully monitored. Some examples of toxicities include: kidney damage caused by aminoglycoside antibiotics, ulcers caused by aspirin, or seizures caused by theophylline.

Drug interactions[5]

When two or more drugs are taken at the same time or in the same time interval, they may interact in ways that can be good or bad. The drugs may interact to be more effective in treating the medical problem. There are three enhancements of drug effects: *additive, synergism,* or *potentiation* activity. An additive response occurs when two or more drugs combine to result in a response that is the **sum** of the drug's individual responses. Synergy occurs when the response is greater than the sum of the individual drugs. *Potentiation* occurs when a drug lacking an effect of its own increases the effect of a second, active drug.

Example:

Additive	$\text{Effect}_{A+B} = \text{Effect}_A + \text{Effect}_B$	(same as $1 + 1 = 2$)
Synergism	$\text{Effect}_{A+B} > \text{Effect}_A + \text{Effect}_B$	(same as $1 + 1 > 2$)
Potentiation	$\text{Effect}_{A+B} > \text{Effect}_A + \text{Effect}_B$	(same as $0 + 1 > 1$)

Drug interactions can also increase the number or severity of adverse effects. Drug interactions can occur between prescription drugs and nonprescription drugs, food, and/or alcohol. It is very important that patients tell their physicians about all of the medicines that they are taking including OTC items, vitamins, alcohol, and any changes in diet. It is recommended that patients get their prescriptions filled at same pharmacy so that the pharmacist can maintain the patient's drug profile and screen for any drug interactions. Patients need to consult their pharmacist when they need an OTC drug, especially when they are also taking prescription medications.

Safety and efficacy[4]

The two goals in drug development are drug efficacy (how well a drug works) and safety. All drugs can cause harm as well as help. The wider the margin of safety, the more useful the agent. This margin of safety is called the therapeutic window and is the distance between the usual effective dose and the dose that will produce a severe or life-threatening side effect.

The best drugs are those that are effective and safe. An example would be penicillin. Except for individuals who are truly allergic to penicillin, it is a very safe drug. Even in large doses it is virtually non-toxic.

The decision to administer a drug to a patient must always be weighed against the risk to the patient who takes that drug. Factors to consider in drug therapy include side effects, toxicities, length of the drug therapy, and the cost. Frequently, the benefits of the drug therapy outweigh the risks involved. However, there may be situations when the drug treatment is more detrimental to the patient than the disease itself. Patients should be included in the decisions about expectations from their drug therapy so that the success or failure of that therapy can be monitored through the physician and pharmacist.

Drug abuse, dependence, and tolerance

Drug abuse can be defined as the excessive or persistent use of a drug for non-therapeutic purposes. Commonly abused drugs include alcohol, marijuana, cocaine, heroin, amphetamines, LSD (lysergic acid diethylamine), and PCP (phencyclidine). Prescription medications may also be abused, and are discussed in Chapter 14 on Pain and Inflammation. Drug dependence occurs when an individual cannot control drug intake due to physiologic or psychologic need. Finally, drug tolerance is an individual's decreased response to the same drug dose when repeated. The person needs to take a higher dose to produce the same effect.

Conclusion

Medication therapy involves using the drugs that will effectively treat a patient based on how the drug acts in the patient's body; how the body absorbs, metabolizes, distributes, and eliminates the drug; and how the patient's individual characteristics affect the drug's activity or disposition. By carefully monitoring a patient's drug therapy, adverse effects, toxicities, and drug interactions can either be avoided or minimized.

References

1. *Pharmacy Law with Rules & Regulations, 1998, California edition*, California State Board of Pharmacy, LawTech Publishing, 1998.
2. American Medical Association, Drug Evaluations Annual, 1993.
3. McEvoy G., editor, *AHFS Drug Information*, American Society of Health-System Pharmacists, 2000.
4. Berkow R., editor-in-chief, *The Merck Manual of Medical Information, Home Edition*, Merck Research Laboratories, New Jersey, 1997.
5. Jacob L.S., editor, *Pharmacology*, 2nd edition, The National Medical Series for Independent Study, 1987.
6. *Pharmacy Certified Technician Training Manual*, 7th edition, Michigan Pharmacists Association, Lansing, MI, 1997.

About the author

Tracey Okabe-Yamamura, Pharm.D., is a clinical pharmacy specialist at Mercy San Juan Medical Center in Carmichael, California. The medical center is part of a multi-facility region of hospitals in the greater Sacramento area and includes services for oncology, trauma, cardiology, and other acute care specialties. Her current responsibilities include pharmacy support for a regional oncology service line, clinical staff development, continuous quality improvement, and preceptorship for pharmacy students and residents. Dr. Okabe-Yamamura is a graduate of the University of California, San Francisco, School of Pharmacy, and completed a clinical pharmacy residency at the University of California Irvine. Her past positions include clinical coordinator at Pacific Hospital of Long Beach and Clinical Pharmacist for FHP, Inc.

Self-assessment questions

1. Which of the following statements regarding a drug is ***not*** correct based on the definition in the United States?
   a. A drug is any substance that affects the body and its processes.
   b. A drug is any substance, other than a food or device, intended for the diagnosis of disease in man or other animals.
   c. A drug is any substance, other than a food or device, intended for the cure of disease in man or other animals.
   d. A drug is any substance, including food, intended to affect the structure or any function of the body of man or other animals.
2. The established (official) United States Adopted Name of a drug is the:
   a. generic name.
   b. chemical name.
   c. brand name.
   d. trade name.
3. The proprietary name of a drug registered to a manufacturer holding the trademark is the:
   a. generic name.
   b. chemical name.
   c. brand name.
   d. technical name.
4. Pharmacodynamics is:
   a. the quantitative aspects of elements of drug disposition: absorption, distribution, metabolism, and excretion.
   b. not only what the drug does to the body but also where the drug works and how the drug works.
   c. when the drug dose exceeds the recommended range, when therapy exceeds the recommended duration, or if a drug is not monitored properly.
   d. when a drug lacking effect of its own increases the effect of a second, active drug.
5. Pharmacokinetics is:
   a. the quantitative aspects of elements of drug disposition: absorption, distribution, metabolism, and excretion.
   b. not only what the drug does to the body but also where the drug works and how the drug works.
   c. when the drug dose exceeds the recommended range, when therapy exceeds the recommended duration, or if a drug is not monitored properly.
   d. when a drug lacking effect of its own increases the effect of a second, active drug.
6. The process that brings a drug from the administration site into the bloodstream is:
   a. absorption.
   b. distribution.
   c. metabolism.
   d. elimination.
7. The alteration of the chemical structure of a drug in preparation for removal from the body is:
   a. absorption.
   b. distribution.
   c. metabolism.
   d. elimination.
8. Which of the following statements is true regarding a nonprescription medication?
   a. It requires the supervision of a healthcare professional licensed to prescribe.
   b. It can be used safely when the consumer follows the manufacturer's directions.
   c. Federal law prohibits dispensing without a prescription.
   d. All of the above statements are true.
9. When two or more drugs combine to provide a response that is greater than the sum of the individual drugs, it is called:
   a. an additive effect.
   b. synergism.
   c. potentiation.
   d. absorption.
10. Two goals in the development of drugs are:
   a. absorption and distribution.
   b. safety and efficacy.
   c. synergism and potentiation.
   d. side effects and toxicities.

Chapter 11

Peripheral Nervous System

Dianne E. Miller, R.Ph., and Caroline Sul, Pharm.D. Candidate

Learning objectives

Upon completion of this chapter, the technician should be able to do the following:

- Differentiate between the general function of the sympathetic and parasympathetic systems.
- Explain the difference between sympathomimetic and sympatholytic drugs.
- Explain the difference between parasympathomimetic and parasympatholytic drugs.
- Define and explain the use of neuromuscular blocking agents and local anesthetics.

Introduction

The peripheral nervous system (PNS), also called the involuntary or autonomic nervous system, is distributed throughout the body and regulates the "autonomic" functions of the body that occur without conscious control. Examples of "autonomic" functions regulated by the peripheral nervous system include respiration, circulation, digestion, body temperature, metabolism, and sweating. The peripheral nervous system is composed of all the nerves outside the central nervous system (brain and spinal cord). It transmits information to and from the brain via chemical and electrical "messages" to other parts of the body. Sensory nerves, or afferent nerves, bring messages to the brain. The brain interprets the incoming afferent message and then sends out a new message via the motor nerves, or efferent nerves, to the rest of the body. These efferent messages then cause a reaction to the initial stimulus.

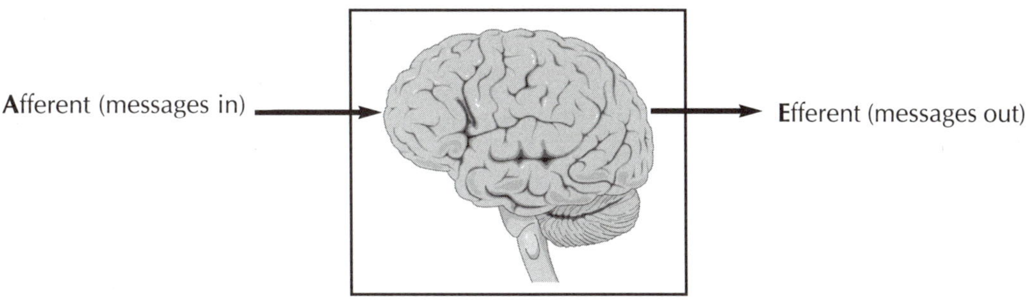

The actions of the efferent nerves can be divided into two groups, which are called the sympathetic nerves and parasympathetic nerves. The sympathetic nerves are often referred to as the "fight or flight" system because they facilitate mobilization of the body for quick action. The parasympathetic nerves are attached to the same organs, but have the opposite action of the sympathetic nerves. They are referred to as the "rest and digest" system because they maintain essential body functions, such as the digestion and elimination processes. The actions of the two systems often oppose each other, allowing for balance between the two.

Receptors and messengers

Neurotransmitters are substances that aid in transmitting impulses between two nerves or a nerve and a muscle. The neurotransmitter released by sympathetic nerve fibers is norepinephrine; the neurotransmitter released by the adrenal medulla (inner part of the adrenal gland located above the kidneys) into the blood is epinephrine. The actions of norepinephrine and epinephrine are described by the term "adrenergic." Norepinephrine is released from sympathetic nerve endings and has excitatory and inhibitory effects known as adrenergic stimulation. Excitatory responses include contraction of the heart and blood vessels; inhibitory responses include relaxation of the muscles of the bronchioles in the lung. Excitatory and inhibitory effects have been observed in different tissues by the same chemical because each tissue will have different receptors. There are two major classes of receptors, alpha (α) and beta (β). There are two subtypes of each category of receptors, which are designated as α_1, α_2, β_1, and β_2 and have different affinities (attraction) for different neurotransmitters. Some organs have only α or β receptors and other organs have both types of receptors. Although an organ can have both receptors, organs tend to have a preference to one type. For example, the blood vessels for skeletal muscles have both α_1, and β_2 receptors, but β_2 receptors are predominant.

Parasympathetic nerve fibers release only acetylcholine as a neurotransmitter. The action of acetylcholine is described by the term "cholinergic." There are two subtypes of cholinergic receptors—muscarinic and nicotinic. Muscarinic receptors were discovered when muscarine, a drug derived from poisonous mushrooms, was found to stimulate cholinergic receptors at the organ. Nicotine, from the tobacco plant, was found to stimulate cholinergic transmission at the ganglia (group of nerve cell bodies in the PNS) and at the skeletal muscle. Therefore, they are referred to as nicotinic receptors. Muscarinic and nicotinic receptors cause the same cholinergic responses; they differ in the location of the receptor.

Table 1 Responses of organs to nerve impulses

Effector organs	Receptor type	Adrenergic response	Cholinergic response
Heart	β_1	increase in heart rate	decrease in heart rate
Blood vessels to:			
Muscle	α and β	contraction, skeletal relaxation	relaxation
Skin	α	contraction	relaxation
Lung (bronchial muscles)	β_2	relaxation	contraction
Stomach motility	α_1, α_2, and β_2	decreased movement	increased movement
Urinary bladder:			
Detrusor muscle	β	relaxation (holds urine)	contraction (urination)
sphincter	α	contraction (holds urine)	relaxation (urination)
Eye			
Radial muscle	α_1	contraction (mydriasis[1])	(none)
Ciliary muscle		(none)	contraction (miosis[2])
Intestine motility	α_1, α_2, β_1, β_2	decrease	increase

[1] contraction which makes the pupil smaller
[2] dialation which makes the pupil appear larger

Sympathomimetics (adrenergic) agents

Drugs that mimic, reinforce, and supplement the messages sent via sympathetic nerves are referred to as sympathomimetic drugs. Direct-acting sympathomimetics will bind directly to the receptors and mimic the effects of epinephrine and norepinephrine. Indirect-acting sympathomimetics facilitate the release of norepinephrine or they block its elimination, so norepinephrine already in the body can interact with the receptor and cause an effect. Sympathomimetics are used in patients with hypertension, shock, heart block, asthma, congestion, and depression.

For example, asthma patients suffer from tightness in the chest and difficulty in breathing due to bronchiole smooth muscle spasm and contraction. Albuterol (Proventil®, Ventolin®) is a sympathomimetic that is selective for β_2 receptors. When administered by inhalation, it produces a bronchodilation effect that occurs rapidly, allowing the patient to breathe easier.

Table 2 Sympathomimetic drugs

Generic	Brand	Main use
epinephrine	Adrenaline®	Bronchospasm (relax bronchial smooth muscle), lower blood pressure in emergency situations
dopamine	Intropin®	Treatment of shock
isoproterenol	Isuprel®	Emergencies to stimulate heart rate (β adrenergic agonist)
albuterol	Ventolin®, Proventil®	Relax bronchial smooth muscle in diseases such as asthma and chronic obstructive pulmonary disease (COPD) (β_2 adrenergic agonist)
salmeterol	Serevent®	Same as albuterol, but longer lasting
phenylephrine	Neosynephrine®	Nasal decongestant and eye drop (α_1 adrenergic agonist)
clonidine	Catapres®	Treatment of hypertension (α_2 adrenergic agonist)
amphetamine	Adderall®	Treatment of attention deficit hyperactivity disorder (ADHD) and narcolepsy[1]
methylphenidate	Ritalin®	Treatment of attention deficit hyperactivity disorder (ADHD) and narcolepsy[1]

[1] Narcolepsy is hypersomnia, or tendency to sleep under conditions not conducive to sleep.

Sympatholytic (anti-adrenergic) agents

Sympatholytic drugs are referred to as adrenergic antagonists or blockers. They prevent epinephrine and norepinephrine from binding to a receptor at the receptor site. Sympatholytics can also be called alpha blockers or beta blockers, depending on what receptor site (α or β) the drug is blocking. They are used in patients with hypertension, heart disease, and migraine headaches.

Propranolol (Inderal®) is the prototype beta blocker that blocks β_1 and β_2 receptors. It is a sympatholytic drug used in the treatment of hypertension. Propranolol blocks β_1 receptors in the heart, which results in a decrease in heart rate. Propranolol blocks beta receptors in blood vessels to cause relaxation of the blood vessels, which leads to a decrease in blood pressure. Propranolol also blocks β_2 receptors in the lungs. This can cause a respiratory crisis in patients with asthma where the patient will be unable to breathe. Propranolol can be used in the treatment of hypertension, but it must not be used in patients who have asthma.

Table 3 Sympatholytic (anti-adrenergic) drugs

α-blockers		
Generic	**Brand**	**Use**
doxazosin	Cardura®	Treatment of hypertension and benign prostate hypertrophy[1]
phenoxybenzamine	Dibenzyline®	Treatment of hypertension in patients with pheochromocytoma[2]
phentolamine	Regitine®	Treatment of hypertension in patients with pheochromocytoma[2] and hypertensive crisis[3]
prazosin	Minipress®	Treatment of hypertension and benign prostate hypertrophy[1]
terazosin	Hytrin®	Treatment of hypertension and benign prostate hypertrophy[1]
β-blockers		
Generic	**Brand**	**Use**
acebutolol	Sectral®	Treatment of hypertension and benign prostate hypertrophy[1]
atenolol	Tenormin®	Treatment of hypertension, myocardial infarction (heart attack) and angina[4]
labetalol	Normodyne®/Trandate®	Use in hypertensive crisis[3]
metoprolol	Lopressor®/Toprol XL®	Treatment of hypertension, myocardial infarction (heart attack) and angina[4]
nadolol	Corgard®	Treatment of hypertension, angina,[4] and arrhythmia[5]
pindolol	Visken®	Treatment of hypertension and angina[4]
propranolol	Inderal®	Treatment of hypertension, angina,[4] migraine headaches, and arrhythmia[5]
timolol	Blocadren®	Treatment of hypertension, myocardial infarction (heart attack), angina,[4] and migraine headache

[1]Benign prostate hypertrophy – non-cancerous, enlargement of the prostate, usually resulting in high blood pressure and decreased urinary flow
[2]Pheochromocytoma – small vascular tumor of the adrenal gland
[3]Hypertensive crisis – situation that occurs when the blood pressure becomes dangerously high, resulting in damage to other parts of the body
[4] Angina – pain in the center of the chest
[5]Arrhythmia – abnormal heart rhythm

Parasympathomimetic (cholinergic) agents

Parasympathomimetic drugs mimic the actions of the parasympathetic nervous system by interacting with parasympathetic receptors. They can be similar in structure and action to acetylcholine and can promote the effects of these nerves, or they inhibit the actions of the enzymes that degrade acetylcholine, therefore prolonging the action of the existing acetylcholine.

Glaucoma is an eye disease that is caused by an increase in pressure in the eye. Pilocarpine (Pilocar®) is a parasympathomimetic drug that causes contraction of the ciliary muscle in the eye. This allows liquid in the eye to drain out, causing a decrease in pressure in the eye. Other clinical uses of cholinergic agents include prevention of postoperative constipation and urinary retention, treatment of high ocular pressure (glaucoma), and treatment of certain cases of rapid heart rate.

Table 4 Parasympathomimetic (cholinergic) drugs

Generic	Brand	Main use
bethanechol	Urecholine®	Treatment of urinary retention, GERD
carbachol	Miostat®	Treatment of glaucoma
pilocarpine	Pilocar®	Treatment of glaucoma
edrophonium	Tensilon®	Diagnosis of myasthenia gravis[1]
neostigmine	Prostigmin®	Treatment of myasthenia gravis[1]
physostigmine	Eserine®	Treatment of glaucoma
pyridostigmine	Mestinon®	Treatment of myasthenia gravis[1]

[1]Myasthenia gravis – chronic disease characterized by severe fatigue and weakness of selected muscles.

Parasympatholytic (anticholinergic) agents

Parasympatholytic drugs block the action of acetylcholine in parasympathetic nerves. They can bind to cholinergic receptors and prevent the binding and action of acetylcholine. There are three types: antimuscarinic; ganglionic blockers, which block nicotinic receptors; and neuromuscular blockers, which are discussed in detail below. Atropine is an antimuscarinic drug that acts at the organ. When applied to the eye, atropine (Atropisol®) blocks all acetylcholine from binding in the eye. This results in the dilatation of the pupil, unresponsiveness to light, and inability to focus for near vision. Optometrists can use atropine eyedrops to look into a patient's eyes in order to see the blood vessels in the eye. Patients with glaucoma should never use this because it will cause the pressure in the eye to increase, making the glaucoma worse. When atropine is taken orally, it can be used to reduce muscle spasms in the stomach and intestine and in the bladder by blocking cholinergic receptors in those organs.

Table 5 Parasympatholytic (anticholinergic) drugs

Generic	Brand	Main use
		Antimuscarinic
atropine	Atropisol®	Diagnosis of eye disease
ipratropium	Atrovent®	Treatment of chronic obstructive pulmonary disease (COPD)
scopolamine	Transderm Scop®	Prevention of motion sickness
cyclopentolate	Cyclogyl®	Diagnosis of eye disease (preferred because shorter duration of action)
benztropine	Cogentin®	Treatment of Parkinson's disease[1]
glycopyrrolate	Robinul®	Pre-anesthesia used to reduce excessive respiratory tract secretions during surgery

[1]Parkinson's disease – disorder of middle-aged and elderly people characterized by involuntary movements resulting in tremors, shaking and rigidity of the extremities.

Table 6 Parasympatholytic (anticholinergic) drugs (Continued)

Generic	Brand	Main use
		Ganglionic blockers
mecamylamine	Inversine®	Alternative treatment for hypertension
nicotine	Nicotrol®	Smoking cessation treatment
trimethaphan	Arfonad®	Alternative treatment for hypertension

Neuromuscular blocking agents

Neuromuscular blocking agents block cholinergic receptors between the nerve and muscle. Curare was used as a poison in South Africa to kill animals because death resulted from paralysis of skeletal muscles. Tubocurarine, the active form of curare, in smaller doses was found to cause temporary paralysis in humans. This results from tubocurarine combining with nicotinic cholinergic receptors and blocking the transmission of acetylcholine. This blockade of nerve impulses between the muscle and nerve causes temporary paralysis. Small, rapidly moving muscles like the eye are affected before the limbs, neck, and trunk. Death occurs when the diaphragm becomes paralyzed, stopping respiration.

Neuromuscular blocking agents are used in combination with surgical anesthesia in order to make the surgery easier. The patient requires less anesthesia, and postanesthesic recovery is shortened. There is another group, central muscle relaxants, that controls spastic muscles for relaxation.

Table 7 Neuromuscular blocking drugs

Generic	Brand	Main use
atracurium	Tracrium®	Used in anesthesia to relax muscles
mivacurium	Miracron®	Used in anesthesia to relax muscles
pancuronium	Pavulon®	Used in anesthesia to relax muscles
rocuronium	Zemuron®	Used in anesthesia to relax muscles
succinylcholine	Anectine®	Used in anesthesia to relax muscles
vecuronium	Norcuron®	Used in anesthesia to relax muscles

Local anesthetics

Local anesthetics are drugs that block nerve transmission when applied locally to nerve tissues in appropriate concentrations. They act on any part of the nervous system and cause sensory and/or motor paralysis in nerves, depending on the amount of anesthetic used. The action is reversible, and there is complete recovery of nerve function once the effects wear off. They are most commonly used in minor surgical procedures, such as stitching deep gashes and dental procedures like extracting teeth. Lidocaine and procaine are commonly used in dental offices for numbing the nerves in the mouth. Epinephrine is sometimes added to local anesthetic preparations to constrict blood vessels. This helps decrease the amount of bleeding and prevents the removal of the drug into the bloodstream.

Table 8 Local anesthetic drugs

Generic	Brand	Main use
bupivacaine	Marcaine®	When local anesthetic of immediate duration is needed (longer action than lidocaine)
lidocaine	Xylocaine®	When local anesthetic of immediate duration is needed
procaine	Novocain®	When local anesthetic of immediate duration is needed (used commonly in dental procedures)
tetracaine	Pontocaine®	Local anesthetic instilled into the eye
cocaine		Topical anesthetic approved only for the upper respiratory tract

Conclusion

Without conscious effort, the peripheral nervous system controls a variety of bodily functions and sends messages to and from the brain. Medications affecting this system can help to send messages throughout the body, block nerve transmission, interact with receptor sites, or block the action of certain chemicals. This typically results in the restoration of regular functioning in organs and the prevention or cessation of pain.

Bibliography

Dox, I., Melloni, B., Eisner, G., Melloni's Illustrated Medical Dictionary, Pearl River, NY, 1993.

Goodman, A., Rall, T., Niles, A., and Taylor, P., The Pharmacological Basis of Therapeutics, New York, NY, 1996, pp. 105-248, 267-294, 331-348.

Mycek, M., PhD., Harvey, R., PhD., Champe, P., PhD., Lippincott's Illustrated Reviews; Pharmacology 2nd edition, Philadelphia, PA, 1997, pp. 27-80.

Van De Graff, K.M., Fox, S., Concepts of Human Anatomy and Physiology, Dubuque, IA, 1988, pp. 472-518.

About the authors

Dianne E. Miller received her bachelor's degrees in pharmacy and applied biology in 1987 from Ferris State University in Big Rapids, Michigan. She has completed a variety of certificate courses and post-graduate training, including the University of Pittsburgh's Smoking Cessation Specialist Certification Program, the National Institute for Pharmacists' Outcomes Osteoporosis Care Certificate Program, University of Tennessee's Asthma Patient Management Certificate Program, American Pharmaceutical Association's Pharmacy-Based Immunization Delivery Certificate Course, and Central Michigan University master's level courses in administration. Miller is the Associate Executive Director at the Michigan Pharmacists Association in Lansing, Michigan. Prior to joining the staff at the association, she was a staff pharmacist for Ingham Regional Medical Center in Lansing, Michigan, where she continues to work as a relief pharmacist.

Caroline Sul of Grosse Pointe Woods, Michigan, is a June 2001 Doctor of Pharmacy Candidate at the University of Michigan College of Pharmacy. Upon graduation, she plans to enroll in a residency program. While at the University of Michigan, Sul was a member of the American Pharmaceutical Association's Academy of Students of Pharmacy chapter, serving as the group's treasurer.

Self-assessment questions

1. The following statements concerning the peripheral nervous system are true *except*:
   a. The peripheral nervous system is called the autonomic nervous system.
   b. The peripheral nervous system regulates respiration, circulation, digestion, body temperature, metabolism, and sweating.
   c. The peripheral nervous system is made up of nerves, the spinal cord, and the brain.
   d. The peripheral nervous system uses afferent nerves to bring messages to the brain and efferent nerves to bring messages out of the brain.

2. Which statement concerning the sympathetic nervous system is correct?
   a. The sympathetic nervous system regulates essential body functions referred to as "rest and digest."
   b. The sympathetic nervous system releases neurotransmitters called norepinephrine and epinephrine.
   c. The sympathetic nervous system has two major classes of receptors, alpha (α) and beta (β) receptors.
   d. The sympathetic nervous system causes the ciliary muscle in the eye to contract.

3. Which one of the following characteristics describes parasympathetic stimulation?
   a. The parasympathetic nervous system causes the heart to beat faster.
   b. The parasympathetic nervous system allows the body to urinate.
   c. The parasympathetic nervous system makes it hard to breathe.
   d. The parasympathetic nervous system prevents food from being digested.

4. What is the difference between sympathomimetic and sympatholytic drugs?
   a. Sympathomimetic drugs imitate the action of acetylcholine, while sympatholytic drugs imitate the action of norepinephrine.
   b. Sympathomimetic drugs act indirectly on receptors, while sympatholytic drugs act directly on the receptor.
   c. Sympathomimetic drugs imitate the message sent through sympathetic nerves, while sympatholytic drugs prevent the message from being sent through sympathetic nerves.
   d. Sympathomimetic drugs work at alpha (α) receptors, while sympatholytic drugs work at beta (β) receptors.

5. Neuromuscular blocking agents:
   a. block nerve transmission when applied locally to nerve tissue.
   b. block epinephrine from binding to sympathetic receptors.
   c. block acetylcholine from binding to parasympathetic receptors in nerves.
   d. block cholinergic receptors between the nerve and muscle.

For questions 6-10, choose the answer that best describes the drug.

6. Atropine:
   a. blocks the action of acetylcholine in parasympathetic nerves.
   b. is used in minor surgical procedures.
   c. affects the lungs as its main action.
   d. is in the same class as clonidine.

7. Propranolol:
   a. blocks nerve transmission when applied locally to nerve tissues.
   b. is used in anesthesia.
   c. affects the kidneys as its main action.
   d. is in the same class as metoprolol.

8. Albuterol:
   a. imitates the effects of norepinephrine in sympathetic nerves.
   b. is used in the diagnosis of eye problems.
   c. affects the liver as its main action.
   d. is in the same class as cocaine.

9. Lidocaine:
   a. blocks norepinephrine from binding to a receptor.
   b. is used when local anesthetic of immediate duration is needed.
   c. affects the stomach as its main action.
   d. is in the same class as nicotine.

10. Pilocarpine:
    a. blocks the action of acetylcholine in parasympathetic nerves.
    b. is used when the patient needs help breathing.
    c. affects the eyes as its main action.
    d. is in the same class as pancuronium.

Chapter 12

Nervous System Disorders

Thomas J. Cali, Pharm.D., and Beverly P. Kershaw, Pharm.M.S.

Learning objectives

Upon completion of this chapter, the technician should be able to do the following:

- Explain how central nervous system (CNS) muscle relaxers work.
- Explain the adverse reactions of muscle-relaxing medications.
- Explain the role of diazepam and baclofen as muscle relaxers.
- Describe the signs and symptoms of Parkinson's disease.
- Explain the medication therapy choices for Parkinson's disease.
- Describe the symptoms of a seizure disorder.
- Discuss the different types of anticonvulsant medications.
- Describe sedative-hypnotic effects of medications used for sleep.

Introduction

Disorders of the human nervous system are treated with medications that have a wide and diverse effect on patients being treated. Drugs used for these disorders may produce stimulation, nervousness, insomnia, drowsiness, and irritability, along with euphoria and anxiety. The disorders discussed in this chapter deal with antagonism of the nervous system as manifested by the various disease states. This chapter will discuss muscle-relaxing medications and drugs used to treat Parkinson's disease and seizure disorders, and medications that enhance sleep.

Muscle-relaxing medications

Painful spasms of the skeletal muscles can occur due to injury, exposure to cold, lack of blood flow to the muscle, and overexertion. These factors can cause additional nerve impulses transmitted to the spinal cord and the brain. The impulses may cause a reflex (involuntary) skeletal muscle contraction or spasm. The spasm causes more sensory impulses, resulting in a cycle of more severe contraction and more painful muscle spasms.

CNS relaxers are used to break the cycle and induce muscle relaxation, resulting in relief of pain. These relaxers are used along with rest and physical therapy. These oral prescription medications include carisoprodol (Soma®), chlorzoxazone (Parafon Forte DSC®), methocarbamol (Robaxin®), metaxalone (Skelaxin®), cyclobenzaprine (Flexeril®), and orphenadrine citrate (Norflex®, Norgesic Forte®). Both methocarbamol and orphenadrine can also be administered parenterally.

CNS relaxers have an onset of action in 30 to 60 minutes. Patients must be warned about the CNS reactions, which include drowsiness, weakness, headache, nightmares, and depression.

CNS relaxers also have anticholinergic effects, including dry mouth, urinary hesitancy, constipation, and visual disturbances. Physical and psychological dependence may result from long term use; stopping this drug may cause severe withdrawal symptoms.

Two other drugs used for skeletal muscle relaxation are diazepam (Valium®) and baclofen (Lioresal®). Diazepam has many uses, including treating spasms in patients with spinal cord injury, cerebral palsy, anxiety disorders, and seizure disorders. Baclofen is the preferred medication for treating muscle spasms from cerebral palsy, for paraplegic patients, or for patients with spinal cord lesions (from trauma or multiple sclerosis). Baclofen is less sedating than diazepam. Although baclofen is effective in reducing the severity of painful muscle spasms, it does not improve manual dexterity or stiff gait. Baclofen's effect can take weeks. Abruptly stopping baclofen can cause hallucinations, seizures, and severe muscle spasms; therefore, slow withdrawal is recommended.

Drugs to treat Parkinson's disease

Parkinson's disease is a disorder with symptoms of complete or partial loss of muscle movement, muscle rigidity, and tremor. The disease is thought to be caused by exposure to neurotoxins, drugs, encephalitis, trauma, or unknown factors. Parkinson's disease usually becomes progressively worse due to ongoing nerve damage.

Two types of medications are used to treat Parkinsonism—anticholinergic or dopaminergic agents. The anticholinergics are benztropine mesylate (Cogentin®), trihexyphenidyl (Artane®), and diphenhydramine (Benadryl®). These medications are often started when the symptoms are mild and the patient's lifestyle is not affected.

The dopaminergic agents are used for a more severe disease state. They include levodopa (Dopar®), the combination drug carbidopa-levodopa (Sinemet®), the antiviral drug amantadine (Symmetrel®), bromocriptine (Parlodel®), pergolide mesylate (Permax®), and selegiline (Eldepryl®). These agents act in the brain to improve motor function by increasing the dopamine concentration or enhancing the action of dopamine in the nervous system. Dopaminergic medications are associated with CNS side effects (i.e., headache, insomnia, hallucinations). Some have GI adverse effects, including nausea and vomiting. Long-term adverse effects can be minimized if the daily doses are kept low and various medications are used with physical therapy and diet. New medications and procedures are being developed for intervention in Parkinson's disease.

Seizure classification

Partial seizures begin in a specific location of the brain. The simple partial seizure is characterized by a sudden onset of clonic jerking (a rhythmic succession of alternating contractions and partial relaxations of muscles) lasting 60 to 90 seconds. Unlike many other types of seizures, simple partial seizures can be remembered by the patient.

The complex partial seizure is characterized by a brief warning sign, followed by a change of consciousness. The patient may stare, fumble, smack his lips and swallow repeatedly. After a minute or two, the patient gradually recovers with no memory of the seizure.

Generalized tonic-clonic (grand mal) seizures are the most dramatic, characterized by muscle rigidity, tremors and massive jerking of the body lasting a couple of minutes. Afterwards, the patient may feel stuporous (dazed) for some time. Generalized tonic-clonic seizures are associated with respiratory depression and a low risk of possible fatality.

Absence seizures (petit mal) begin in childhood and can occur hundreds of times per day. These seizures usually start and end abruptly (less than 10 seconds duration). During the seizure the patient is not responsive (absent) and may have mild jerking of the extremities or eyelids.

Medications to treat seizure disorders

The goals of anticonvulsant therapy are to prevent and control seizures. The medication chosen depends on the type of seizure being treated. A seizure is an episode of brain dysfunction resulting from an abnormal transmission in the nervous system. Causes of seizures include head injury, disease, infection, cancer, high body temperature (febrile seizure), or unknown causes. Seizures can also be caused by toxic drug concentrations (cocaine, certain antibiotics, etc.).

Phenytoin

The anticonvulsant activity of phenytoin (Dilantin®) has been known since 1938. Phenytoin is effective against partial seizures and generalized tonic-clonic seizures. It blocks the repetitive stimulation of the neurons and suppresses seizure spread. Phenytoin is most effective when the dose produces a therapeutic serum concentration between 10 and 20 micrograms per milliliter (mcg/ml). At higher serum concentrations, further dosage increases result in disproportionately higher serum concentrations; therefore, these increases must be made cautiously. Side effects can include nausea, lethargy, swollen gums (gingival hyperplasia), ataxia (dizziness), and coarsening of facial features. Many medications interact with phenytoin, resulting in decreased or increased serum concentrations. Phenytoin also affects the heart and is used for some heart rhythm disturbances.

Carbamazepine

Effective for partial seizures and tonic-clonic seizures, carbamazepine (Tegretol®) inhibits the spread of seizure activity and neuromuscular transmission (similar to phenytoin). It may be used with phenytoin in patients with seizures that are difficult to control. Carbamazepine has the most effect with least side effects when the dose produces a therapeutic serum concentration of four to eight mcg/ml just before the morning dose. Many medications interact with carbamazepine, resulting in decreased or increased serum concentrations. Carbamazepine is sometimes used to relieve neurologically related pain such as the pain of trigeminal neuralgia (tic douloureux) and the behavioral disturbances associated with dementia in geriatric patients.

Phenobarbital

Barbiturates are relatively safe but are not often used because of the sedation they cause. Barbiturate anticonvulsants include phenobarbital, mephobarbital (Mebaral®), and primidone (Mysoline®). While barbiturates are useful in most types of seizures, phenobarbital is often used with phenytoin to stop continuous seizures and as prophylaxis for febrile (high temperature) seizures seen in infants. Many medications interact with barbiturates, resulting in an increase or decrease of barbiturate serum concentration.

Ethosuximide

Absence seizures are most often treated with three related medications—ethosuximide (Zarontin®), methsuximide (Celontin®), and phensuximide (Milontin®). Ethosuximide remains the preferred medication for absence seizures, because it is effective with few side effects, and because the alternative is valproic acid, which is sometimes associated with liver toxicity and carries a rare risk of pancreatitis. Ethosuximide interacts with valproic acid, resulting in higher and potentially toxic ethosuximide serum concentrations.

Valproic acid and derivatives

Like phenytoin and carbamazepine, valproic acid (Depakene®), valproate acid (Depacon®), and divalproex sodium (Depakote®) are effective for partial seizures and tonic-clonic seizures and are useful in absence seizures. Valproic acid and its derivatives are monitored for therapeutic concentrations of valproate, ranging from 50 to 100mcg/ml. Many medications interact with valproate. It is also used for psychiatric disorders and for disturbed behavior associated with dementia in geriatric patients.

Benzodiazepine agents

Four benzodiazepine medications are considered anticonvulsant because they are capable of inhibiting the development and spread of seizure in the CNS. Diazepam (Valium®) given intravenously is highly effective for stopping continuous seizure activity, but the duration of control is often less than one hour. In acute situations, diazepam may be administered by the rectal route. Lorazepam (Ativan®) may be given intravenously and lasts somewhat longer than diazepam. Clonazepam (Klonopin®) is an oral, long-acting and potent anticonvulsant, but also causes marked sedation. Clorazepate (Tranxene®) is available as a short-acting or prolonged absorption (Tranxene-SD®) oral product and has been useful for seizure control. Many medications interact with the benzodiazepine class of medications. Benzodiazepines are classified as Schedule IV drugs by the Drug Enforcement Agency (DEA).

Miscellaneous medications

Felbamate (Felbatol®)was marketed in the United States and resulted in extremely severe adverse effects (aplastic anemia, death). The use of this medication is limited to patients who have failed on all other medications but are responding to felbamate. Gabapentin (Neurontin®), used for partial seizures, is known to cause sedation and interacts with many other medications. Gabapentin also has usage in disturbed behavior, pain from neurological causes, and other neurological syndromes. Lamotrigine (Lamictyl®) is effective for partial seizures and is similar in action to phenytoin.

Teratogenicity

Children born to mothers taking anticonvulsant medications have an increased potential for birth defects. Phenytoin, phenobarbital, and carbamazepine have all been associated with congenital birth defects. Valproate has been implicated in the malformation spina bifida. Even though most neurologists agree that a definite cause and effect relationship has not been established between anticonvulsant medications and birth defects, they still believe that it is important to minimize exposure to the anticonvulsants while treating maternal seizures.

Medications to treat sleep disorders

Sedative medications reduce anxiety and provide a calming effect while causing some degree of CNS sedation. A hypnotic medication produces drowsiness and encourages the onset and continued state of sleep. Sedative-hypnotics are indicated for short-term use (seven to 14 days) because dosing these drugs beyond seven to 14 days may produce tolerance to the sedation and/or possible drug dependence, and discontinuing the medication may cause rebound insomnia. Sedative-hypnotics should be used along with good sleep hygiene practices such as proper diet, avoidance of late-night exercise, avoiding stimulants, and consistent, regular bedtimes.

The benzodiazepine class of medications are the most common sedative-hypnotics used for sleep disorders. Benzodiazepines produce anticonvulsant activity, muscle relaxation, dose-related amnesia, depression of breathing, and change in consciousness. With continued use, a decreased effectiveness and increased physical and psychological dependence occurs. Sedation on the day following medication administration is more common with long-acting flurazepam (Dalmane®). The opposite problem of early-morning awakening may occur with a short-acting drug such as triazolam (Halcion®). Temazepam (Restoril®) has a medium duration of action. Benzodiazepines are classified as Schedule IV by the DEA, and their action is reversed by flumazenil (Romazicon®).

Other hypnotics include chloral hydrate (Noctec®) and barbiturates such as pentobarbital (Nembutal®) and secobarbital (Seconal®). Zolpidem (Ambien®) and zaleplon (Sonata®) are structurally different from benzodiazepines, but have a similar mechanism of action and the same effectiveness as triazolam. Their action is also reversed by flumazenil (Romazicon®).

Table 1 Drugs to treat nervous system disorders

Skeletal muscle relaxants
baclofen (Lioresal®)
carisoprodol (Soma®)
chlorphenesin (Maolate®)
chlorzoxazone (Parafon Forte®)
cyclobenzaprine (Flexeril®)
dantrolene (Dantrium®)
diazepam (Valium®)
methocarbamol (Robaxin®)
metaxalone (Skelaxin®)
orphenadrine (Norflex®)
tizanidine (Zanaflex®)

Anti-Parkinson's
amantadine (Symmetrel®)
benztropine (Cogentin®)
biperiden (Akineton®)
bromocriptine (Parlodel®)
carbidopa (Lodosyn®)
diphenhydramine (Benadryl®)
entacapone (Comtan®)
ethopropazine (Artane®)
levodopa (Dopar®)
pergolide (Permax®)
procyclidine (Kemadrin®)
selegiline (Eldepryl®)
tolcapone (Tasmar®)
trihexyphenidyl (Artane®)

Seizure disorders
ethotoin (Peganone®)
fosphenytoin (Cerebyx®)
mephenytoin (Mesantoin®)
phenytoin (Dilantin®)

Succinimides
ethosuximide (Zarontin®)
methsuximide (Celontin®)
phensuximide (Milontin®)

Sulfonamides
zonisamide (Zonegran®)

Oxazolidinediones
paramethadione (Paradione®)
trimethadione (Tridione®)

Benzodiazepines
carbamazepine (Tegretol®)
clorazepate (Tranxene®)
clonazepam (Klonopin®)
diazepam (Valium®)
oxcarbazepine (Trileptal®)

Adjunctive agents
felbamate (Felbatol®)
gabapentin (Neurontin®)
lamotrigine (Lamictal®)
levetiracetam (Keppra®)
primidone (Mysoline®)
tiagabine (Gabitril®)
topiramate (Topamax®)

Valproic acid derivatives
divalproex sodium (Depakote®)
valproic acid (Depakene®)

Miscellaneous agents
acetazolamide (Diamox®)
magnesium sulfate (Magnesium Sulfate®)
mephobarbital (Mebaral®)
phenobarbital (Phenobarbital®)
pramipexole (Mirapex®)
ropinirole (Requip®)

Sleep aides
acetylcarbromal (Paxarel®)
apobarbital (Alurate®)
butabarbital (Butisol®)
chloral hydrate (Noctec®)
estazolam (ProSom®)
ethchlorvynol (Placidyl®)
flurazepam (Dalmane®)
glutethimide (Doriden®)
mephobarbital (Mebaral®)
pentobarbital (Nembutal®)
phenobarbital (Phenobarbital®)
paraldehyde (Paral®)
propiomazine (Largon®)
quazepam (Doral®)
secobarbital (Seconal®)
temazepam (Restoril®)
triazolam (Halcion®)
zaleplon (Sonata®)
zolpidem (Ambien®)

Conclusion

Medications used to relax muscles, treat Parkinson's disease and seizure disorders, and enhance sleep produce a variety of effects; therefore, patients taking these medications need to be counseled regarding the possible side effects. Additionally, because many medications interact with the drugs discussed in this chapter, having complete patient profiles on such patients is imperative to ensure serum concentrations of the medications remain ideal.

About the authors

Thomas J. Cali earned both his bachelor's degree and Doctor of Pharmacy degree from the Philadelphia College of Pharmacy and Science in Pennsylvania. Dr. Cali is an independent clinical practitioner with his own practice, Thomas J. Cali & Associates. His previous experience includes serving as vice president of clinical affairs with Managed Care Resources, Inc. of Chesapeake, Virginia; director of clinical services for FACS for Long-Term Care in San Francisco, California; an assistant professor at the University of Maryland Hospital School of Pharmacy, the Hospital of the University of Pennsylvania, and the Philadelphia College of Pharmacy and Science; and in various consulting positions. Dr. Cali has been published extensively and has delivered numerous continuing education presentations. He was named Teacher of the Year of the University of Maryland School of Pharmacy in 1982 and received the 1994 George F. Archambault Award from the American Society of Consultant Pharmacists, which is the society's highest honor, for his outstanding contributions to consultant pharmacy.

Beverly P. Kershaw is the assistant director of pharmacy at William Beaumont Hospital in Royal Oak, Michigan. Kershaw received both her bachelor's and master's degrees in pharmacy from Wayne State University in Detroit, Michigan. She has served as an officer and board member the Michigan Society of Health-System Pharmacists (MSHP), the Southeastern Michigan Society of Health-System Pharmacists, and the Macomb County Pharmacists Association, as well as on numerous professional committees. As a member of the American Society of Health-System Pharmacists, Kershaw served on the Council for Educational Affairs from 1999 through 2001.

Self-assessment questions

1. Which of the following statements describes the mechanism of action of skeletal muscle-relaxing medications?
   a. They break the cycle of sensory impulses and reflex muscle contractions.
   b. They produce anticholinergic effects resulting in muscle relaxation.
   c. They induce peripheral nervous system sedation, which produces skeletal muscle relaxation.
   d. They have an onset of action of 30-60 minutes.

2. Which of the following medications is classified as a skeletal muscle relaxer?
   a. Cogentin®
   b. Lioresal®
   c. Benadryl®
   d. Phenytoin

3. Which of the following is a dopaminergic medication used to treat Parkinson's disease?
   a. Benztropine
   b. Procyclidine
   c. Levodopa
   d. Diphenhydramine

4. A seizure which begins in a specific location of the brain and is characterized by a sudden onset of clonic jerking lasting 60-90 seconds is a:
   a. partial seizure.
   b. generalized seizure.
   c. petit mal seizure.
   d. grand mal seizure.

5. Which of the following anticonvulsants may be used to treat generalized seizures?
   a. Phenytoin
   b. Carbamazepine
   c. Phenobarbital
   d. All of the above

6. Phenytoin is most effective at a serum concentration of:
   a. greater than 20 micrograms per liter.
   b. 10 - 20 milligrams per milliliter.
   c. 10 - 20 micrograms per milliliter.
   d. less than 10 micrograms per milliliter.

7. The preferred medication for treating absence seizures is:
   a. phenytoin.
   b. carbamazepine.
   c. phenobarbital.
   d. ethosuximide.

8. Side effects related to phenytoin may include:
   a. nausea.
   b. gingival hyperplasia.
   c. coarsening of facial features.
   d. all of the above.

9. A hypnotic medication:
   a. reduces anxiety and provides a calming effect while causing some degree of CNS sedation.
   b. produces drowsiness and encourages the onset and continued state of sleep.
   c. induces muscle relaxation and relief of pain.
   d. acts in the brain to improve motor function by increasing the dopamine concentration or enhancing the action of dopamine in the nervous system.

10. Which medication class is the most common sedative-hypnotic used for sleep disorders?
    a. Benzodiazepines
    b. Barbiturates
    c. Chloral hydrate
    d. Carbamazepine

Chapter 13

Affective Disorders

Thomas J. Cali, Pharm.D., and Beverly P. Kershaw, Pharm.M.S.

Learning objectives

Upon completion of this chapter, the technician should be able to do the following:

- Describe the clinical symptoms for which antidepressant and antimanic medications would be indicated.
- Discuss the use of tricyclic antidepressants and monoamine oxidase inhibitors (MAOIs).
- Explain the role of selective serotonin reuptake inhibitors (SSRIs) in the treatment of affective disorders.
- Describe the use of lithium in the treatment of affective disorders.
- Discuss the clinical indications for antipsychotic medications.
- Identify the medications used as antipsychotic agents.
- Explain the importance of early detection of adverse effects such as dystonia and tardive dyskinesia.

Introduction

Affective disorders are those arising from or influenced by emotions or feelings. Since the early antidepressant prototypes, such as imipramine, were introduced in the 1940s, many new mood-elevating agents have been introduced by the pharmaceutical manufacturers. Medications used to treat depression and psychosis will be reviewed in this chapter.

Drugs used to treat depression and mania

Depression, one of the most common psychiatric disorders, is estimated to affect 10 percent of people at some time in their life. Depression is characterized by the presence of several of the following signs or symptoms for weeks: poor appetite, sleep disturbance, agitation, fatigue, feelings of worthlessness, loss of interest in activities, slowed thinking, difficulty with concentration, thoughts of death, and suicide ideation. Mania is characterized by euphoria, rapid speech, flight of ideas, reduced need for sleep, and hyperactivity. Of people who are diagnosed with depression, approximately 90 percent have common depression (unipolar) and 10 percent have mania-depression (bipolar).

The cause of these disorders is uncertain and thought to be related to genetic factors, chemical neurotransmitter imbalances, psychological factors, or unknown causes. The neurotransmitters serotonin and norepinephrine are diminished in depression and excessive in mania. Medication treatments aim to adjust these neurotransmitters over time. Depression is treated with tricyclic antidepressants, monoamine oxidase inhibitors (MAOIs), selective serotonin reuptake inhibitors (SSRIs), and other antidepressants.

Tricyclic antidepressants

Tricyclic antidepressants are so named because of the three rings in their chemical structures. Examples of tricyclic antidepressants include amitriptyline (Elavil®), clomipramine (Anafranil®), desipramine (Norpramine®), doxepin (Sinequan®), and nortriptyline (Pamelor®). Norepinephrine and serotonin increase in the brain and symptoms of depression diminish beginning after one to two weeks of therapy using these medications; these effects may not become maximal for months. Daily dosing is possible after the patient has adjusted to the medication. Tricyclic antidepressants are usually taken at bedtime to reduce the effects of the sedation and hypotension that may occur after the dose.

Because adverse reactions differ among the tricyclic medications, switching to another may reduce or eliminate the reaction. For example, if doxepin causes low blood pressure, the patient can be switched to nortriptyline, which is less likely to cause this reaction. Besides treatment of depression, tricyclic drugs have been useful in treatment of bed-wetting (enuresis) and chronic pain from neurological causes. These agents can cause heart arrhythmias and may prove fatal in very high doses. Tricyclic medications are known to interact with many other medications and may produce fatality in overdose situations.

Monoamine oxidase inhibitors (MAOIs)

Monoamine oxidase inhibitors inhibit the enzyme that normally metabolizes tyramine, norepinephrine, and serotonin. The enzyme is called monoamine oxidase (MAO). The resulting increased concentrations of norepinephrine and serotonin relieve the symptoms of depression. MAO inhibitors (MAOIs) include phenelzine (Nardil®) and tranylcypromine (Parnate®). These medications are considered for treating depression when the tricyclic drugs have failed or when the depression is accompanied by anxiety or phobias.

The inhibition of MAO can continue for a week after the last dose of an MAOI. A seven- to 10-day "wash out" period after the last dose of an MAOI is recommended before a patient starts to use or ingest a medication or food that interacts with MAOIs. Because life-threatening reactions (hypertensive crisis, high temperature, seizure, and death) can occur, patients receiving an MAOI must be extra cautious in using any other medication. Some drugs known to interact with MAOIs are meperidine (Demerol®), decongestants (e.g., pseudoephedrine), cough suppressants (e.g., dextromethorphan), and other antidepressants (e.g., serotonin reuptake inhibitors or tricyclic drugs). Foods with high tyramine content will interact with an MAOI to cause a hypertensive crisis. Foods high in tyramine include Chianti and burgundy wines, beer, aged cheeses, and meats. The patient should consult a complete list of foods and substances that interact with MAOIs.

Selective serotonin reuptake inhibitors (SSRIs)

By inhibiting the reuptake of serotonin, the increased serotonin concentrations relieve the symptoms of depression. Selective serotonin reuptake inhibitors (SSRIs) are very effective, have fewer side effects than the tricyclic drugs, and have great patient acceptance despite adverse effects such as headache or nausea. SSRIs include fluoxetine (Prozac®), paroxetine (Paxil®), sertraline (Zoloft®), fluvoxamine (Luvox®), and citalopram (Celexa®). While these agents are safe when used alone, if a patient is switched to an MAOI, a sufficiently long "wash out" period is needed. Besides treatment of depression, SSRIs are useful in panic disorder, obsessive-compulsive disorders, eating disorders, and attention deficit disorder. The SSRIs may produce adverse reactions secondary to serotonin excess concentrations.

Second generation antidepressants

Some antidepressants are considered "second generation" after the tricyclic drugs and have also been grouped as the "heterocyclic" antidepressants. These agents include amoxapine (Asendin®), bupropion (Wellbutrin®), maprotiline (Ludiomil®), trazodone (Desyrel®), nefazodone (Serzone®), and venlafaxine

(Effexor®). As with antidepressants, heterocyclic antidepressants may have adverse effects, may be lethal in overdoses, and commonly interact with other medications. Venlafaxine is similar to SSRIs and must not be used with an MAOI.

Lithium

Lithium (Lithobid®, Eskalith®) is often used for manic-depressive (bipolar) disorders; its success rate is reported at 60 percent to 80 percent. It is sometimes called a "mood stabilizer." Although lithium's mechanism of action is unclear, at very specific serum concentrations it is effective in relieving symptoms of mania. Lithium toxicity occurs when medication serum concentrations exceed 1.5 milliequivalents (mEq)/liter. Symptoms of toxicity include slurred speech, confusion, and seizures. Lithium may be used with antidepressant therapies. Many medications are known to interact with lithium.

Drugs used to treat psychosis

Psychosis is a general term used for a variety of mental disorders, including schizophrenia and schizo-affective disorders. The agents used for treatment of psychosis are called *antipsychotic major tranquilizers,* because they reduce symptoms of psychosis and help calm an agitated patient. These medications are used to reduce anxiety, internal voices, delusional beliefs, incoherence, illogical thinking, agitation, hostility, paranoia, and hallucinations. While not a cure for schizophrenia or other psychoses, tranquilizers help control psychotic episodes and restore orderly thought.

The older, conventional antipsychotics—which include the phenothiazines, chlorpromazine (Thorazine®), thioridazine (Mellaril®), and mesoridazine (Serentil®)—cause more sedation and dry mouth than fluphenazine (Prolixin®), perphenazine (Trilafon®), or trifluoperazine (Stelazine®). There are numerous conventional antipsychotic agents, all with individual characteristics.

Several medications act similarly to the phenothiazines, but with less sedation. These medications include thiothixene (Navane®), haloperidol (Haldol®), loxitane (Loxapine®), and molindone (Moban®). Several other atypical drugs are noted for treating the symptoms of schizophrenia (i.e., lack of motivation, isolation). These atypical medications are clozapine (Clozaril®), risperidone (Risperdal®), olanzapine (Zyprexa®), and quetiapine (Seroquel®). Only a seven-day supply of clozapine is dispensed at a time, after the patient's white blood cell (WBC) count is confirmed as normal. Approximately 1 percent to 2 percent of patients have the adverse effect of lowered WBC count. Rarely, an absence of WBCs and fatalities have occurred.

The antipsychotic medications are central nervous system (CNS) depressants; therefore, patients should be warned of drowsiness that may impede driving or operating hazardous machines. Alcoholic beverages will worsen the drowsiness. A patient experiencing hypotension when standing (light headedness) may relieve it by sitting or lying down. Adverse neurological effects may occur with these medications. Dystonia, which is characterized by spasms of the tongue, face, neck, and back, requires a decreased drug dosage and treatment with diphenhydramine (Benadryl®) or benztropine (Cogentin®). Tardive dyskinesia (characterized by involuntary lip smacking, tongue darting, and movements of the arms or legs) may appear after several months or years of antipsychotic medication treatment. The offending antipsychotic drug should be stopped immediately upon the appearance of these symptoms because there is no effective treatment known, and the effects are usually irreversible.

Table 1 Drugs to treat affective disorders

Tricyclic antidepressants	Second generation antidepressants
amitriptyline (Elavil®)	amoxapine (Asendin®)
amoxapine (Asendin®)	bupropion (Wellbutrin®)
clomipramine (Anafranil®)	maprotiline (Ludiomil®)
desipramine (Norpramin®)	mirtazapine (Remeron®)
doxepin (Sinequan®)	trazodone (Desyrel®)
imipramine (Tofranil®)	venlafaxine (Effexor®)
nortriptyline (Pamelor®, Aventyl®)	**Antipsychotic agents**
protriptyline (Vivactil®)	chlorpromazine (Thorazine®)
trimipramine (Surmontil®)	fluphenazine (Prolixin®)
MAOIs	mesoridazine (Serentil®)
phenelzine (Nardil®)	perphenazine (Trilafon®)
isocarboxazid (Marplan®)	prochlorperazine (Compazine®)
loxapine (Loxitane®)	promazine (Sparine®)
tranylcypromine (Parnate®)	thioridazine (Mellaril®)
SSRIs	thiothixene (Navane®)
citalopram (Celexa®)	trifluoperazine (Stelazine®)
fluoxetine (Prozac®)	triflupromazine (Vesprin®)
fluvoxamine (Luvox®)	**Phenylbutylpiperadine derivatives**
nefazodone (Serzone®)	haloperidol (Haldol®)
paroxetine (Paxil®)	pimozide (Orap®)
sertraline (Zoloft®)	**Dihydroindolone derivative**
	molindone (Moban®)
	Dibenzapine derivatives
	clozapine (Clozaril®)
	loxapine (Loxitane®)
	olanzapine (Zyprexa®)
	quetiapine (Seroquel®)
	Benzisoxizole derivative
	risperidone (Risperdal®)
	Other
	lithium (Eskalith®, Lithobid®)

Conclusion

The newer SSRIs and second-generation antidepressants offer many advantages over the early prototype medications. Nevertheless, pharmacists and technicians need to be aware of the adverse reactions associated with medications used to treat affective disorders.

About the authors

Thomas J. Cali earned both his bachelor's degree and Doctor of Pharmacy degree from the Philadelphia College of Pharmacy and Science in Pennsylvania. Dr. Cali is an independent clinical practitioner with his own practice, Thomas J. Cali & Associates. His previous experience includes serving as vice president of clinical affairs with Managed Care Resources, Inc. of Chesapeake, Virginia; director of clinical services for FACS for Long-Term Care in San Francisco, California; an assistant professor at the

University of Maryland Hospital School of Pharmacy, the Hospital of the University of Pennsylvania, and the Philadelphia College of Pharmacy and Science; and in various consulting positions. Dr. Cali has been published extensively and has delivered numerous continuing education presentations. He was named Teacher of the Year of the University of Maryland School of Pharmacy in 1982 and received the 1994 George F. Archambault Award from the American Society of Consultant Pharmacists, which is the society's highest honor, for his outstanding contributions to consultant pharmacy.

Beverly P. Kershaw is the assistant director of pharmacy at William Beaumont Hospital in Royal Oak, Michigan. Kershaw received both her bachelor's and master's degrees in pharmacy from Wayne State University in Detroit, Michigan. She has served as an officer and board member the Michigan Society of Health-System Pharmacists (MSHP), the Southeastern Michigan Society of Health-System Pharmacists, and the Macomb County Pharmacists Association, as well as on numerous professional committees. As a member of the American Society of Health-System Pharmacists, Kershaw served on the Council for Educational Affairs from 1999 through 2001.

Self-assessment questions

1. What is one of the most common affective disorders?
   a. Anxiety disorder
   b. Depression
   c. Mania
   d. Bipolar disorder
2. Which of the following medications is a tricyclic antidepressant?
   a. Phenelzine
   b. Fluoxetine
   c. Amitriptyline
   d. Buproprion
3. A patient prescribed a tricyclic antidepressant should be cautioned about:
   a. sedative effects.
   b. weight gain.
   c. agitation.
   d. enuresis.
4. Which of the following may interact with a monoamine oxidase inhibitor?
   a. Meperidine
   b. Pseudoephedrine
   c. Dextromethorphan
   d. All of the above
5. Which of the following medications is classified as a selective serotonin reuptake inhibitor?
   a. Desipramine
   b. Fluoxetine
   c. Phenelzine
   d. Trazodone
6. Which of the following medications is often used to treat manic-depressive disorder?
   a. Desipramine
   b. Fluoxetine
   c. Phenelzine
   d. Lithium
7. Which affective disorder is associated with hearing internal voices and delusional beliefs?
   a. Depression
   b. Mania
   c. Bipolar disorder
   d. Schizophrenia
8. Which of the following medications is an antipsychotic?
   a. Sertraline
   b. Chlorpromazine
   c. Venlafaxine
   d. Fluvoxamine
9. Which of the following medications requires monitoring of the white blood cell count?
   a. Resperidone
   b. Clozapine
   c. Olanzapine
   d. Lithium
10. Which of the following is ***not*** true about tardive dyskinesia?
    a. It is characterized by involuntary lip smacking, tongue darting, and movements of the arms or legs.
    b. It may appear after several months or years of treatment with an antipsychotic medication.
    c. It is characterized by spasms of the tongue, face, neck, and back.
    d. It has no effective treatment and it is usually irreversible.

CHAPTER
14

PAIN AND INFLAMMATION

Livia L. Franchina, R.Ph.

Learning objectives

Upon completion of this chapter, the technician should be able to do the following:

- ♦ Describe the actions of narcotic analgesics.
- ♦ Describe the actions of tramadol and acetaminophen.
- ♦ Describe the actions of salicylates and nonsteroidal anti-inflammatory drugs.
- ♦ Explain the common uses of nonsteroidal anti-inflammatory drugs.
- ♦ Discuss the treatment of gout.

Introduction

Pain usually occurs as a result of injury, disease, or surgery. Signals from the site of pain are sent along nerves to the spinal cord, then up to the brain. Once the brain receives the message that something is causing pain, the sensation is felt. Medications that are used to treat pain, known as analgesics, are primarily focused on decreasing the signals coming from the site of pain or stopping the signals from getting to the brain. For example, medications that decrease inflammation (swelling, heat, redness) can decrease the signals coming from the pain site. Medications that alter the levels of chemicals in the nervous system or behave like them can affect whether pain signals get to the brain.

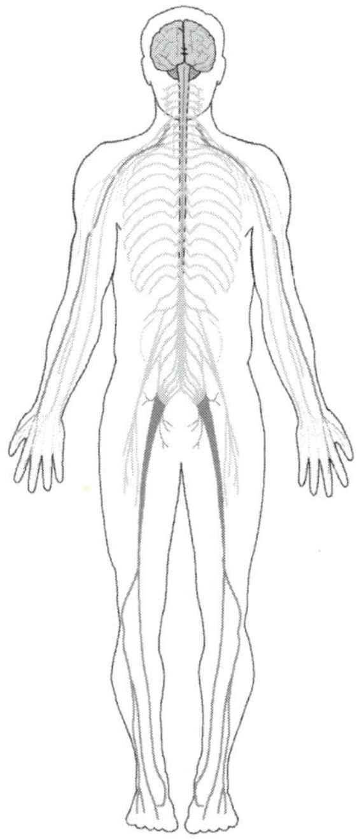

The nervous system

Narcotic analgesics

Narcotic analgesics, or opioids, raise the pain threshold and increase pain tolerance by binding with opioid receptors in the nervous system. They behave like the naturally occurring chemicals in the nervous system called endorphins and enkephalins. Narcotics are used to relieve pain in acute, chronic, and terminal illness. They also decrease preoperative anxiety and are used to relieve diarrhea and cough. Narcotics are classified according to their potential for addiction and abuse. Schedule I drugs are those that have no medicinal use and are often abused, such as heroin. Schedule II medications are primarily potent narcotics used for severe pain. Schedule III and IV medications are narcotics in combination with other medications, such as acetaminophen or aspirin. Schedule V medications also include opioid combinations that are used to treat cough, such as guaifenesin plus codeine (Robitussin AC®).

Equianalgesic dosage

The pain relief achieved with 10mg of intramuscular (IM) morphine is the standard to which other narcotics are compared to determine the dosage needed for the same level of pain relief (equianalgesic: equal pain relief). This is helpful when a patient must be switched from one narcotic to another. There are also differences in dosage when switching from an IM or intravenous (IV) narcotic to the same drug in oral form. (See Table 1.)

Table 1 Equianalgesic doses

Narcotic	Approximate IM doses	Approximate oral doses
codeine	120mg	200mg
hydromorphone	1.5mg	7.5mg
meperidine	75-100mg	300mg
morphine	10mg	30-60mg
methadone	10mg	20mg

The narcotic analgesics are central nervous system (CNS) depressants, and patients should be warned about possible drowsiness. Alcoholic beverages usually worsen the drowsiness. As the dose is increased, side effects also increase, which include respiratory depression (contact a physician if fewer than 10 breaths per minute), nausea, vomiting, and sedation. Often these side effects will decrease with continued use. Constipation is a common side effect that does not resolve and may require treatment with stool softeners or laxatives. Patients do develop physical dependence after long-term use of narcotics. Because of this, the dose will have to be reduced gradually if the medication is no longer needed in order to avoid withdrawal effects. However, dependence does not automatically imply that a patient is addicted.

Acetaminophen

It is not known exactly how acetaminophen works, but it does have effects in the central nervous system. Acetaminophen (Tylenol®) is an effective analgesic and antipyretic (reduces fever) drug. For children, acetaminophen is the drug of choice to treat fever and flu-like symptoms. Acetaminophen is often found in combination with other medications, too, such as narcotics, antihistamines, and other cough and cold medications. Acetaminophen has **no** anti-inflammatory activity, so it is not as useful for pain of inflammatory origin, such as rheumatoid arthritis. However, it is very effective for pain associated with osteoarthritis, which does not usually involve inflammation. Acetaminophen has **no** antiplatelet activity, so prolonged bleeding is not a concern. Neither does it cause the degree of gastrointestinal (GI) discomfort seen with other analgesics. Very high doses (or continued use) of acetaminophen can cause kidney and liver damage. Adult patients should not exceed four grams of acetaminophen per day. Since it is available in so many combination products, patients may not be aware of the amount of acetaminophen being consumed.

Tramadol

Tramadol (Ultram®) is a unique analgesic because it works in two ways. It is classified as a central analgesic because it works in the CNS. It has some weak binding effects with an opioid receptor, which gives it some properties similar to narcotics. In addition, it affects the levels of two chemicals in the nervous system, serotonin and norepinephrine, which are involved in decreasing pain. It is used primarily to treat chronic pain, such as pain due to osteoarthritis or nerve damage. It has no anti-inflammatory effects. Side effects include nausea, vomiting, lightheadedness, and constipation. It is also associated with an increased risk of seizures, particularly if the dose exceeds the recommended maximum of 400mg per day (300mg if the patient is over 75). The potential for dependency is much less than that seen with narcotics.

Salicylates

Salicylates have anti-inflammatory, analgesic, and antipyretic effects. The analgesic and anti-inflammatory effects take place through inhibition of cyclooxygenase, an enzyme needed for formation of prostaglandins. Some of the prostaglandins are involved in causing pain and inflammation, while others are important for regular bodily functioning, like protecting the stomach from damage. Aspirin is a salicylate derivative and is found in many over-the-counter (OTC) medicines for colds, pain relief, and influenza treatments. Children should not be given aspirin for viral symptoms because of the association with Reye's Syndrome, a potentially fatal disorder that is characterized by vomiting, lethargy, and belligerence and may progress to delirium and coma. Aspirin inhibits blood platelets from the first steps in blood clot formation (aggregation), and is used to prevent clots associated with heart attacks and stroke.

Other salicylates are available with analgesic, antipyretic, and anti-inflammatory properties. These salicylates do not affect platelet aggregation and may cause less GI distress than aspirin. They are mostly used to relieve pain and reduce the inflammation of arthritis. Common adverse effects associated with long-term use of salicylates include GI distress (nausea, vomiting, pain, peptic ulcer formation, GI bleeding), allergic reactions, hearing loss, and dizziness.

Nonsteroidal anti-inflammatory drugs (NSAIDs)

Nonsteroidal anti-inflammatory drugs (NSAIDs) are a large group of structurally different acids. They have anti-inflammatory, analgesic, and antipyretic properties that are similar to aspirin. Like aspirin, they also inhibit cyclooxygenase and the formation of prostaglandins. Recently, new NSAIDs have been developed that primarily inhibit only one form of cyclooxygenase, known as COX-2, so the prostaglandins that are needed to protect the stomach are not affected. These NSAIDs, celecoxib (Celebrex®) and rofecoxib (Vioxx®), appear to cause much less GI distress and damage. Only ketorolac (Toradol®) is available for intramuscular (IM) or intravenous (IV) administration.

While NSAIDs are similar, a patient may have a variable response to different products. If one NSAID does not produce a therapeutic effect within two to four weeks, another NSAID can be tried. NSAIDs are used for rheumatoid arthritis (affecting muscles and joints), osteoarthritis, ankylosing spondylitis (a rheumatoid disease involving the backbone and sacroiliac joints), dysmenorrhea (menstrual pain), headache, and many other pain problems. Many NSAIDs are now available without a prescription (e.g., ibuprofen, ketoprofen, naproxen) and are useful for any mild to moderate pain relief. They are included in nonprescription cough and cold products, and many other combination pain relievers. Ibuprofen is often used to treat high fevers in children. The most common adverse reactions from NSAIDs include GI distress (abdominal pain, nausea, gastric and duodenal ulcers, bleeding) and CNS reactions (headache, confusion, drowsiness). They may cause fluid retention and increase blood pressure. Liver abnormalities and kidney damage may also occur.

Drugs used to treat gout

Gout is a disease in which the inability of the body to metabolize uric acid causes an excess of the acid and its salts to accumulate in the bloodstream and joints. Intensely painful episodes of gout result from inflammation in the joints caused by uric acid crystals depositing there. Usually hyperuricemia (high blood levels of uric acid) accompanies gout. Hyperuricemia can be a clue to identifying persons likely to experience gout. Hyperuricemia is often caused when too much uric acid is produced or uric acid cannot be eliminated. Probenecid (Benemid®) and sulfinpyrazone (Anturane®) are called uricosurics because they work to eliminate uric acid through the urine instead of allowing it to crystallize in the joints. Patients taking these medications should avoid aspirin and other salicylates because they counteract the effects of the uricosurics. Colchicine is used to reduce the immediate inflammatory response. Allopurinol (Zyloprim®) is used to inhibit the making of uric acid, resulting in lower blood and urine levels of uric acid. Indomethacin, naproxen, and sulindac are also used to treat the pain and inflammation of gout. Nausea and vomiting is commonly seen with all the agents used to treat gout.

Table 2 Selected drugs to treat pain and inflammation

Narcotic analgesics

Schedule II

alfentanil (Alfenta®)
codeine
fentanyl (Sublimaze®, Duragesic®, Fentanyl Oralet®, Actiq®)
hydromorphone (Dilaudid®)
levorphanol (Levo-Dromoran®)
meperidine (Demerol®)
methadone (Dolophine®)
morphine (MSIR®, MS Contin®, Oramorph SR®, Kadian®, Roxanol®)
oxycodone (OxyContin®, OxyIR®, Roxicodone®)
oxycodone + acetaminophen (Percocet®, Tylox®)
oxycodone + aspirin (Percodan®)
oxymorphone (Numorphan®)
sufentanil (Sufenta®)

Schedule III

codeine + acetaminophen (Tylenol No.3®)
hydrocodone + acetaminophen (Vicodin®, Lortab®)
hydrocodone + ibuprofen (Vicoprofen®)

Schedule IV

butorphanol (Stadol®, Stadol NS®)
pentazocine (Talwin®)
pentazocine + acetaminophen (Talacen®)
pentazocine + naloxone (Talwin NX®)
propoxyphene (Darvon®)
propoxyphene + acetaminophen (Darvocet N-100®)
propoxyphene + aspirin (Darvon Compound®)

Schedule V

buprenorphine (Buprenex®)

Unscheduled

nalbuphine (Nubain®)

Central analgesics

acetaminophen (Tylenol®*, Panadol®*, Tempra®*, and in combination with narcotic analgesics as noted above)
tramadol (Ultram®)

Salicylates

aspirin (Bayer®*, Ecotrin®*, ZORprin®, Ascriptin®*, Bufferin®*,and in combination with narcotic analgesics as noted above)
choline magnesium trisalicylate (Trilisate®)
choline salicylate (Arthropan®*)
diflunisal (Dolobid®)
salsalate (Disalcid®)

Nonsteroidal anti-inflammatory drugs (NSAIDs)

celecoxib (Celebrex®)
diclofenac (Cataflam®, Voltaren®)
diclofenac + misoprostol (Arthrotec®)
etodolac (Lodine®)
fenoprofen (Nalfon®)
flurbiprofen (Ansaid®)
ibuprofen (Advil®*, Motrin®, Motrin IB®*, Nuprin®*)
indomethacin (Indocin®)
ketoprofen (Actron®*, Orudis®, Orudis KT®*, Oruvail®)
ketorolac (Toradol®)
mefenamic acid (Ponstel®)
meloxicam (Mobic®)
nabumetone (Relafen®)
naproxen (Aleve®*, Anaprox®, Naprosyn®, EC-Naprosyn®)
oxaprozin (Daypro®)
piroxicam (Feldene®)
rofecoxib (Vioxx®)
sulindac (Clinoril®)
tolmetin sodium (Tolectin®)

Agents for gout

allopurinol (Zyloprim®)
colchicine
probenecid (Benemid®)
sulfinpyrazone (Anturane®)

*indicates nonprescription status

Conclusion

Every person experiences some sort of physical pain throughout his or her lifetime, whether a simple headache or a chronic, debilitating pain associated with certain disease states. There seems to be a growing number of people in whom pain has unfortunately become part of their daily lives. For some, the pain they experience prohibits them from functioning normally. One of the main goals of pain management is to treat patients' pain in such a manner that it will enable them to enjoy the highest possible quality of life with the least amount of pain.

Bibliography

Aronson, M.D., "Nonsteroidal Anti-Inflammatory Drugs, Traditional Opioids, and Tramadol: Contrasting Therapies for the Treatment of Chronic Pain," *Clinical Therapeutics*, Vol. 19, No. 3, pp. 420-432, 1997.

Bjorkman, D.J., "The Effect of Aspirin and Nonsteroidal Anti-Inflammatory Drugs on Prostaglandins," *The American Journal of Medicine*, Vol. 105 (1B), pp. 8S-12S, July 27, 1998.

Pharmacy Certified Technician Training Manual, 7th edition, Michigan Pharmacists Association, Lansing, MI, 1997, pp. 187-190.

Drug Facts and Comparisons, St. Louis, Missouri, January 2000, pp. 369-375, 784-813, 817-848.

Stacey, B.R., "Effective management of chronic pain – The analgesic dilemma," *Postgraduate Medicine*, Vol. 100, No. 3, pp. 281-296, September 1996.

Turturro, M.A. and Paris, P.M., "Oral narcotic analgesics," *Postgraduate Medicine*, Vol. 90, No. 7, pp. 89-95, November 15, 1991.

Acknowledgment

The author and publisher wish to acknowledge Beverly P. Kershaw, Pharm.M.S., for her extensive contributions to this chapter in the previous edition of this manual.

About the author

Livia L. Franchina earned her bachelor's of science degree in pharmacy from Wayne State University College of Pharmacy & Allied Health Professions in 1978. She is a clinical pharmacy specialist at the Gertrude Levin Pain Center, Hutzel Hospital, Detroit Medical Center in Detroit, Michigan. Her job functions involve patient medication histories and evaluations, therapy recommendations, and patient monitoring. She provides medication information to the medical staff and medical residents who are on rotation at the Pain Center. She also serves as preceptor for portions of the ambulatory care rotation for doctor of pharmacy students from Wayne State University. Franchina is also an adjunct instructor at Wayne State University College of Pharmacy & Allied Health Professions in Detroit. She was employed as a staff pharmacist at Harper Hospital from 1978–1990 with experience in pharmacokinetic dosing, patient drug monitoring, patient consultation, and nutrition support service.

Self-assessment questions

1. How do narcotic analgesics decrease pain?
   a. They inhibit the production of uric acid.
   b. They bind with opioid receptors.
   c. They inhibit cyclooxygenase.
   d. They increase serotonin and norepinephrine.

2. Which of the following is ***not*** a medical use for a narcotic analgesic?
   a. Decrease pain
   b. Suppress cough
   c. Treat constipation
   d. Alleviate preoperative anxiety

3. The standard for pain relief against which other narcotics are compared is:
   a. Morphine 10mg IM
   b. Morphine 100mg IM
   c. Hydromorphone 10mg IM
   d. Meperidine 25mg IM

4. Which of the following is ***not*** a therapeutic effect of salicylates and NSAIDs?
   a. Antipyretic
   b. Uricosuric
   c. Analgesic
   d. Anti-inflammatory

5. Which of the following should ***not*** be used to treat flu and fever symptoms in children?
   a. Aspirin
   b. Codeine
   c. Acetaminophen
   d. Ibuprofen

6. Which of the following is ***not*** true of the actions of tramadol?
   a. May cause seizures
   b. Has anti-inflammatory properties
   c. Is a central analgesic
   d. Is useful in pain due to osteoarthritis

7. Which of the following would be an appropriate drug for chronic treatment of the inflammation associated with rheumatoid arthritis?
   a. Meperidine
   b. Acetaminophen
   c. Naproxen
   d. Cochicine

8. Which of the following drugs may be used to reduce the immediate inflammatory response of gout?
   a. Colchicine
   b. Probenecid
   c. Allopurinol
   d. Sulfinpyrazone

9. Uricosurics should ***not*** be used in combination with which class of medications?
   a. Narcotic analgesics
   b. Salicylates
   c. NSAIDs
   d. Central analgesics

10. Celecoxib and rofecoxib have been associated with a lower occurrence of which side effect commonly seen with NSAIDs?
   a. Elevated blood pressure
   b. Kidney damage
   c. Drowsiness
   d. Gastric ulcers

Chapter 15

Cardiac Function

Lynette Moser, Pharm.D.

Learning objectives

Upon completion of this chapter, the technician should be able to do the following:

- Describe the normal function of the cardiovascular system, including route of blood flow, muscular contraction, coronary blood flow, electrical activity, and vascular pressure.
- Explain the risks associated with hypertension.
- Discuss the risk factors for developing ischemic heart disease.
- Compare and contrast the characteristics of angina and myocardial infarction.
- Describe the symptoms associated with congestive heart failure.
- Define *cardiac arrhythmia*.
- Explain the indications and adverse effects associated with each of the following drug classes: angiotensin converting enzyme inhibitors, alpha blockers, angiotensin II receptor antagonists, antiarrhythmics, beta blockers, calcium channel blockers, digoxin, diuretics, glycoprotein IIb/IIIa receptor antagonists, nitrates, thrombolytics, and vasodilating drugs.

Figure 1 Blood flow through the heart

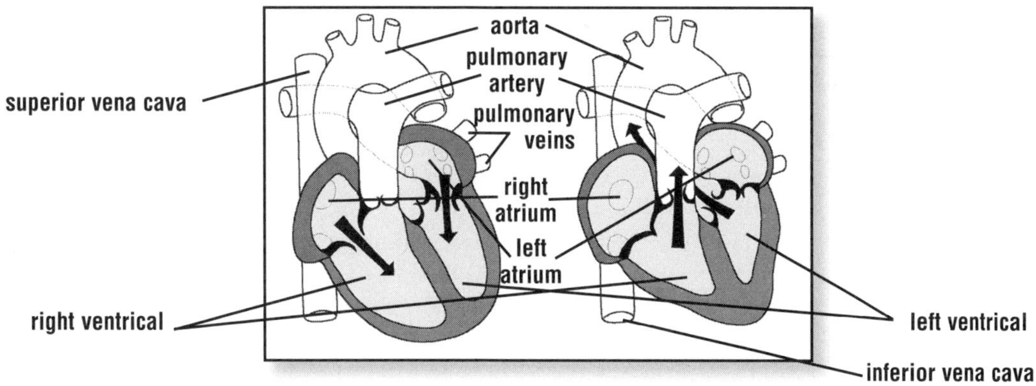

Introduction to normal cardiovascular physiology

The function of the heart is to supply oxygen and nutrients to the organs of the body. The whole system can be described and understood as a pump and pipes. (See Figure 1.) The pump is the heart itself and the pipes are all of the blood vessels which deliver the blood either to the organs and tissues of the body or back to the heart after oxygen and nutrients have been delivered.

The heart requires electrical stimulation, muscle contraction, and energy to do its job. The electrical stimulation in the heart is generated in the sinoatrial (SA) node and, under normal circumstances, travels through the heart in an organized manner. This electrical activity is sensed by an electrocardiogram (ECG or EKG) and defines a person's heart rate. The result of electrical stimulation in the heart is contraction of the heart muscle. This contraction pushes blood through the heart, to the lungs, and finally to the blood vessels and the body. The normal path of blood through the heart is illustrated in Figure 1. Blood returns from the body through veins and enters the right atrium of the heart. The blood flows from the right atrium down into the right ventricle. When the right ventricle pumps (contracts), the blood is sent flowing into the lung where it picks up oxygen. The blood returns from the lung to the left atrium and passes down into the left ventricle, which contracts and sends blood through the aorta to the rest of the body. Normally, the heart pumps about one-half of the blood it holds with each beat. The heart gets its energy from blood supplied by the coronary arteries. These arteries fill with blood when the heart is at rest. When the heart beats faster, it requires more oxygen. The heart is functioning normally when the electrical system is stimulating the muscle to contract and the coronary arteries are supplying sufficient energy and oxygen (from the blood).

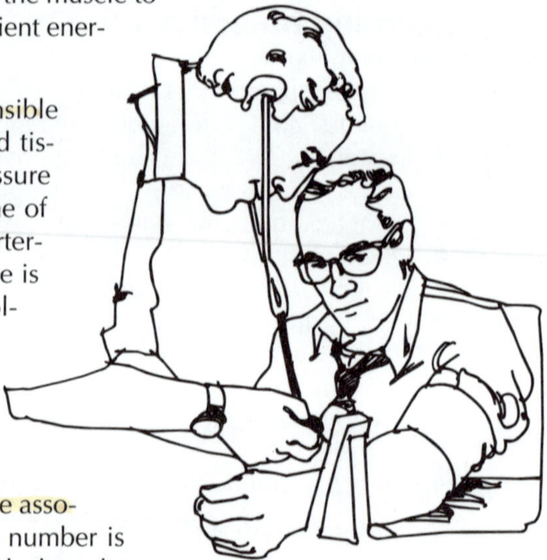

The arteries of the cardiovascular system are responsible for supplying oxygen and nutrients to the organs and tissues of the body. As in any system of pipes, the pressure is dependent upon the force of the pump, the volume of fluid, and the size of the pipes. The pressure in the arteries is referred to as the blood pressure. Blood pressure is dependent upon several factors. Heart rate, blood volume, hormones, and the nervous system can all affect blood pressure, which affects the size of the arteries and how hard the heart pumps. Blood pressure is commonly referred to using two numbers; for example, 120/70 (which is read as "120 over 70"). The top number is the systolic pressure, or the pressure associated with the contraction of the heart. The bottom number is the diastolic pressure, or the pressure associated with the relaxation of the heart.

Hypertension

Hypertension (high blood pressure) is a common condition in the United States and is referred to as the "silent killer" because the patient experiences few, if any, symptoms and is at a higher risk of experiencing a myocardial infarction (heart attack), stroke, and kidney failure. It usually occurs in patients between 30 and 50 years of age and is slowly progressive. In 95 percent of patients, no cause of hypertension can be determined and is called essential hypertension. Factors that increase the risk of developing hypertension include obesity, high salt intake, severe stress, poor diet, genetic factors, and kidney disease.

The Joint National Committee on Prevention, Detection, Evaluation, and Treatment of High Blood Pressure provides guidelines for the diagnosis and management of hypertension. The committee has updated and published their guidelines for healthcare professionals multiple times to keep up with progress in the field of hypertension. The committee also focuses on informing the public about the risks of hypertension and increasing screening and treatment in the community.

Blood pressure is categorized as optimal, normal, high-normal, and hypertension. There are three stages of hypertension, indicating an increased risk of developing heart attack, stroke, or kidney disease. The diagnosis of hypertension is based on an average of two or more blood pressure readings.

Table 1 Classification of blood pressure

Category	Systolic (mmHg)	Diastolic (mmHg)
Optimal	<120	<80
Normal	<130	<85
High-normal	130-139	85-89
Hypertension		
Stage 1	140-159	90-99
Stage 2	160-179	100-109
Stage 3	≥180	≥110

Lifestyle modification is the first step of treating any patient with hypertension. This includes losing weight if the patient is overweight, limiting alcohol intake to a moderate level, increasing physical activity, decreasing sodium intake, and stopping smoking.

The decision to start drug therapy for hypertension is based on the patient's response to lifestyle modifications and the level of blood pressure elevation. Antihypertensive drugs act on one or more of the mechanisms that regulate blood pressure. Drug therapy is generally started at low doses and increased as necessary to reach the desired blood pressure. The categories of medications used to treat high blood pressure include beta blockers, diuretics, angiotensin converting enzyme (ACE) inhibitors, angiotensin II receptor antagonists, calcium channel blockers, direct blood vessel dilators, and alpha blockers. The therapies of choice for patients with high blood pressure are beta blockers and diuretics. However, the drugs of choice may change depending on the patient's other disease states. Patients with diabetes mellitus, a history of heart attack, or heart failure may be started on ACE inhibitors because of additional benefits for these diseases. Calcium channel blockers may be the drugs of choice in patients with some abnormal heart rhythms. If the patient's blood pressure is not controlled with one drug, a drug from a different class may be substituted or added to current therapy. Drugs from different categories may work together to decrease blood pressure and cause less side effects. There are numerous combination products available which are designed to take advantage of this effect.

Ischemic heart disease (coronary artery disease) and myocardial infarction (MI)

Ischemia means "deficiency of blood in a part of the body, due to functional constriction or actual obstruction of a blood vessel." When the coronary arteries are constricted or obstructed, it results in a decrease of blood supply to the heart muscle (myocardium). The symptom most commonly associated with this decrease in blood supply is chest pain, which may be described as an uncomfortable pressure, crushing pain or radiating pain to the jaw or shoulder. This is referred to as *angina pectoris.* It may be difficult to distinguish this pain from heartburn; however, if the patient gives a good history of symptoms, it will be possible to tell the difference because of precipitating factors (exercise versus a big meal), relieving factors, and duration.

Blockages in the coronary arteries are made up of cholesterol and other blood components and are referred to as coronary plaques. This disease process is known as atherosclerosis and can be found in many of the arteries in the body (including the brain, kidneys, and legs). Patients who have plaques that cover more than 75 percent of their coronary arteries may experience chest pain when their heart works hard enough to cause a greater demand of oxygen. This is called *stable angina*. Plaques may rupture and cause a clot (thrombus) to form in the coronary artery, which will lead to complete closure of the artery. *Unstable angina* is occurring if the thrombus does not block the entire artery and the patient's symptoms last less than 20 minutes. If this is prolonged (more than 30 minutes) it will lead to death of the myocardial cells that are supplied with oxygenated blood by this artery. This is a heart attack or *myocardial infarction (MI)*. When a patient is having an MI, it is extremely important for him or her to seek medical attention as quickly as possible. Once the patient is under medical care, efforts will be made to increase blood flow to the damaged area of the heart as quickly as possible. Increased blood flow to the area will minimize the amount of damage to the heart muscle and decrease the risk of further cardiac problems in the future. Blood flow can be re-established by using either medications (thrombolytics, which are discussed later) or performing a percutaneous coronary intervention (PCI). PCI refers to procedures that involve a catheter being placed in the coronary arteries and a balloon being blown up to remove blockages. Other causes of coronary ischemia include spasms of the artery, obstruction of atherosclerosis, anemia or increased work of the heart, as from exertion.

Recognizing risk factors and modifying them are the cornerstones to preventing ischemic heart disease. The risk factors have been well described and include: 1) men ≥45 years old or women ≥55 years old, 2) family history of MI or sudden death before age 55 in a male relative and age 65 in a female relative, 3) elevated total or LDL cholesterol, 4) current cigarette smoking, 5) hypertension, 6) low HDL cholesterol (< 35 mg/dl), and 7) diabetes mellitus. An HDL cholesterol ≥60 mg/dl is considered to be protective against the development of ischemic heart disease and is listed as a "negative risk factor."

The medical treatment of coronary artery disease (CAD) can be divided into several different areas: 1) treating chest pain, 2) preventing chest pain, 3) decreasing the risk of having an MI, 4) slowing the growth of or breaking down a blood clot in the situation of plaque rupture (during an MI), and 5) decreasing the risk of death or reinfarction after an MI. Every patient who has CAD should be receiving 75mg to 325mg of aspirin every day. This has been shown to reduce the risk of having an MI. Aspirin has also been shown to decrease the risk of dying in patients who are having an MI.

Nitroglycerin is used to treat patients who are actually having chest pain. It is available in several different forms and is used either as a sublingual tablet, spray, or intravenous solution when patients are experiencing pain. In patients who have been having pain for longer than 20 to 30 minutes and may be experiencing an MI, morphine should also be used because it helps to decrease anxiety and relieve pain.

Beta blockers, calcium channel blockers, and nitrates are the medications used to prevent chest pain in patients with stable angina. Beta blockers are the drugs of choice, but the other classes may be used in patients who have side effects with beta blocker use or who don't have enough control of their chest pain. These medications may be used in combination because they will provide greater benefit without producing as many side effects as using higher doses of just one medication. When a medication is started to prevent chest pain, it is usually started at a low dose and increased as necessary.

The therapy of unstable angina and MI is much more aggressive than for stable angina. The risk of dying or developing other disease states (arrhythmias, congestive heart failure) is much greater at these times. Thrombus formation is the primary problem in both unstable angina and MI. The therapies for these conditions are aimed at the thrombus. Heparin, thrombolytics, and glycoprotein (GP) IIb/IIIa receptor antagonists are used in MI. Heparin and GP IIb/IIIa receptor antagonists are used in patients with unstable angina. The decision to use these medications is usually made in the emergency room or on an urgent basis, and they are all given as a short (one- or two-day) infusion or a one-time intravenous dose.

Patients who have had an MI are at an increased risk of dying or having another MI. Beta blockers, ACE inhibitors, aspirin and cholesterol-lowering medications have all been shown to prolong life after an MI. These medications are usually used in some combination. The goal is to use high doses of ACE inhibitors and beta blockers, unless the blood pressure is too low.

Congestive heart failure (CHF)

Congestive heart failure (CHF) occurs when the heart is unable to pump enough oxygen-rich blood to supply the needs of the body. This usually happens because the ventricle cannot contract strongly enough and pumps much less blood with each beat. Patients may be tired and confused because their muscles and brain are not getting enough oxygen. Because less blood can enter the ventricle, blood backs up into other body organs. As a result, blood and fluids may collect or pool in the lungs causing shortness of breath. Fluid also may cause swelling in the abdomen, legs, ankles, and feet. CHF may be caused by a previous heart attack, a heart muscle disorder (cardiomyopathy), high blood pressure, or heart valve disease.

CHF patients are at risk of dying from an abnormal heart rhythm or decreased oxygen to vital body organs. The symptoms of CHF are distressing to patients, for they feel that they cannot breathe. Fatigue and shortness of breath limit their normal activities.

The goals of treating CHF are primarily to help the heart pump better, decrease how hard the heart has to work, improve the patient's quality of life by decreasing symptoms, and prolong life span. High heart rate, blood vessel constriction, and increased blood volume make the heart work harder to contract. Increased fluids cause most of the symptoms of CHF. Diuretics are the primary medications given to decrease the amount of fluid in the patient. The heart has to do less work if the pipes (blood vessels) are larger (dilated). Vasodilators and ACE inhibitors are important in therapy because they decrease the work of the heart by making the vessels larger and prolong the life of the patient. Digoxin may be used to improve the pumping of the heart and is usually used in sicker patients. Beta blockers are the most recent class of drugs to be used for the treatment of CHF. These drugs are used in patients who are not short of breath and have been shown to prolong life.

CHF is a progressive disease. Drugs may increase the life span and help relieve symptoms, but they do not cure the disease itself. Patients with severe CHF may need to be placed on a breathing machine and may receive medications intravenously which will help the heart pump and increase the blood pressure. These medications are called positive inotropes and vasopressors.

Arrhythmias

Abnormalities of cardiac electrical activity, called arrhythmias, are diagnosed with an ECG (EKG). Arrhythmias are abnormal heart contractions from abnormal electrical impulses. Abnormalities may take place either in the atria or the ventricles. Arrhythmias can reduce the heart's ability to pump blood and, in some cases, stop the pumping entirely. It is important to convert the arrhythmias back to a contraction pattern that is as near normal as possible (called cardioversion) and maintain the pattern using antiarrhythmic drugs. Some of the more common arrhythmias include the following:

- Bradycardia: a very slow contraction pattern of the heart
- Tachycardia: a very rapid contraction pattern of the heart
- Flutter: a fast rate with a small amount of disorganized contraction
- Fibrillation: a very rapid, disorganized contraction, no effective pump action
- Heart Block: the electrical impulse is slowed, or blocked, causing disorganized contraction

There are several classes of antiarrhythmic medications, based on their effects on the electrical pathway and the heart muscle. These medications may be used either to change the rhythm from abnormal to normal (e.g., from ventricular tachycardia to normal sinus rhythm) or to maintain a normal rhythm in someone who is at risk of returning to an arrhythmia. Arrhythmias in the ventricles (ventricular tachycardia and ventricular fibrillation) are considered medical emergencies and intravenous medications are given. Arrhythmias in the atria (atrial fibrillation or supraventricular arrhythmias) are usually stable and can be treated with oral medications.

Medications used to treat cardiac diseases

Angiotensin converting enzyme (ACE) inhibitors

The class of medications that inhibit the angiotensin converting enzymes (ACE), called ACE inhibitors, are effective in relaxing blood vessels and making it easier for the heart to pump. ACE inhibitors are used in the treatment of high blood pressure, CHF, and in patients after a heart attack. In fact, in patients who have had a heart attack or with CHF, ACE inhibitors have been proven to prolong life.

ACE inhibitors cause very few side effects. However, patients on ACE inhibitors may not eliminate potassium well, resulting in hyperkalemia (above normal potassium in the blood). Other side effects include cough, skin rash, swelling, kidney problems, and low blood pressure. None of the ACE inhibitors should be used in pregnant women.

There are many ACE inhibitors on the market. Many people believe that they are interchangeable, but this remains controversial. ACE inhibitors are listed in Table 2.

Table 2 ACE inhibitors

Tip: Generic names for ACE inhibitors usually end in "pril."
benazepril (Lotensin®)
captopril (Capoten®)
enalapril (Vasotec®)
fosinopril (Monopril®)
lisinopril (Zestril®, Prinivil®)
moexipril (Univasc®)
quinapril (Accupril®)
ramipril (Altace®)
trandolapril (Mavik®)

Alpha blockers

Alpha blocking drugs, including prazosin (Minipress®), terazosin (Hytrin®), and doxazosin (Cardura®) cause vasodilation. Benign prostatic hypertrophy (BPH) is the primary use of these agents. Alpha blockers may be used to treat high blood pressure, but they are usually used only after other medications have failed. These medications may cause too much lowering of blood pressure after the first dose and should be taken at bedtime. Some dizziness and headaches occur as side effects. As with other vasodilators, the body may compensate by increasing heart rate and retaining sodium and water. *Tip: Generic names for alpha blockers usually end in "sin."*

Angiotensin II receptor antagonists

Angiotensin II receptor antagonists act by blocking the effect of angiotensin II (a powerful vasoconstrictor) at its site of action. These medications include losartan (Cozaar®), irbesartan (Avapro®), and Valsartan (Diovan®). Angiotensin II receptor antagonists are used to treat high blood pressure. They may be used as an alternative to ACE inhibitors for CHF in patients with an unacceptable cough.

These medications may cause high potassium levels, kidney problems and swelling. *Tip: Generic names for angiotensin II receptor antagonists usually end in "sartan."*

Antiarrhythmics

The antiarrhythmic medications fall into several different classes. All of these medications have numerous side effects. The most serious side effect which is caused by *all* of the antiarrhythmics is new or worsened arrhythmias. This is referred to as "proarrhythmia." See Table 3 for more information about the antiarrhythmics.

Table 3 Antiarrhythmics

Class	Drugs	Uses	Most common adverse effects
IA	quinidine (Quinaglute®, Quinidex®, Cardioquin®)	Atrial arrhythmias	Diarrhea
	procainamide (Procan SR®, Pronestyl®)	Atrial and ventricular arrhythmias	Systemic lupus
	disopyramide (Norpace®)	Atrial arrhythmias	Urinary retention
IB	lidocaine (Xylocaine®)	Ventricular arrhythmias	Numbness and seizures
	mexiletine (Mexitil®)		
IC	flecainide (Tambocor®)	Atrial arrhythmias	Visual distrubances
	propafenone (Rythmol®)	Atrial and ventricular arrhythmias	Dizziness, nausea and vomiting, unusual taste
II	beta blockers	Some atrial arrhythmias	See beta blocker section.
III	amiodarone (Cordarone®)	All arrhythmias	Pulmonary fibrosis, thyroid disorders, skin discoloration, liver toxicity
	bretylium (Bretylol®)	Ventricular arrhythmias	Decreased blood pressure
	ibutilide (Corvert®)	Atrial fibrillation	
IV	verapamil (Calan®, Isoptin®) diltiazem (Cardizem®)	Some atrial arrhythmias	See calcium channel blocker section.

Beta blockers

Beta blockers are effective for the treatment of high blood pressure, some atrial arrhythmias, ischemic heart disease, and for congestive heart failure, as well as after a heart attack. These medications have been shown to prolong life in multiple disease states and are used widely in many cardiac patients. The doses are commonly started low and increased as the patient can tolerate them. Beta blockers should be used carefully in patients with lung diseases (asthma and chronic obstructive pulmonary disease [COPD]), heart blocks, peripheral vascular disease, and severe diabetes mellitus.

Beta blockers may be associated with low blood pressure, slow heart rate, and depression. Patients with asthma or COPD may develop difficulty in breathing. Less serious side effects are insomnia, fatigue, and decreased ability to exercise. Beta blockers should not be stopped too quickly. If someone has been on these medications for at least a month, the dose should be decreased slowly over one or two weeks to assure the blood pressure and heart rate do not increase too much.

Numerous beta blockers are available on the market. The differences between them include: 1) number of times taken per day, 2) effects on the mood, 3) elimination from the body, and 4) duration of effect. Beta blockers are listed in Table 4.

Table 4 Beta blockers

Tip: Generic names for beta blockers usually end "lol."
acebutolol (Sectral®)
atenolol (Tenormin®)
betaxolol (Kerlone®)
bisoprolol (Zebeta®)
carteolol (Cartrol®)
carvedilol (Coreg®)
esmolol (Brevibloc®)
labetalol (Normodyne®, Trandate®)
metoprolol (Lopressor®, Toprol XL®)
nadolol (Corgard®)
penbutolol (Levatol®)
pindolol (Visken®)
propranolol (Inderal®)
timolol (Blocadren®)

Calcium channel blockers

Calcium channel blockers treat high blood pressure, ischemic heart disease, and some atrial arrhythmias. Calcium ions moving into the cells of the heart help the muscles and the electrical conduction system of the heart to function. Calcium channel blockers act by hindering calcium ions from entering the smooth muscle of the heart, thereby relaxing the blood vessels and the heart muscle, which then lowers the blood pressure and improves the supply of blood to the heart. Calcium channel blockers are separated into two groups, dihydropyridines and non-dihydropyridines. The non-dihydropyridines are diltiazem and verapamil, which are the only agents used in atrial arrhythmias. Decreased blood pressure, decreased heart rate, edema, and worsening CHF are side effects associated with most of these medications. Verapamil may cause constipation. A list of calcium channel blockers is presented in Table 5.

Table 5 Calcium channel blockers

Tip: Generic names for calcium channel blockers usually end "ipine."
diltiazem (Cardizem®, Dilacor®)
verapamil (Isoptin®, Calan®, Verelan®)
amlodipine (Norvasc®)
felodipine (Plendil®)
isradipine (Dynacirc®)
nicardipine (Cardene®)
nifedipine (Procardia®, Adalat®)
nisoldipine (Sular®)

Digoxin

Digitalis medications, including digoxin (Lanoxin®, Lanoxicaps®), increase the force of heart contraction. Digoxin is added to CHF therapy when ACE inhibitors and diuretics are not enough to control the patient's symptoms. If the dose of digoxin is too high, side effects such as low heart rate, nausea, vomiting, depression, or visual disturbances may occur. Digoxin interacts with many other medications, and all drug interactions should be checked when digoxin is started.

Diuretics

Diuretics decrease blood volume and body sodium. This is beneficial in patients with high blood pressure and CHF. Diuretics fall into three groups. The potassium-sparing diuretics are not as strong, but they do not cause as much potassium loss (as implied by their name) as the others. These include amiloride (Midamor®), spironolactone (Aldactone®), and triamterene (Dyrenium®). The thiazide diuretics are used most commonly for high blood pressure and include chlorthalidone (Hygroton®), hydrochlorothiazide (HydroDIURIL®, Microzide®, Esidrix®), indapamide (Lozol®), and metolazone (Zaroxolyn®). The loop diuretics are the most potent and are used primarily in patients with CHF. They include bumetanide (Bumex®), ethacrynic acid (Edecrin®), furosemide (Lasix®), and torsemide (Demadex®). The choice of diuretic is based on the patients' potassium needs and the severity of their disease. Metolazone is sometimes used in combination with the loop diuretics to get a more powerful effect.

Diuretics may cause decreases in potassium and magnesium. Many patients who are receiving diuretics will usually be on supplemental potassium. A low potassium level can put patients at risk of arrhythmias. Other side effects of diuretics include increased levels of blood glucose, calcium, cholesterol, and uric acid. Patients on intravenous loop diuretics may suffer from hearing loss if these drugs are administered too quickly.

Glycoprotein (GP) IIb/IIIa receptor antagonists

The GP IIb/IIIa receptor antagonists are a relatively new group of medications used intravenously for 24 to 96 hours for unstable angina or myocardial infarction. The glycoprotein IIb/IIIa receptor is important in clot formation, so these medications decrease the size of a clot and decrease the risk of a patient having an MI. The agents available include abciximab (Reopro®), eptifibatide (Integrilin®), and tirofiban (Aggrastat®). The main side effect of these medications is bleeding and a decrease in the number of platelets.

Nitrates

Nitrates work to relax the coronary arteries, allowing more oxygenated blood to reach the heart muscle. The nitrates are a group of medications that may be administered in various ways. When given under the tongue (nitroglycerin sublingual), patients are usually instructed to dissolve one tablet under the tongue every five minutes for three doses. If angina persists, they should contact their doctor. Nitroglycerin can also be applied as a paste or skin patch (Nitrodur® patch, Transderm-Nitro®), sprayed into the mouth (Nitrospray®) or swallowed.

The oral nitrate products include isosorbide dinitrate (Isordil®), isosorbide mononitrate (Ismo®, Imdur®), and nitroglycerin (Nitrobid®). The oral preparations may be used to prevent chest pain in patients with stable angina. A throbbing headache and low blood pressure may occur as a side effect of nitrates. Patients should have a period of eight to 12 hours every day when there is no nitrate in their body (a "nitrate free period"), so the body doesn't become tolerant and the drug does not lose its effect. To prevent loss of potency, the nitrate container should be kept tightly closed.

Thrombolytics

Patients who are having an MI need to be treated quickly and aggressively to try to dissolve the clot that has formed in the coronary artery and is preventing blood from getting to part of the heart muscle. This can be done with a class of drugs call thrombolytics. *Thrombolytic* means to break down a blood clot. These medications will decrease the number of people who die from heart attacks if they are given in the first six to 12 hours after the chest pain begins. Because these medications break down blood clots, the most common side effect is bleeding. These patients may bleed into the stomach, urine, or brain. They are also at risk of developing large bruises around intravenous access sites. The thrombolytics include streptokinase (Streptase®), anistreplase (Eminase®), alteplase (Activase®), and reteplase (Retavase®).

Vasodilating drugs

Relaxing the smooth muscles in the blood vessels creates vasodilation or a widened space for the blood to flow through. This concept is similar to a high flow of water through a narrow closed loop of garden hose, causing great pressure in the system, versus the same water flow through a larger diameter hose, producing less pressure in the system. In the body, extreme high blood pressure can be an emergency, treated with fast-acting drugs such as nitroprusside (Nipride®), labetalol (Trandate®, Normodyne®), or enalapril (Vasotec®) given intravenously.

For long-term vasodilator therapy of hypertension, oral medications include hydralazine (Apresoline®), minoxidil (Loniten®), calcium channel blockers, and ACE inhibitors. The body reacts to vasodilators by increasing the heart rate and holding sodium and water. The addition of diuretics and beta blockers will counteract these effects and also treat hypertension.

Miscellaneous drugs

The central nervous system plays a role in increasing blood pressure as part of the sympathetic system that constricts blood vessels. Methyldopa (Aldomet®), clonidine (Catapres®), guanabenz (Wytensin®), and guanfacine (Tenex®) are all centrally acting antihypertensives. These medications have side effects related to the central nervous sytem activity that include tiredness, lack of mental concentration, and nightmares. Clonidine may cause life-threatening hypertension if the drug is stopped abruptly and, therefore, should be gradually reduced to prevent this.

Conclusion

The cardiovascular system is a very intricate system that can be impacted by numerous classes of medications. It is important for pharmacy technicians to know that different classes of cardiovascular medications may be used to treat a single cardiovascular disease, especially when entering new medications into a patient profile. Often when more than one medication is used, the goals are to maximize pumping force of the heart, get the most blood volume circulating throughout the body, and have the patient experience the least amount of side effects.

Bibliography

Pharmacy Certified Technician Training Manual, 7th edition, Michigan Pharmacists Association, Lansing, MI, 1997, pp. 143-150.

About the author

Lynette Moser received her Doctor of Pharmacy degree from the University of Illinois at Chicago. She then completed a residency and fellowship in cardiovascular pharmacotherapy at the University of Utah in Salt Lake City, Utah. Since that time, she has been an assistant clinical professor at Wayne State University College of Pharmacy & Allied Health Professions in Detroit, Michigan. Dr. Moser maintains a clinical practice in the cardiac intensive care unit at St. John Hospital in Detroit.

Self-assessment questions

1. Which of the following shows the electrical activity of the heart?
   a. EKG
   b. Echocardiogram
   c. Cardiac catheterization
   d. Blood pressure

2. Patients with hypertension are at greater risk of developing:
   a. diabetes.
   b. stroke.
   c. hyperthyroidism.
   d. increased cholesterol.

3. Angina pectoris may be caused by:
   a. a damaged heart valve.
   b. a cholesterol plaque in the coronary artery.
   c. not eating enough.
   d. taking aspirin.

4. Which of the following is true about someone having an MI?
   a. The pain goes away with rest.
   b. The pain goes away after taking one sublingual nitroglycerin.
   c. The pain lasts longer than 20 to 30 minutes.
   d. The pain occurs after a large meal.

5. Which of the following medications is a beta blocker?
   a. Atenolol
   b. Amiodarone
   c. Furosemide
   d. Nifedipine

6. A common side effect of diuretic therapy is:
   a. fluid accumulation.
   b. loss of potassium.
   c. high potassium levels.
   d. severe cough.

7. Angina, or lack of oxygenated blood flow to the coronary arteries, is best relieved with:
   a. nitrates.
   b. digoxin.
   c. diuretics.
   d. methyldopa.

8. Which of the following medications is an angiotensin converting enzyme inhibitor?
   a. Propranolol
   b. Amiodarone
   c. Furosemide
   d. Enalapril

9. Which of the following medications is a beta receptor blocker?
   a. Prozosin
   b. Hydrocholorthiazide
   c. Hydralazine
   d. Propranolol

10. Which of the following medications is an antiarrhythmic?
    a. Furosemide
    b. Procainamide
    c. Methyldopa
    d. Capropril

Chapter 16

Blood Disorders

Kevin G. Przybylski, Pharm.D.

Learning objectives

Upon completion of this chapter, the technician should be able to do the following:

- Discuss the medications used for anemia and the hematopoietic (hĕm″-ă-tō-poy-ĕt′-ik) growth factors (pertaining to the production and development of blood cells).
- Discuss the different types of antiplatelet medications.
- Describe the different types of anticoagulants and thrombolytics.
- Explain the differences between water-soluble vitamins and fat-soluble vitamins.
- List some minerals found in oral and parenteral nutrition products.

Introduction

Blood disorders can occur in anyone from infants to the elderly. A couple of these disorders include anemia and blood clots. Many medications, vitamins, and minerals are currently available to help treat and prevent these problems. This chapter will review these disorders and their treatments.

Anemia

Red blood cells (RBCs) transport oxygen into tissues throughout the body. Anemia is defined as a reduction in the number of circulating red blood cells per cubic millimeter. Anemia is associated with certain nutritional deficiencies and both acute and chronic disease, and may also be drug induced. There can be several causes of anemia, including decreased red blood cell production, increased red blood cell destruction, or increased red blood cell loss.[1,2]

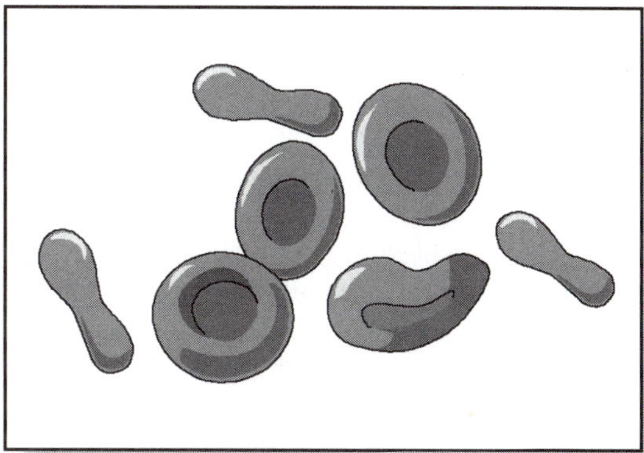

Red blood cells

Erythropoiesis (ĕ-rĭth″-rō-poy-ē′-sĭs) is the normal production of RBCs. Red cell formation in the adult takes place in the red bone marrow, principally in the vertebrae, ribs, sternum, and proximal ends (nearest the point of attachment) of the humerus (bone of the arm from the elbow to the shoulder joint) and femur (bone that extends from the hip to the knee). Iron, Vitamin B12, and folic acid are essential nutrients that are required for erythropoiesis. Normally these nutrients are found in a well-balanced diet. If the body is deficient of one of these nutrients, a severe anemia can result. Iron is required for hemoglobin production. Hemoglobin is the iron-containing pigment of the RBCs. Its function is to carry oxygen from the lungs to the tissues. If there is not enough iron, very small RBCs are formed with insufficient hemoglobin, which is called microcytic hypochromic anemia. If there is not enough Vitamin B12 or folic acid present in the body, the precursor cells (immature blood cells that eventually lead to the formation on RBCs) do not mature correctly, resulting in a megaloblastic anemia (large-sized, abnormal red blood cells).

Erythropoietin is a hormone which is found in the body in very tiny quantities. It is required to stimulate the production of RBCs. For treatment of patients with chronic anemia, such as seen with renal disease, erythropoietin/epoetin alfa (sometimes referred to as EPO) is available in pharmacies for parenteral administration to stimulate RBCs.

Treatment of anemia

Most body iron is present in hemoglobin in the RBCs; therefore, anemia is the most prominent feature of iron deficiency. Hemoglobin is a protein structure that allows for reversible binding of oxygen. By binding oxygen in the lungs, the RBCs travel throughout the body and transport the oxygen to tissue where the oxygen is released. Iron normally comes from foods such as meat, eggs, greens, and dried fruit. Deficiency of iron may result from inadequate ingestion, decreased absorption or utilization, blood loss (including menstruation), or increased requirements (infants and adolescents have increased iron needs during rapid growth periods).

Iron therapy is given in the form of iron salts or iron complexes. Iron products are available orally as ferrous fumurate (Feostat®), ferrous gluconate (Fergon®) and ferrous sulfate (Feosol®). Ferrous salts are the iron preparations of choice because they appear to be the most readily absorbed from the gastrointestinal (GI) tract (approximately 60 percent absorption in the iron-deficient patient). Adverse effects of the oral iron preparations include constipation, diarrhea, dark stools, nausea, and occasional gastrointestinal pain in up to 20 percent of patients. To help absorb more oral iron from the GI tract, ascorbic acid (Vitamin C) may be administered concurrently with the iron. The average length of iron therapy for anemia is six months.

Parenteral iron dextran (Imferon®) is used in the treatment of iron deficiency when oral iron preparations are ineffective or cannot be used. Fatal anaphylactic reactions (an allergic hypersensitivity reaction of the body to a foreign protein or drug) have occurred with iron dextran and; therefore, it should be reserved for patients in whom a clearly established indication exists.[1,2]

Antacids, coffee, tea, and milk decrease iron absorption, and iron may interfere with absorption of tetracycline and some other drugs. Oral iron should be given between meals and at least two hours before an antacid. Liquid iron preparations may be taken through a straw to prevent staining of teeth.

Vitamin B12 and folic acid are chemically unrelated vitamins that are essential. Deficiencies lead to impaired DNA synthesis, inhibited cell mitosis (division), and abnormal maturing and function of cells. These problems are most often seen in cells that undergo rapid cell division, such as in the GI tract and bone marrow. Severe anemia is seen in Vitamin B12 and folic acid deficiencies, along with GI symptoms and pancytopenia (low production of RBCs, white blood cells, and platelets). Oral Vitamin B12 is considered an *extrinsic factor* that must combine with an *intrinsic factor*, found in the GI tract, for absorption. The intrinsic factor is a glycoprotein (compound consisting of a carbohydrate and protein) that is normally present in the gastric juice. The complex is absorbed through the ileum (lower portion of the small intestine) via a transport system. Vitamin B12 is transported to many tissues and any extra is stored in the liver. Vitamin B12 given by injection (cyanocobalamin or hydroxocobalamin) avoids absorption problems and can be given daily to replenish body stores and then once a month for maintenance. There is no evidence that Vitamin B12 injections have any benefit in persons who do not have a deficiency.

Folic acid is found in fresh green vegetables, meat, and eggs. Folic acid is given orally to treat a deficiency or to prevent deficiencies in patients who have liver failure, alcoholism, skin diseases, or renal failure. In addition, folic acid may be administered to pregnant women who are folate deficient. Parenteral folic acid is usually reserved for reversing the effects of certain cancer chemotherapy.

Erythropoietin is a hormone that regulates the production of red blood cells and is used for the treatment of renal failure patients with significant anemia. In addition, erythropoietin may be used for the treatment of anemia in cancer patients who are receiving chemotherapy. It is intended to decrease the need for transfusions in patients who will be receiving chemotherapy for a minimum of two months. Epoetin alpha (Epogen®, Procrit®) is available for subcutaneous injection up to three times per week. The most common adverse effects include hypertension and thrombosis (blood clots). Epoetin is being studied for treatment of zidovudine-induced anemia in HIV-infected patients and for anemia in premature infants.

Prevention and treatment of blood clots and hemostatic agents

When a blood vessel becomes damaged and begins to bleed, the vessel will immediately begin to spasm (vasospasm). Within seconds, platelets adhere to the damaged area and to each other (aggregation). Platelets lose their individual membranes and form a gelatinous mass to plug the damaged vessel. Fibrin then reinforces the platelet plug. Red blood cells and other substances become trapped with the platelets and fibrin to form a red thrombus. Clotting factors in the blood become activated and continue to build the clot, forming a long thrombotic tail. If the tail breaks off and travels through the blood stream it is called an emboli. When the emboli goes into a small vessel, it may block or occlude blood flow causing painful lack of oxygen to tissues. If the patient has clots or is prone to repeated clots, medications are given to prevent the clot formation or counteract the coagulation in process. These medications include antiplatelet drugs, anticoagulants, and thrombolytics. When the opposite problem occurs (blood clotting is impaired), hemostatic medications are used to stop bleeding. These medications include systemic drugs like antihemophiliac factor (AHF) or aminocaproic acid (Amicar®).

Antiplatelet drugs

Antiplatelet medications interfere with platelet aggregation, the initial step in blood clot formation. Oral antiplatelet drugs include aspirin, dipyridamole (Persantine®), sulfinpyrazone (Anturane®), ticlopidine (Ticlid®), clopidogrel (Plavix®), and nonsteroidal anti-inflammatory drugs (NSAIDs) such as ibuprofen (Advil®, Motrin®) and indomethacin (Indocin®). The parenteral antiplatelet drugs include dextran and the glycoprotein IIb/IIIa receptor antagonists, including abciximab (Reopro®), eptifibatide (Integrilin®), and tirofiban (Aggrastat®).

Aspirin is the prototype for the antiplatelet drugs. In a low dosage (325 mg), aspirin has been shown to prevent first heart attacks. It may also reduce risk of other vascular events like stroke or transient ischemic attack (temporary interference with blood supply to the brain). Aspirin is also recommended at the first sign of a heart attack. Patients should chew and swallow non-enteric coated aspirin (160mg to 325mg) as soon as possible after the clinical impression of an acute myocardial infarction (heart attack) has been formed. The dose of aspirin should be repeated daily, indefinitely. Aspirin may be used along with anticoagulants in patients with various heart arrhythmias or recurrent strokes. Aspirin interacts with the anticoagulant to increase the risk of bleeding. If aspirin causes upset stomach when taken daily, patients can take it with food, milk, or antacids to diminish this upset. Also, enteric coated aspirin will not dissolve until it gets to the small intestine, reducing stomach discomfort. Hypersensitivity reactions to the antiplatelet medications may occur and include rash, asthma-like bronchospasm, and even anaphylaxis.[3]

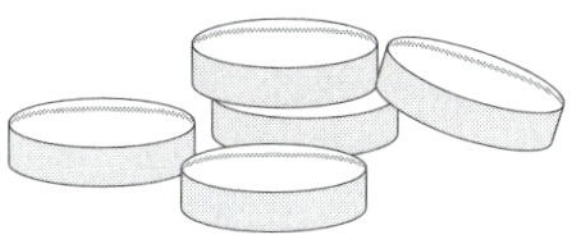

Anticoagulant medications

Anticoagulant medications stop or slow the clotting process. Heparin is an anticoagulant that inhibits coagulation by preventing conversion of prothrombin to thrombin and prevents further formation of a clot. Thrombin is an enzyme that helps form the basis of a blood clot. Heparin itself cannot dissolve clots; the body's own process must do this over time. The anticoagulant effect of heparin is monitored with a laboratory test on the blood called a partial thromboplastin time (PTT). Heparin is given subcutaneously or by continuous intravenous (IV) infusion (at rates ranging from 300 to 2,000 or more units per hour, based on the patient's weight). If the patient bleeds or becomes over-anticoagulated, heparin's effect can be neutralized by protamine sulfate given by the IV route. Another serious adverse effect of heparin is thrombocytopenia (a decrease in the number of blood platelets). Thrombocytopenia requires heparin therapy to be discontinued. Low molecular weight (LMW) fractions of heparin such as enoxaparin (Lovenox®) and dalteparin (Fragmin®) have been approved for subcutaneous administration to treat some blood clots and also to prevent the start of clots when patients are at risk (e.g., after hip or knee replacement surgery). The LMW heparins, when compared to regular heparin, have similar effects and similar bleeding rates, with less frequent dosing (once or twice daily) and no laboratory testing.

In addition to heparin and the low molecular weight heparins, warfarin is also used to help treat and prevent blood clots. Warfarin (Coumadin®) is an oral anticoagulant that prevents the activation of the clotting factors requiring Vitamin K. These clotting factors include Factors II, VII, IX, and X. The anticoagulant effects occur when circulating clotting factors become depleted. The full anticoagulation effects from warfarin are not seen for at least five days after commencing therapy. The warfarin dose is then adjusted to the prothrombin time (PT) (a laboratory blood test) and the calculated international normalized ratio (INR). The INR is a standardized way of monitoring warfarin therapy in patients that was introduced by the World Health Organization (WHO) in 1983. The oral anticoagulant is the preferred medication for preventing clotting in patients with deep vein thrombosis, prosthetic heart valves, diseased heart valves, and chronic atrial fibrillation. The duration of warfarin therapy can be as short as one month (for atrial fibrillation converted to normal sinus rhythm) or as long as the patient remains alive (for chronic atrial fibrillation or heart valve replacement).

Warfarin should not be given to pregnant patients because it can cross the placenta and damage the fetus. Heparin does not cross the placenta and may be used in pregnancy. Warfarin is known to interact with many medications (e.g., antibiotics, aspirin), causing an increased bleeding risk. Careful monitoring of the patient's INR is necessary when interacting medications with warfarin are added or discontinued. Diet also plays a role in warfarin therapy. Vitamin K or Vitamin K-rich foods may interfere with the effects of warfarin. A consistent diet is recommended to patients who are taking warfarin therapy.

Thrombolytic agents

To dissolve a newly formed clot, a thrombolytic, such as streptokinase (Streptase®), anistreplase, (Eminase®), or urokinase (Abbokinase®), can be administered. Another group of thrombolytic agents are classified as tissue plasminogen activators (tPA). The tPAs, alteplase (Activase®), reteplase (retavase®), and tenecteplase (TNKase®), exert their thrombolytic action through the activation of plasminogen to plasmin. Plasimin, in turn breaks down fibrin in the thrombus. These medications may be used to dissolve clots that block off an IV catheter, cause stroke, or cause heart attacks. When the emboli is dissolved quickly, blood flow is re-established to bring oxygen to tissue that could otherwise die. Thrombolytic agents interact with anticoagulants, anti-platelet drugs, and NSAIDs, causing an increased risk of bleeding.[3]

Hemostatics

Deficiencies of coagulation factors can cause bleeding and hemophilia (condition where blood fails to clot and abnormal bleeding occurs). Certain factors found in normal plasma are available for the treatment of these deficiencies. Antihemophilic Factor (AHF), also known as Factor VIII, can temporarily correct the coagulation defect of patients with classical hemophilia (Hemophilia A). Patients who have a Factor IX deficiency in their blood can be administered Human Factor IX complex. The downfall of these blood products, however, is the fear of spreading viral hepatitis or AIDS. This has spurred the interest in synthesized recombinant factor replacements. Aminocaproic acid, which also encourages coagulation, has been used for therapy of hemophilia or after surgeries known to cause bleeding. Aprotinin (Trasylol®), is also a hemostatic drug used to protect a patient's platelets during open-heart surgery.

Vitamins

The term *vitamin* refers to substances that are necessary for normal body functions. (A complete discussion of vitamins and minerals is found in Chapter 18.) Vitamins are usually obtained from a balanced diet or in a tablet supplement. They are divided into two types—fat-soluble (such as Vitamins A, D, E, and K) or water-soluble (such as B-complex and C vitamins). Accumulation of fat-soluble vitamins in the body can cause adverse effects. Water-soluble vitamins do not accumulate in the body.

Vitamin A is necessary for healthy skin, vision in dim light, and normal growth and reproduction. Vitamin D regulates calcium and phosphorus balance for healthy teeth and bones. Vitamin K is synthesized by intestinal bacteria and is needed for blood clotting factors. Vitamin E is an antioxidant that may be useful in protecting against heart disease and environmental pollutants.

Thiamine (Vitamin B1) is involved in energy production from dietary carbohydrates. It is needed for growth and functioning of nerve tissue. Thiamine deficiency, known as beri-beri, affects the nervous system and heart. Cyanocobalamin (Vitamin B12) is needed for normal development of RBCs. Since the body stores Vitamin B12, it takes years to become deficient if no supplements are taken. Most Vitamin B12 comes from animal products; therefore, strict vegetarians may need to take Vitamin B12 supplements. Riboflavin (Vitamin B2) is used for energy production and synthesis of fat and protein. A riboflavin deficiency may have symptoms of skin and mouth lesions. Pyridoxine (Vitamin B6) is used for RBC synthesis and for proper functioning of the immune system, nervous system, and brain. Other members of the B-complex group of vitamins are niacin or nicotinic acid (Vitamin B3). Ascorbic acid (Vitamin C) is an essential vitamin necessary for the formation and the maintenance of collagen (a fibrous insoluble protein found in the connective tissue, including skin, bone, ligaments, and cartilage).

Fat-soluble vitamins may cause adverse reactions such as nausea and vomiting. Vitamin A may cause yellow or orange skin changes. Vitamin D may cause hypercalcemia. Severe allergic-like reactions, including anaphylaxis, have been associated with Vitamin K administered by an IV push. Therefore, when administering Vitamin K by the IV route, it should be diluted in 25 to 50 milliliters of normal saline or dextrose 5% in water and given over 15 to 30 minutes. Vitamin K can also be administered subcutaneously and orally. The water-soluble vitamins are usually considered nontoxic and do not accumulate in the body. They may, however, cause nausea and vomiting, flushing, or rash. Vitamins can be taken with food to lessen nausea and vomiting.

Minerals

The inorganic chemicals that are components of all living cells are called *minerals*. Minerals are not synthesized by the body and must be provided through supplements or diet. Minerals include chromium, copper, fluoride, iodine, manganese, molybdenum, selenium, and zinc. Deficiencies of these minerals may especially occur in patients receiving only parenteral nutrition. IV supplements of these minerals are added to parenteral nutrition. Many oral vitamin supplements include minerals in trace quantities.

Table 1 Medications used for treatment of various blood disorders

Treatment of Anemia

Iron Products
- ferrous fumurate (Feostat®)
- ferrous gluconate (Fergon®)
- ferrous sulfate (Feosol®)
- iron dextran (InFeD®, DexFerrum®) – parenteral preparation

Others
- cyanocobalamin (Vitamin B12)
- erythropoietin (Epogen®, Procrit®)
- folic acid

Antiplatelet Medications
- anagrelide (Agrylin®)
- aspirin
- clopidogrel (Plavix®)
- dextran
- dipyridamole (Persantine®)
- dipyridamole + aspirin (Aggrenox®)
- glycoprotein IIb/IIIa receptor antagonists – abciximab (ReoPro®), eptifibatide (Integrilin®), and tirofiban (Aggrastat®)
- nonsteroidal anti-inflammatory agents - ibuprofen (Advil®, Motrin®), indomethacin (Indocin®)
- sulfinpyrazone (Anturane®)
- ticlopidine (Ticlid®)

Anticoagulants
- dalteparin (Fragmin®)
- danaparoid (Orgaran®)
- enoxaparin (Lovenox®)
- heparin
- tinzaparin (Innohep®)
- warfarin (Coumadin®)

Thrombolytic agents
- alteplase (Activase®)
- anistreplase (Eminase®)
- reteplase (Retevase®)
- streptokinase (Streptase®)
- tenecteplase (TNKase®)
- urokinase (Abbokinase®)

Hemostatics
- aminocaproic acid (Atnicar®)
- antihemophilic factor (AHF) or Factor VIII (Monoclate-P®, Recombinate®)
- aprotinin (Trasylol®)
- human Factor IX (Konyne 80®, Proplex T®)

Vitamins

Fat-soluble
- Vitamins A, D, E, K

Water-soluble
- ascorbic acid (Vitamin C)
- cyanocobalamin (Vitamin B12)
- nicotinic acid (Vitamin B3)
- pyridoxine (Vitamin B6)
- riboflavin (Vitamin B2)
- thiamine (Vitamin B1)

Minerals
- Chromium
- Copper
- Fluoride
- Iodine
- Manganese
- Molybdenum
- Selenium
- Zinc

Conclusion

There are different types of anemia. It needs to be determined first what type of anemia a patient has to determine the appropriate treatment. Blood clots can be treated with IV heparin or subcutaneous low molecular weight heparin in addition to warfarin. Close monitoring of the INR is necessary for patients on warfarin therapy. Many vitamins are necessary for normal body function. If vitamins are not obtained in the diet, supplements must be taken.

Acknowledgment

The author and publisher wish to acknowledge Beverly P. Kershaw, Pharm.M.S., for her extensive contributions to this chapter in the previous edition of this manual.

References

1. Peterson, C.W., Applied Therapeutics: The Clinical Use of Drugs, Vancouver, WA, 1995, pp. 89-1-89-14.
2. Lindenbaum, J., Cecil Textbook of Medicine, Philadelphia, PA, 1996, pp. 823-831.
3. Dalen, J.E., Fifth ACCP Consensus Conference on Antithrombotic Therapy (1998): Summary Recommendations, Chest, Northbrook, IL, 114 (suppl): 439S-769S.

Bibliography

Pharmacy Certified Technician Training Manual, 7th edition, Michigan Pharmacists Association, Lansing, MI, 1997, pp. 171-176.

About the author

Kevin G. Przybylski received his Doctor of Pharmacy degree from the University of Michigan College of Pharmacy in Ann Arbor, Michigan, in 1993. He then completed a general practice residency with a focus on critical care at Detroit Receiving Hospital in Detroit, Michigan. Dr. Przybylski is currently the Clinical Coordinator of Critical Care and the Outpatient Anticoagulation Clinic Supervisor at MidMichigan Medical Center (MMC) in Midland, Michigan. MMC's Outpatient Anticoagulation Clinic manages more than 600 patients receiving anticoagulant therapy.

Self-assessment questions

1. Microcytic hypochromic anemia is the result of:
   a. Vitamin B12 deficiency.
   b. folic acid deficiency.
   c. iron deficiency.
   d. folate deficiency.

2. Which of the following stimulates red blood cell production to treat chronic anemia?
   a. Intrinsic factor
   b. Erythropoietin
   c. Extrinsic factor
   d. InFeD®

3. Which of the following is the parenteral form of iron?
   a. Feostat®
   b. Imferon®
   c. Fergon®
   d. Feosol®

4. The effect of aspirin on red blood cells is best described as:
   a. antiplatelet.
   b. anticoagulant.
   c. hemostatic.
   d. thrombolytic.

5. An injectable anticoagulant that accelerates the process of Antithrombin III is:
   a. tissue plasminogen activator.
   b. dextran.
   c. warfarin.
   d. heparin.

6. The anticoagulant of choice to prevent clotting in patients with chronic atrial fibrillation or deep vein thrombosis is:
   a. tissue plasminogen activator.
   b. warfarin.
   c. heparin.
   d. enoxaparin.

7. A thrombolytic which dissolves a newly formed blood clot is:
   a. tissue plasminogen activator.
   b. warfarin.
   c. heparin.
   d. enoxaparin.

8. Which of the following is a fat-soluble vitamin?
   a. Vitamin C
   b. Vitamin K
   c. Vitamin B6
   d. Vitamin B1

9. Vitamin B6 is also known as:
   a. thiamine.
   b. cyanocobalamin.
   c. riboflavin.
   d. pyridoxine.

10. Which of the following is not a mineral?
    a. Fluoride
    b. Copper
    c. Pyridoxine
    d. Chromium

CHAPTER 17

GASTROINTESTINAL TRACT FUNCTION

Pramodini B. Kale-Pradhan, Pharm.D.

Learning objectives

Upon completion of this chapter, the technician should be able to do the following:

- Describe the action of antiflatulence drugs.
- Describe the action of antidiarrheal drugs.
- Explain the difference between laxatives and stool softeners.
- Explain which antiemetic drugs are available over-the-counter (OTC) or by prescription.
- Explain peptic ulcer formation.
- Describe the drug treatments for peptic ulcers.
- Describe the role of antibiotics in ulcer treatment.

Figure 1 The digestive system

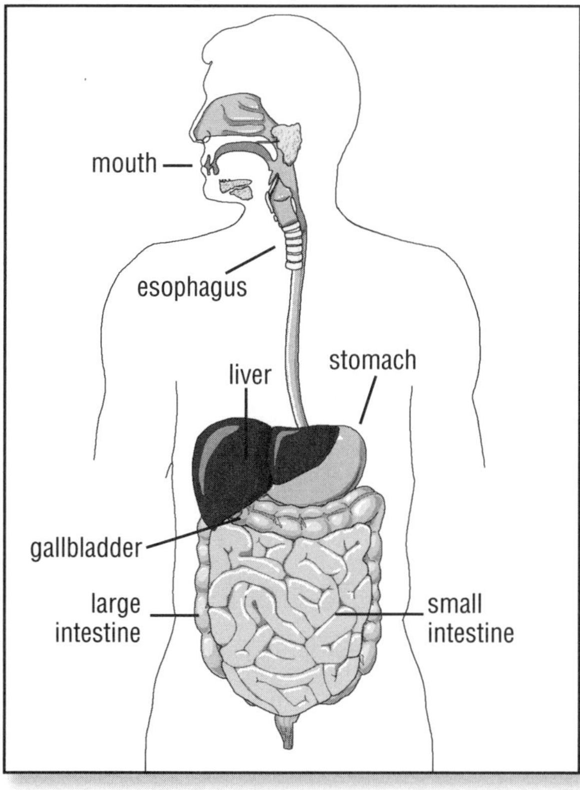

Introduction

The gastrointestinal (GI) tract is comprised of the stomach and the intestines and is part of the digestive system (see Figure 1). This system is a series of connected organs that help us break down the food and beverages we consume so that the body can use their nutrients. This chapter will discuss common disorders of the GI tract and the medications used to treat them.

Drugs used to treat flatulence

Flatulence is gas in the GI tract that can cause discomfort and pain. To treat flatulence, the over-the-counter (OTC) drug simethicone is used. It provides defoaming action by producing a film on the intestines that collapses the gas bubbles and prevents the trapping of these bubbles in the GI tract. Simethicone is available alone or in combination with antacid preparations and is chewed well before swallowing. Simethicone may be used to treat conditions of excess gas, bloating, and infant colic.

Drugs used to treat diarrhea

Diarrhea refers to the increased frequency and liquid nature of stools produced by rapid movement of fecal matter through the large intestine. Drugs to treat diarrhea are categorized as antimotility, adsorbent, antisecretory, and others.

Antimotility agents include diphenoxylate with atropine (Lomotil®), loperamide (Imodium AD®), paregoric, opium tincture, and diphenoxin with atropine (Motofen®). These are absorbed into the bloodstream and act systemically to depress peristalsis (contractions of the intestinal muscle). Diphenoxylate and diphenoxin are related to meperidine (Demerol®), and are classified as Schedule V drugs because of their potential for dependence and abuse. Atropine is combined with diphenoxylate and diphenoxin to discourage abuse of the narcotic agent. Some of the adverse effects include blurred vision, dry mouth, and urinary hesitancy.

Adsorbents such as kaolin and pectin mixture (Kapectolin®), polycarbophil (Fibercon®), and attipulgite (Kaopectate®) act locally on the intestine mucosa to bind with bacteria, toxins, and other irritants that cause diarrhea. These products are given following a loose stool for symptomatic relief.

Antisecretory agents, such as bismuth subsalicylate (Pepto Bismol®) and octreotide (Sandostatin®), work by inhibiting intestinal secretion (intestinal discharge which causes diarrhea) and stimulating intestinal absorption. Bismuth subsalicylate is mainly used for traveler's diarrhea. Bismuth subsalicylate may interfere with warfarin and some antibiotics (such as tetratcylines). Octreotide is used for diarrhea caused by cancer.

Other agents used to treat diarrhea include lactase and bacterial replacement, such as *lactobacillus*. Lactase is an enzyme that digests carbohydrates. Individuals who are lactose intolerant are deficient in this enzyme, which leads to osmotic diarrhea (solutes that cannot be absorbed remain in the bowel) when dairy products are consumed. Replacement of lactase prevents this type of diarrhea. *Lactobacillus* preparations replace normal colonic bacteria; therefore, suppressing bacteria that cause disease. *Lactobacillus* may be replaced by dietary intake of yogurt.

Drugs used to treat constipation

Constipation is the difficulty or infrequent passing of stool. Constipation may be treated with bulk-forming laxatives, emollients, stimulant laxatives, and other agents.

Bulk-Forming Laxatives—Eating a high fiber diet and drinking plenty of fluids are the most natural ways of preventing or treating constipation. In place of natural fiber, bulk-forming laxatives are available OTC. These may take up to three days for the desired effects to be seen. Bulk-forming laxatives include methycellulose (Citrucel®), polycarbophil, and psyllium (Metamucil®), and are used to treat simple constipation and manage irritable bowel syndrome and diverticulitis (inflammation of a sac or pouch that has formed in the colon).

Emollients are stool softeners that work slowly over several days, allowing for the absorption of water into the stool and making the formed stool soft and easier to pass. This helps to avoid straining during defecation. Stool softeners include mineral oil (Agoral Plain®), glycerin suppositories (Sani-Supp®), and the different salts of docusate (Colace®).

Stimulant laxatives increase bowel movements; they include bisacodyl (Dulcolax®), cascara sagrada, casanthranol/docusate (Peri-Colace®), and senna (Senokot®). Peristalsis is stimulated within six to eight hours after oral administration. Stimulant laxatives are preferred for emptying the bowel in preparation of gastrointestinal surgery or tests. Habitual use may lead to dependence on laxatives.

These laxatives are slightly absorbed and distributed to body tissues, including breast milk, and should be avoided when nursing.

Other laxatives include lactulose (Duphalac®), magnesium salts (Milk of Magnesia®), and sodium biphosphates (Fleet Phospho-Soda®). They draw water into the intestine, causing the bowel to distend from fluid accumulation and promote peristalsis. This takes effect in approximately one hour for sodium biphosphate or one day for lactulose.

Drugs used to treat nausea and vomiting

Nausea and vomiting (also called emesis) may occur for a variety of reasons including pregnancy, motion sickness, GI obstruction, peptic ulcer, drug toxicity, heart attack, kidney failure, or chemotherapy. Overall, the vomiting center in the brain integrates the nausea response and coordinates the resulting vomiting reflex. Various antiemetics are used to control nausea and vomiting. This condition may be treated with antihistamines, phenothiazines, butyrophenones, cannabinoids, corticosteroids, benzodiazepines, selective serotonin receptor antagonists, and other medications.

Antihistamines/Anticholinergics are effective in decreasing nausea, vomiting, vertigo (dizziness), and motion sickness through effects on the nervous system. To prevent nausea of motion sickness, the patient takes the first dose 30 minutes before exposure to motion. These agents can cause sedation and include the OTC products such as dimenhydrinate (Dramamine®), diphenhydramine (Benadryl®), cyclizine (Marezine®), and meclizine (Antivert®). Others requiring a prescription include trimethobenzamide (Tigan®) and hydroxyzine (Atarax®). Scopolamine (Transderm-Scop Patch®)is the most effective drug for motion sickness. It is available as a patch placed behind the ear for up to 72 hours.

Phenothiazines are another class of antiemetics. This class works by blocking dopamine receptors. Prochlorperazine (Compazine®) and promethazine (Phenergan®) are the most commonly prescribed antiemetics in this class. Their use is limited due to the sedation they cause and the possible side effect of involuntary muscle jerking (dystonia).

Butyrophenones work by blocking the action of dopamine in the brain. Some examples of drugs in this class include droperidol (Inapsine®) and haloperidol (Haldol®). These agents may cause sedation and dsytonic reactions.

Cannabinoids such as dronabinol (Marinol®) are derivatives of marijuana. They are used for vomiting associated with chemotherapy.

Corticosteroids such as dexamethasone (Decadron®) are another agent that is used to treat chemotherapy-induced nausea and vomiting. The exact mechanism of action is unknown. The most common adverse effects include mood changes, metallic taste, and stomach upset.

Benzodiazepines such as lorazepam (Ativan®) or diazepam (Valium®) are used to treat anticipatory nausea and vomiting due to chemotherapy agents. They are given one to two hours before the course of treatment.The most common adverse effects of these agents include drowsiness, hypotension, urinary retention, and hallucinations.

Selective serotonin receptor antagonists (5HT3 antagonists) such as ondansetron (Zofran®), granisetron (Kytril®), and dolasetron (Anzemet®) are used in the treatment of chemotherapy and in anesthesia-induced nausea and vomiting. These agents commonly cause headache, dizziness, diarrhea, or constipation.

Miscellaneous antiemetics include benzquinamide (Emete-Con®) (only by injection) and metoclopramide (Reglan®). They are used for nausea and vomiting associated with surgery, anesthesia, and chemotherapy.

Table 1 Drugs used to treat flatulence, diarrhea, constipation or vomiting

Antiflatulence
simethicone (Mylicon®)*

Antidiarrheal
attapulgite (Kaopectate®, Donnagel®)*
bismuth subsalicytate (Pepto Bismol®)*
diphenoxin with atropine (Motofen®)
diphenoxylate with atropine (Lomotil®)
kaolin and pectin (Kapectolin®)*
loperamide (Imodium AD®, Kaopectate II®)*
octreotide (Sandostatin®)
polycarbophil (Fibercon®)*

Stool softeners
docusate sodium (Colace®)*
docusate calcium (Surfak®)*
glycerin suppositories (Sani-Supp®)*
mineral oil (Agoral Plain®, Fleet Mineral Oil®)*

Laxatives
bisacodyl (Dulcolax®)*
casanthrol/docusate (Peri-Colace®)*
cascara (Cas-Evac®)*
lactulose (Cephulac®, Chronulac®)*
magnesium salts (Milk of Magnesia®, magnesium citrate®)*
methylcellulose (Citrucel®)*
polycarbophil (Fibercon®)*
psyllium (Metamucil®, Fiberall®, Effersyllium®)*
senna (Senokot®)*
sodium biphosphate (Phosphosoda®)*

Nausea and vomiting

Antihistamines/Anticholinergics
cyclizine (Marezine®)*
dimenhydrinate (Dramamine®)*
diphenhydramine (Benadryl®)*
hydroxyzine (Atarax®, Vistaril®)
meclizine (Antivert®, Bonine®, Dramamine II®)*
scopolamine (Transderm-Scop Patch®)
trimethobenzamide (Tigan®)

Phenothiazine
chlopromazine (Thorazine®)
prochlorperazine (Compazine®)
promethazine (Phenergan®)

Butyrophenones
droperidol (Inapsine®)
haloperidol (Haldol®)

Cannabinoids
dronabinol (Marinol®)

Corticosteroids
dexamethasone (Decadron®)

Benzodiazepines
diazepam (Valium®)
lorazepam (Ativan®)

Selective serotonin receptor antagonists
alosetron (Lotronex®)
dolasetron (Anzemet®)
granisetron (Kytril®)
ondansetron (Zofran®)

Others
benzquinamide (Emete-Con®)
metoclopramide (Reglan®)

* indicates nonprescription status in certain strengths

Drugs used to treat acid-peptic disease

An open lesion, or ulcer in the lining of the lower esophagus, stomach, or intestines is called a *peptic ulcer*. The GI tract has mechanisms in place to prevent the acid and digestive enzymes from damaging its lining. When the protective mechanisms fail or are overcome, peptic ulcers can form. Factors that encourage ulcer formation include an excess of acid, the presence of the bacteria *Helicobacter pylori*, or the use of aspirin, nonsteroidal anti-inflammatory drugs (NSAID), or corticosteroids. Neutralizing the acidic nature of the stomach and treating *Helicobacter pylori* have been shown in studies to lead to healing of ulcers and preventing recurrence.

Antacids

Eating a meal will stimulate an outpouring of gastric acid. A dose of an antacid, given an hour after a meal, will neutralize the acid for about two hours. Antacids are effective in healing ulcers when the dose is sufficient and are given one to three hours after a meal and at bedtime. Most antacids contain magnesium (Mag-Ox 400®) or aluminum (Alu-Cap®). Magnesium may cause diarrhea, and aluminum may cause constipation. A combination of these two drugs helps offset the side effects. Calcium carbonate (Tums®) is another antacid, which also may cause constipation. Magnesium- or calcium-containing products should be used cautiously in a patient with kidney failure as they may cause toxicities.

Antacids are available as oral suspensions, oral tablets, chewable tablets, and soft chews that are like gum. These drugs are also used to relieve symptoms of refluxing of acid into the esophagus, acid indigestion, heartburn, and upset stomach. Antacids mostly stay in the GI tract and are eliminated in the stool. They often absorb other drugs, reducing their effect; therefore, spacing the doses of other drugs far apart is important. Patients may be reluctant in using antacids due to frequent dosing, their chalky taste, and their consistency.

Table 2 Liquid antacid dose for similar acid-neutralizing effect

Trade name	Generic name	Dose
AlternaGEL®	Aluminum hydroxide	44ml
Gelusil®	Aluminum & magnesium hydroxides & simethicone	64ml
Maalox TC®	Aluminum & magnesium hydroxides	33ml
Mylanta DS®	Aluminum & magnesium hydroxides & simethicone	39ml

Histamine-2 receptor antagonists

Cimetidine (Tagamet®), famotidine (Pepcid®), nizatidine (Axid®), and ranitidine (Zantac®) are included in the group of histamine-2 (H_2) receptor antagonists. These drugs promote the healing of ulcers by blocking the H_2 receptors in the GI tract, in turn reducing the production of acid from other cells. Many studies have proven the effectiveness of H_2 receptor antagonists in the healing of stomach and duodenal (small intestine) ulcers, and with continued use, preventing recurrence. All are equally effective and capable of more than a 90 percent reduction in food-stimulated, resting, or nocturnal acid production. These drugs may also be prescribed to treat conditions of acid hypersecretion (Zollinger-Ellison Syndrome) and to prevent stress-related ulcers in severely ill patients, upper GI bleeding, or acid reflux into the esophagus.

The H_2 receptor antagonists are well tolerated with few side effects. In addition to prescription strength, there are lower-dose, nonprescription versions of these drugs. Original dosing recommendations were at least twice a day, but studies show that a single bedtime dose may be effective for ulcer healing and may result in better compliance. This class of drugs is known to interact with many drugs. Cimetidine is known to interact (causing increased blood levels of the target drug) with warfarin, theophylline, diazepam, and phenytoin.

Proton pump inhibitors

By inhibiting the hydrogen ion pump (the last step in the production of gastric acid), omeprazole (Prilosec®), lansoprazole (Prevacid®), rabeprazole (Acephex®), and pantroprazole (Protonix®) can block almost 100 percent of gastric acid secretion. These agents are better than the H_2 receptor antagonists in reducing acid. These drugs are given once or twice daily for the treatment of an ulcer and are effective for patients with acid reflux into the esophagus. These drugs are used in combination with antibiotics to treat the ulcer-producing bacteria, *Helicobactor pylori*.

Miscellaneous drugs

Misoprostol (Cytotec®) protects the lining of the gastrointestinal tract and is used to prevent ulcers caused by NSAIDs. The most frequent side effect is diarrhea, especially in higher doses. It can also cause menstrual disorders and miscarriage of pregnancy. A pregnancy test should be done and contraceptives begun before starting misoprostol in a woman of child-bearing age.

Sucralfate (Carafate®) works by binding to the ulcer and is minimally absorbed. It requires an acid media to form a paste-like substance to be effective. Therefore, sucralfate should not be given with antacids, H_2 receptor antagonists, or proton pump inhibitors. The dose of sucralfate is 1 gram, four times daily on an empty stomach (at least one hour before meals).

Helicobactor pylori has been implicated as the cause of gastric ulcers in some patients. Eradication of this bacteria may be the focus of ulcer treatment. The most current recommendations for the treatment of this infection include a combination of antibiotics and a proton pump inhibitor. Antibiotics shown to be effective include tetracycline, amoxicillin, metronidazole, erythromycin, and clarithromycin.

Bismuth, like sucralfate, also binds to the ulcer, coating it and protecting it from acid. Bismuth subsalicylate has been successful in combination with other drugs in the treatment of *Helicobactor pylori* bacterial infections.

Table 3 Selected drugs used to treat peptic ulcer

Antacids
aluminum/magnesium hydroxide (Maalox®, Mylanta®)*
calcium carbonate (Tums®, Titralac®)*
magaldrate (Riopan®)

Histamine-2 receptor antagonists
cimetidine (Tagamet®, Tagamet-HB®)*
famotidine (Pepcid®, Pepcid-AC®)*
nizatidine (Axid®, Axid-AR®)*
ranitidine (Zantac®, Zantac-75®)*

Proton pump inhibitors
lansoprazole (Prevacid®)
omeprazole (Prilosec®)
pantoprazole (Protonix®)
rabeprazole (Aciphex®)

Miscellaneous peptic ulcer agents
bismuth subsalicylate (Pepto-Bismol®)*
misoprostol (Cytotec®)
sucralfate (Carafate®)

Antibiotics
amoxicillin (Polymox®, Amoxil®)
clarithromycin (Biaxin®)
erythromycin (EES®, ERYC®, Erytab®)
metronidazole (Flagyl®)
tetracycline (Achromycin®, Sumycin®)

*indicates nonprescription status

Conclusion

The GI tract is affected not only by what the body consumes, but also by disease states in the body and the treatment of those diseases. Technicians in all practice settings need to be knowledgeable of the various types of medications that are used to treat the disorders affecting this portion of the digestive system.

Acknowledgment

The author and publisher wish to acknowledge Beverly P. Kershaw, Pharm.M.S., for her extensive contributions to this chapter in the previous edition of this manual.

About the author

Pramodini B. Kale-Pradhan received her bachelor's degree in pharmacy from the University of Wisconsin-Madison College of Pharmacy in 1981 and her Doctor of Pharmacy degree from the Philadelphia College of Pharmacy and Science in Philadelphia, Pennsylvania, in 1989. Dr. Kale-Pradhan completed an advanced residency in infectious diseases and surgery at the University of Illinois at Chicago (UIC) College of Pharmacy in 1990 and became a Fellow in Infectious Diseases and Surgery from that institution in 1991. Presently, she is an assistant professor of pharmacy practice at Wayne State University College of Pharmacy & Allied Health Professions in Detroit, Michigan. Her previous experience includes serving as a clinical pharmacist in the infectious diseases and Dapsone® clinics at UIC. Dr. Kale-Pradhan has delivered several presentations on topics related to the gastrointestinal system. She was the recipient of the 1998 Hoffman LaRoche Hospital Preceptor of the Year Award and the 1992-1993 Southeastern Michigan Society of Hospital Pharmacists Preceptor of the Year Award. Her professional memberships include the American Association of Colleges of Pharmacy, the American Colleges of Clinical Pharmacy, the American Society of Health-System Pharmacists, and the Southeastern Michigan Society of Health-System Pharmacists.

Self-assessment questions

1. The antiflatulent simethicone acts by:
   a. some unknown means.
   b. producing a film that collapses gas bubbles and prevents the bubbles from being trapped in the GI tract.
   c. stimulating intestinal absorption.
   d. binding with bacteria on the intestinal mucosa.

2. A drug that acts systemically to treat diarrhea by suppressing peristalsis is:
   a. diphenoxylate.
   b. kaolin.
   c. attipulgite.
   d. bismuth subsalicylate.

3. The difference between stimulant laxatives and emollient laxatives is:
   a. while both promote peristalsis, a stimulant laxative increases bowel motility and promotes bowel evacuation, while emollient laxatives draw water into the intestine, causing the bowel to distend from fluid accumulation.
   b. a stimulant laxative is a stool softener that works over several days, allowing water to be absorbed into the stool and making the formed stool soft and easier to pass, while an emollient laxative increases bowel motility and promotes bowel evacuation through increased peristalsis.
   c. a stimulant laxative draws water into the intestine, causing the bowel to distend from fluid accumulation and promotes peristalsis, while emollient laxatives are stool softeners that work over several days, allowing water to be absorbed into the stool and making the formed stool soft and easier to pass.
   d. a stimulant laxative increases bowel motility and promotes bowel evacuation through increased peristalsis, while emollient laxatives are stool softeners that work over several days, allowing water to be absorbed into the stool and making the formed stool soft and easier to pass.

4. Which of the following is a stimulant laxative?
   a. Glycerin
   b. Bisacodyl
   c. Docusate sodium
   d. Mineral oil

5. Which of the following drugs used as an antiemetic does ***not*** require a prescription?
   a. Ondansetron
   b. Granisetron
   c. Diphenhydramine
   d. Metoclopramide

6. A peptic ulcer:
   a. is an excess of gas in the GI tract that causes pain and discomfort.
   b. causes the increased frequency and liquid nature of stools.
   c. is an open lesion in the mucosal lining of the lower esophageal, stomach, or intestines.
   d. results from a lack of acid in the stomach.

7. Which of the following has ***not*** been shown to encourage peptic ulcer formation?
   a. Excess of gastric acid
   b. Aspirin
   c. Spicy foods
   d. *Helicobacter pylori*

8. Which of the following drugs is classified as a proton pump inhibitor?
   a. Omeprazole
   b. Misoprostol
   c. Ranitidine
   d. Sucralfate

9. Which of the following drugs is classified as an H_2-receptor antagonist?
   a. Lansoprazole
   b. Misoprostol
   c. Ranitidine
   d. Sucralfate

10. Antibiotics are used to treat peptic ulcers caused by:
    a. *Staphylococcus aureus.*
    b. *Haemophilus influenza.*
    c. *Haemophilus ducreyi.*
    d. *Helicobacter pylori.*

Chapter 18

Nutritional Deficiencies

James "Mike" Sadler, R.Ph, C.C.N., and Pamela M. Sadler, R.N., B.S.N., C.C.N.

Learning objectives

Upon completion of this chapter, the technician should be able to do the following:

- Realize the importance of good nutrition to proper health.
- Identify the major nutrients and the role they play in good health.
- Identify the top 20 categories of prescription medications and what nutrients they deplete.
- Identify signs of nutrient depletions.

Introduction

The endocrine system is comprised of a group of organs and body tissues that produce, store and secrete hormones directly into the bloodstream. Among their functions, the organs of the endocrine system regulate metabolism, regulate the body's growth and development, and support reproductive functions. This chapter will focus on the pancreas, the thyroid gland, and the organs of the female reproductive system, which are part of the endocrine system.

Receiving proper nutrition is very important, but it is often not considered in our fast-paced, fast-food society. The 1988 Surgeon General's Report stated that two-thirds of all deaths are associated with imbalances in diet and nutrition. Stress, environmental pollutants, and poor diet all contribute to the depletion of nutrient levels in the body.[1,4] Considering these facts, it is probably safe for most people to take a multivitamin. However, the research surrounding supplementation, both in favor of and against, can make the issue confusing. Some of the reasons for the confusion surround the quality of research, the amounts of supplements given in a research project, and the synergistic and antagonistic properties of supplements. To date, it has been very difficult to design a study that incorporates all of these variables.

Consider vitamins, minerals, and other nutrients as instruments of an orchestra. When all the instruments are present, you have optimal sound, excitement, and vibrancy. The same principal applies to the body—when all the nutrients are present in adequate amounts, optimal health is achieved. The person is energetic, thinks clearly, and is rarely, if ever, sick.

There is much controversy regarding nutrition and nutritional supplementation. Currently the most quoted official guideline is the Recommended Daily Allowance or RDA. Many experts agree that these daily allowances need to be changed, but they disagree on what changes need to be made.

This chapter will explain the different nutrients, their sources, safety, side effects, signs of deficiencies and excess, as well as prescriptions that cause depletions of specific nutrients. Much is still not known as far as drug depletion, but this chapter will discuss the most common occurrences of nutrient deficiencies caused by medications.

Antioxidants are nutrients that help protect cells from unstable, or free oxygen molecules. During normal metabolism of the body, free radical oxygen molecules are produced in a process called oxidation. These free radicals cause damage to the cells and can affect genetic material. Antioxidants help protect against free radical damage. Nutrient antioxidants include Vitamins A, C, E, beta-carotene, and others. Other substances called "bioflavonoids," a class of water-soluble plant pigments, can help the antioxidants to work.

Protein is made up of combinations of 22 different amino acids. The body makes most of the amino acids. There are nine essential amino acids that a body needs to obtain from food. Protein is used to not only to build muscle, but also to make enzymes, hormones, and organs. Meats are called "complete proteins" because they contain all of the amino acids. Plants, except for soy, are incomplete proteins, but they can be made complete by eating a complementary protein during the day. An example of this is rice and beans. Soy is a complete protein.

Enzymes, simplistically, are complex proteins that are capable of producing or speeding up chemical changes in the body. From digesting food to changing chemicals in the cell, the function of enzymes can be greatly changed by nutrient depletions. Many minerals and some vitamins act as co-factors (helpers) to these reactions. Their reaction can also depend upon the acidity or alkalinity of the environment in which they are located.

Carotenoids (red and yellow pigments found in plants and animals) by themselves are thought to prevent cancer and protect against heart disease. Specific carotenoids, lutein and zeoxanthine, may protect against macular degeneration. Lycopene may protect against prostate cancer. There is no RDA for carotenoids, and there is no known toxicity associated with them. There has been a study showing that beta-carotene may increase lung cancer risk in smokers, possibly because of the low levels of Vitamin C that are often found in smokers.

Vitamins

Vitamin A (beta-carotene, retinol) is important for vision, the immune system function, and reproductive health, plus it helps maintain epithelial tissues (skin and mucous membranes). Night blindness (an inability to see at night or in dim light) may occur if a person gets too little of this vitamin.

Vitamin A is a fat-soluble vitamin, so it is possible to consume too much of it. The body can store excess amounts of fat-soluble vitamins to be used when they are needed at a later time. However, if excessive amounts of fat-soluble vitamins are stored in the body, toxic levels of the vitamin can accumulate in places such as the liver, which can lead to potentially dangerous and long-term physical problems. An excess of Vitamin A may cause fatigue, headaches, hair loss, drying of mucous membranes, itchy scaly skin, and liver damage.

Vitamin A can be found in organ meats, fish, and egg yolks. Milk is fortified with Vitamin A. Dark green, orange, and red vegetables are good sources of carotenoids, which the body can convert to Vitamin A.

Vitamin B6 (all B vitamins are water soluble) is actually three B vitamins: pyridoxine, pyridoxal, and pyridoxamine. These nutrients are responsible for more than 100 chemical reactions. They play an essential role in protein production, immune function, sugar metabolism, and manufacture of neurotransmitters. They work with B12 and folic acid to prevent a buildup of homocysteine (an amino acid that needs to be eliminated from the body to protect the heart). Elevated homocysteine can lead to atherosclerosis (plaque buildup in the arteries).

It is very common to be deficient in Vitamin B6. According to the Second National Health and Nutrition Examination Survey (NHANES II), 71 percent of men and 90 percent of women consumed less than the RDA of Vitamin B6. Deficiency can cause not only elevated homocysteine, but weakness, irritability, nervousness, insomnia, and dermatitis. In infants, it can lead to convulsions.

Vitamin B6 is destroyed by heat and other food processing methods. Whole wheat products contain Vitamin B6, but refined flours do not. (If a bread says it is "enriched," it has been refined. Vitamin B6 is not required to be put back.) Fish, poultry, beets, bananas, and avocados are good sources of Vitamin B6.

Vitamin B12 (cyanocobalmin) is the only water-soluble vitamin that is stored in the body. It is stored in the liver. In general, the body cannot store water-soluble vitamins to any great extent. This vitamin is important for forming red blood cells, producing DNA, helping convert folic acid into an active form, and forming myelin (the fatty sheath that surrounds nerves). Vitamin B12 is found only in animal products.
A Vitamin B12 deficiency may be caused by poor absorption. Vitamin B12 must bind with a particular protein in order to be absorbed. Some people may lack that protein due to a normal decrease in its production with age, surgery, or a genetic defect. Strict vegetarians (those who don't consume animal products such as eggs and cheese) may also become deficient. Deficiency can cause pernicious anemia (which is characterized by defective production of red blood cells and the presence of abnormal precursors to red blood cells in the bone marrow), neurological problems, and contribute to an elevated homocysteine level. Deterioration of myelin may also occur, causing nerve damage. Signs of damage can include numbness and tingling of the hands and feet, poor coordination, moodiness, depression, and confusion. It may also be responsible for memory loss and senility in older people. This may be mistaken for Alzheimer's disease.

Vitamin C (ascorbic acid) is needed for proper functioning of the immune system, provides structure to capillary and cell walls, is needed to produce collagen, helps form hemoglobin, enhances iron absorption and wound healing, helps prevent bruising, and is involved with the production of the neurotransmitters serotonin and norepinephrine. Humans are one of the only mammals that do not produce their own Vitamin C; we must get it from our food. Vitamin C is found in many fruits and vegetables. The darker green the vegetable, the more Vitamin C it contains.

Vitamin C can be used up more rapidly if a person is under a lot of stress, either physical or emotional. Smokers require more Vitamin C. Fatigue, poor wound healing, bleeding gums, bruising, and reduced immune function can be caused by too little Vitamin C. The optimal daily dose of Vitamin C may actually be 200mg, which is four times the current RDA for the vitamin. Any amount of Vitamin C taken above that is probably excreted, although a person may take it in divided doses to avoid excretion of the vitamin. An excess of Vitamin C can cause diarrhea in some people.

Vitamin E's (tocopherol) benefits are well accepted for promoting normal growth and development, protecting tissues against oxidation, and promoting the normal formation of red blood cells. It has also been suggested that it helps delay the development of cataracts, helps immune function, reduces cancer risk, prevents angina, slows the progression of Alzheimer's disease, protects against toxins, and postpones aging. More studies need to be done on Vitamin E, but many look promising. Vitamin E deficiency can lead to neurological damage. There are not many serious side effects that result from taking too much Vitamin E, even though this is a fat-soluble vitamin. If someone is on an anticoagulant medication, Vitamin E may prolong clotting time; therefore, these individuals should consult a physician if they want to take this vitamin.

"Mixed tocopherols" are the best choice for a Vitamin E supplement. Synthetic Vitamin E is poorly utilized by the body, so it is important to use natural Vitamin E. Synthetic Vitamin E will say "dl-alpha tocopheryl" on the ingredient list. Vitamin E is found in vegetable oils, nuts, green leafy vegetables, and whole grains. Olive oil is a poor source, however.

Vitamin K (phytonadione) is needed for blood clotting and helps with bone building. It is given to newborns at birth. Vitamin K is manufactured by normal intestinal bacteria; therefore, people on long courses of antibiotics can become deficient. Deficiencies can also be present in people with malabsorption syndromes or liver disease. Blood thinners interfere with production of Vitamin K. The body normally manufactures most of its necessary supply. Vitamin K is found in green, leafy vegetables such as broccoli and brussels sprouts.

Folic Acid (Vitamin B9) is important for making genetic material in cells and hemoglobin, as well as cell reproduction. It aids in lowering homocysteine along with Vitamins B6 and B12.

Deficiencies in pregnant women lead to neural tube defects such as spina bifida. Since the defects form in the first two weeks of pregnancy, it is important that women of childbearing age consume adequate amounts of folic acid. Megoblastic anemia (the presence of abnormal precursors to red blood cells in the bone marrow), glossitis (inflammation and soreness of the tongue), poor growth, and gastrointestinal problems may also occur in folic acid deficiency. A high intake of folic acid may mask a Vitamin B12 deficiency in the blood. This can lead to nerve damage related to the Vitamin B12 deficiency.

Niacin (Vitamin B3) helps energy to be released from foods and is important for maintaining health in the skin and the nervous and digestive systems. Physicians sometimes prescribe 1.5 grams to 6 grams per day to lower LDL (bad) cholesterol and raise HDL (good) cholesterol. Some people will experience flushing and stomach upset from these high doses. Megadoses of niacin may also cause rash, liver damage, or ulcers. Too little niacin may cause dry, scaly skin in areas exposed to the sun (pellagra). Diarrhea, inflamed mucous membranes, depression, headache, memory loss, and dementia may also be indicative of low niacin levels. Niacin can be found in protein foods and enriched grains. Do not give niacin with "statin" (cholesterol-lowering) drugs because it increases the risk of liver damage.

Pantothenic Acid (Vitamin B5) helps release energy from foods and is a precursor to acetylcholine, which is used in the transmission of nerve impulses. It also plays a role in fat metabolism. Signs of deficiency include headache, fatigue, numbness and tingling of the hands and feet. The only side effect known of too much pantothenic acid is diarrhea. The best sources are organ meats, fish, poultry, whole grains, yogurt, and legumes.

Riboflavin (Vitamin B2) is essential for enzyme function. This contributes to energy resources, as well as the proper use of Vitamin B6, niacin, folic acid, and Vitamin K. It also has an antioxidant function in regard to the fat content in cell membranes. A deficiency is rarely seen by itself, but it may occur in conjunction with other B-vitamin deficiencies. Some thyroid and adrenal abnormalities, as well as some antidepressants and cancer drugs, may interfere with riboflavin use. Mouth soreness, eye irritation, fatigue, and skin irritation, particularly in the vulva in women and the scrotum in men, are signs of deficiency. Any excess riboflavin is excreted in the urine. The best sources of riboflavin include dairy products, liver, poultry, fish, and eggs.

Thiamin (Vitamin B1) is found in the bran and germ of rice and other grains. However, it is removed in the milling process. This caused the disease beriberi in Japanese sailors in the 1880s when they were fed white rice. Beriberi is characterized by muscle paralysis and nerve damage leading to death. Thiamin is necessary for food to release its energy and for proper sugar metabolism and nervous system functioning. Deficiency causes depression, irritability, poor concentration, and fatigue. It is common for alcoholics to be deficient and is often given to them intravenously upon admission to the hospital. Raw fish, shellfish, beets, brussels sprouts, red cabbage, tea, coffee, and antacids all lead to thiamin deficiency. Few foods contain an abundant amount of thiamin, although lean pork, whole grains, dried beans, nuts, fish, and enriched breads and cereals are good sources.

Biotin (Vitamin H) is important for making digestive enzymes and forming antibodies. It aids in the metabolism of fatty acids, amino acids, and carbohydrates. It also helps the body use other B vitamins. Weight loss, nausea, vomiting, depression, dermatitis, hair loss, and high cholesterol can occur when there is a biotin deficiency. There are no known toxic effects. Some biotin is synthesized in the gastrointestinal tract by the normal bacteria residing there. Antibiotics can kill this bacteria, causing a depletion of biotin. Tegretol® and Dilantin® also interfere with absorption. Sources of biotin are yeast, corn, soybeans, egg yolks, liver, cauliflower, peanut butter, and mushrooms.

Vitamin D (cholecalciferol) is produced in the body by a response to sunlight. Technically this is a hormone and is normally found in few foods. Getting 10 to 15 minutes of midday sun, two to three times per week, supplies the body with adequate amounts of Vitamin D. The ability to produce Vitamin D declines with age. Sunscreen does not interfere with absorption of Vitamin D. Without Vitamin D, the body cannot use calcium and phosphorus. This has ramifications for bone health, as well as other functions for which these minerals are needed. Insufficient Vitamin D causes rickets (a disease where the bones are not hardened and are malformed) in children. It may also be important for immune and reproductive health, as well as insulin secretion. Vitamin D may also have a role in slowing osteoarthritis and preventing colon cancer. Foods containing Vitamin D are fatty fish, such as salmon, fortified milk, cereals, grains, and flours.

It is hard to get an excess of Vitamin D unless the vitamin is taken in supplements. An excess of Vitamin D may cause hypercalcemia, which results in loss of appetite, nausea, weight loss, and slow growth.

Minerals

Calcium is important for bone health throughout life. Building up enough bone mass when you are young will help protect a body against osteoporosis as it ages. There are different types of calcium, and absorption of this mineral by the body varies by type. One can increase calcium absorption by using calcium citrate or microcrystalline hydroxyapatite; however, note that the RDA was formulated based on calcium carbonate, which is absorbed at a lower rate. Vitamin D, boron, magnesium, and silica help in the absorption and utilization of calcium. A good calcium supplement to treat or prevent osteoporosis will include these nutrients.

Calcium is essential for the proper functioning of muscles (including the heart muscle) and transmission of nerve impulses. It controls cell membrane permeability (so substances can flow in and out of cells) and is involved in several enzyme reactions. It is also an important factor in blood clotting.

Calcium can be found in dairy products, kale, swiss chard, broccoli, almonds, sardines, and firm tofu. To help increase absorption, a calcium supplement is best taken twice daily with meals, each time with the dose being half the desired total intake. Diuretics and drugs that inhibit stomach acid can lead to calcium depletion. Soft drinks will increase phosphorus levels in the body, resulting in calcium depletion. Excess calcium is deposited in organs and soft tissues causing kidney and heart damage.

Copper is part of at least 15 proteins, but the body contains only 1/250 ounce of copper. Copper is part of many biochemical reactions in the body, including reactions using oxygen. For instance, copper oxidizes iron so it can be transported to different sites in the body where it is needed. It is also used to promote healthy blood vessels, connective tissue, hair, skin pigmentation, and several neurotransmitters. It also aids fertility and immunity.

Copper deficiency is rare, but it would cause anemia and a decrease in white blood cell production. Too much copper may cause vomiting and diarrhea, liver damage, coma, and even death. The majority of toxicity issues involve people who work with pesticides containing copper. No toxic effects from oral intake of copper have been noted. There is a rare genetic disorder called Wilson's Disease that causes abnormal storage of copper that could eventually lead to liver failure if left untreated for years.

Shellfish, organ meats, legumes, nuts, and seeds are good sources of copper. Copper and zinc have a balancing effect with each other in the body. Taking megadoses of zinc, which has become a popular trend during cold season, can deplete copper.

Iron is an essential component of hemoglobin. Hemoglobin is the part of the red blood cell that carries oxygen. Of the iron in the body, 70 percent is found in the red blood cells. Iron is also part of myoglobin, which stores oxygen in muscles to provide energy for muscle contractions. The body will reuse much of its iron, so little is excreted, except during menstruation, childbirth, and injury.

The body regulates iron absorption according to need, unless a person has the genetic disease called hemochromatosis in which the body keeps absorbing iron whether or not it is needed. **Iron is the number one cause of poisoning *death* in children under 6 years of age;** therefore, supplements containing iron should be kept out of a child's reach. As few as five high potency, over-the-counter supplements may cause death in a child.

Liver, beef, lamb, pork, poultry, and fish all have iron, though the first three have the most amounts. Dried beans and peas; green, leafy vegetables; nuts; and seeds are also good sources. Vitamin C helps the absorption of iron. Acidic foods cooked in cast-iron pots will also absorb iron.

According to the NHANES II survey, 9 percent of toddlers and adolescent girls and 11 percent of women between the ages of 20-49 are deficient in iron. Deficiency in infants can cause irritability; in children it can hamper learning and the capacity for problem solving. Anemia with fatigue and weakness eventually occurs in iron deficiency, reducing the oxygen supply to cells.

Magnesium is essential to many processes in the body. It is used in more than 300 enzymatic reactions. It helps convert carbohydrates, fat, and protein into energy. It is a major component of bones and teeth, is involved in the proper functioning of nerves and muscles, and helps regulate heart rhythm. Magnesium may help prevent coronary artery disease. Those with a magnesium deficiency may suffer from constipation, heart irregularities, weakness, irritability, muscle tremors, spasms, and mental derangement. It is common to become deficient in magnesium as we age. Alcoholics are also especially prone to deficiency. Thiazide diuretics may also cause deficiency.

The kidneys are efficient in regulating magnesium by excreting excess amounts. Those with kidney disease should use magnesium with caution. Hypermagnesium signs include diarrhea, nausea, abdominal cramping, muscle weakness, drowsiness, confusion, heart abnormalities, and, eventually, respiratory arrest.

Whole grains, nuts, seeds, legumes, cocoa, and green, leafy vegetables are high in magnesium. Flour that has been refined and then enriched will not contain magnesium since magnesium is only contained in the bran and germ of grains. Many nutritional supplements contain magnesium oxide, which is not a very absorbable form of magnesium.

Manganese is important for the formation maintenance of bones and connective tissue and for proper brain formation and function. It has a lot of enzymatic functions, including the formation of urea (a chief component of urine), the production of fats and cholesterol, and the metabolism of carbohydrates for energy. It also aids in the production of an antioxidant enzyme, superoxide dismutase. Deficiency has not been proven in humans, only animals. Magnesium can take over many of manganese's functions. It would be difficult to consume too much manganese, though chemical toxicity (through inhaling manganese in an industrial setting) has caused central nervous system complications, iron deficiency, and reproductive problems. Nuts, shellfish, and whole grains are good sources of manganese.

Phosphorus is linked with calcium in that 85 percent of each mineral is found in the bones and teeth. A lack of phosphorus is detrimental to bone health. Phosphorus is also involved in energy production in that it is part of the adenosine triphosphate (ATP) cycle (an energy cycle in the cell). It also helps transport nutrients into and out of cells and is needed to produce the genetic materials DNA and RNA. Phosphorus deficiency is very uncommon because it is in many foods, including processed foods, soft drinks, and high-protein foods. Those with a deficiency would experience fragile bones, fatigue, weakness, loss of appetite, stiff joints, and increased susceptibility to infections. Premature infants need more phosphorus than what is found in breast milk or they may develop rickets. Excess phosphorus may inhibit the absorption of calcium.

Potassium, an electrolyte, works opposite sodium in balancing intracellular (inside cells) and extracellular (outside cells) fluids. Potassium also helps transport electrical impulses such as nerve transmissions and muscle movement. Potassium is found mostly inside the cells where it is part of many metabolic functions. It is also outside the cells in smaller amounts where it helps to regulate the heartbeat, muscle contraction, and blood pressure. Adequate potassium intake may help lower blood pressure in patients with hypertension. It will not lower a normal blood pressure.

Thiazide diuretics cause potassium deficiencies; therefore, a supplement is usually prescribed along with the diuretic. Potassium is found in a wide variety of foods, so deficiencies are not common. If a potassium deficiency does occur, it can result in weakness, fatigue, paralysis, abnormalities of heart contractions, and cardiac arrest.

ACE inhibitors may increase potassium levels, so people taking them should have their serum potassium levels monitored. Signs of too much potassium include weakness, paralysis, abdominal distension, and a rapid heartbeat. This is rare because the kidneys closely regulate electrolyte balance.

Fruits and vegetables are excellent sources of potassium, especially dehydrated fruits such as sulfured apricots and peaches (1 cup), sardines (1 can), and avocados (1 medium), which all have more than 1,000mg of potassium. One medium banana has 467mg. Meats and fish are also good potassium sources.

Selenium's availability in food depends on where the food is grown. Some areas in the United States have high selenium levels in the soil. Selenium is found in Brazil nuts, meats, poultry, seafood, grains, and grain products.

Selenium is being studied for protectant affects in cancer and heart disease and perhaps even rheumatoid arthritis and AIDS. It works synergistically with Vitamin E and is important for proper thyroid function. It also is a part of glutathione peroxidase, an antioxidant enzyme present in all cells.

Too little selenium may impair the immune system, as well as the ability of the body to neutralize toxic substances it is exposed to, such as certain drugs and chemicals. In China, where soil selenium levels are lower than anywhere in the United States, deficiency has been linked to enlargement of the heart and osteoarthritis in children. Low selenium levels may also decrease thyroid function.

There is a narrower margin of safety with selenium compared to other nutrients. Serous side effects have been reported at less than 1,000mcg. Excess selenium can cause nausea, diarrhea, fatigue, and nerve damage in the hands and feet, as well as hair and fingernail loss. It also produces garlic odor of the breath.

Sodium is an electrolyte mostly located extracelluarly and helps maintain fluid balance with potassium. A body will retain sodium if it needs it and excrete it if it does not. If one retains sodium, water will be retained along with it. The kidneys, brain, adrenal glands, and heart work together to monitor sodium balance.

Sodium deficiencies are rare because it is so abundant in the diet. However, with severe vomiting and diarrhea, or profuse sweating that goes with sustained and strenuous exercise, sodium levels can be severely depleted. If this happens, a hormone called aldosterone is secreted to promote sodium retention. When sodium falls dangerously low, cardiovascular complications, coma, and even death may occur.

Too much sodium makes a person thirsty to encourage water consumption in order to increase urine production and help excrete the excess sodium. Some people are sodium-sensitive, which increases their blood pressure. (Some people are chloride-sensitive, causing hypertension. Table salt is "sodium chloride.") Sodium sensitivity may increase with age. Too much sodium may also cause increased calcium loss, thus promoting osteoporosis. Other sources of sodium include baking soda, baking powder, sodium nitrate, sodium phosphate, sodium saccharin, and monosodium glutamate (MSG). Also brine, garlic salt, kelp, onion salt, sea salt, and soy sauce contain sodium.

The National Academy of Science recommends an intake of 500mg of sodium per day. A single serving of many processed foods has double this amount. Limiting intake then becomes more important. (On "Nutritional Facts" labels on foods, the recommended maximum amount of sodium intake is 2,400mg per day.) Low-sodium foods are fresh fruits, vegetables, meats, and eggs. Many packaged and canned foods are high in sodium.

Zinc is an integral part of the enzymes used to produce RNA and DNA and is used for cell duplication. It is necessary for proper growth and is important for protein metabolism, especially collagen. It aids wound healing; helps the body utilize Vitamin A; maintains the ability to taste, smell, and use insulin; and strengthens the immune system. It is also important for prostate health.

Zinc deficiency may cause skin problems such as acne and increased scarring from wounds. It will inhibit growth and sexual maturation in children, and even mild deficiencies will dull the sense of taste, causing poor appetite and growth. Some experts believe it plays a role in anorexia. In pregnancy, zinc deficiency can result in low-birth-weight babies. Fiber and phytates (a chemical present in some grains like wheat) can inhibit zinc absorption.

Too much zinc can interfere with copper absorption. Large doses of zinc can impair blood cell formation, depress the immune system, and decrease HDL (good cholesterol). Nausea, vomiting, and diarrhea may be caused by zinc excess.

Zinc is found in red meat, shellfish (especially oysters), legumes, nuts, and organ meats. It is in some grains, but the body does not absorb zinc well from them.

Boron helps maintain cell membrane structure, is involved with the metabolism of several minerals (calcium in particular), and may enhance the effects of estrogen. It may also help regulate brain function. There are probably other roles yet to be discovered as not much research was done until the late 1980s. Too much boron (more than 50mg daily) can cause gastrointestinal upset, skin problems, and seizures. Insufficient amounts of boron may affect motor and cognitive function and put postmenopausal women at risk for osteoporosis. Some experts believe that 1mg of boron per day is sufficient. Boron is found in nuts, legumes, dried beans and leafy, green vegetables.

Chromium is very important for sugar metabolism. The body needs it to use insulin in order to make glucose available to cells. It is also important in burning carbohydrates and metabolizing fats and some proteins. A lack of chromium may cause high blood cholesterol, and low HDL (good) cholesterol. Chromium is not known to cause adverse reactions. It comes in several forms, however, and in one study chromium picolinate caused damage to cells in hamsters, raising the question of whether it might be implicated in cancer. Other forms of chromium did not cause this damage.

Chromium is found in whole grains, brewer's yeast, prunes, peanut butter, potatoes, and seafood. Vitamin C aids absorption of chromium. Cooking acidic foods in stainless steel pots may draw chromium into the foods.

Iodine is most noted for its importance in the manufacturing of thyroxine in the thyroid. The thyroxine governs metabolism and growth. It may also help convert beta-carotene to Vitamin A, synthesize protein and cholesterol, and absorb carbohydrates. It is also essential for reproduction. A lack of iodine will cause the thyroid gland to enlarge. Once this enlargement becomes visible, it is called a goiter. This was a common problem before iodine was added to salt.

Low iodine levels cause decreased thyroid function. It also leads to fatigue, skin changes, an increase in lipids, hoarseness, delayed reflex reactions, and reduced mental functioning. A lack of iodine in pregnant women causes cretinism, a form of severe mental retardation. In children, it can adversely affect mental ability.

Extremely high doses of iodine can also cause a goiter, but usually there is no adverse reaction in doses 10 to 20 times the RDA.

Besides iodized salt, iodine is present in saltwater fish, shellfish, and dairy products, as well as some fruits and vegetables, depending upon the levels of iodine present in the soil in which they were grown.

Molybdenum has been studied very little. It is known that it is essential (you need to eat it). It is needed to produce enzymes that aid in other chemical reactions in the body, particularly the excretion of urea. Molybdenum is also involved in reactions that include copper and sulfur. Megadoses can interfere with copper absorption, causing a copper deficiency. Side effects of a molybdenum deficiency are not known. It is found in milk, legumes, grains, and cereals. The molybdenum content of plant food depends upon the soil in which it was grown.

Fats are an important dietary consideration and a very complex subject. Most experts concur that the total intake of fats should be 30 percent of calories, of which less then 10 percent should be from saturated fats.[1,2,3] Saturated fats are biologically inactive since their molecules are already saturated with hydrogen. They are solid at room temperature. Polyunsaturated fats are more active because of their ability to give and take hydrogen molecules. These fats are generally liquid at room temperature. All fats contain nine calories per gram.

Fats (lipids) are in every cell in our body. They store energy; support cell walls; store and circulate fat-soluble Vitamins A, D, E, and K; help regulate cholesterol levels; and are important for healthy skin and hair. They are important for cellular communication and proper hormone production, including prostaglandins. Prostaglandins are important for controlling blood pressure, blood clotting, inflammation, as well as other functions.

The body can manufacture most of the kinds of fat it needs if it gets enough of the essential linoleic acid (ELA) and alpha-linoleic acid (ALA). These fatty acids can be found in the highest quantity in high-fat, cold water fish (salmon, sardines, mackerel, and trout) and in flaxseed. It is very common for people not to get enough of these kinds of fats. If someone is deficient in B vitamins or zinc, fish oil is the best source of fat.

Too much fat and the wrong kind of fat contribute to high cholesterol, high blood pressure, heart disease, cancer, obesity, and decreased immune function.

Probiotics is a term used for the beneficial bacteria that reside in the gastrointestinal tract. There are many different beneficial organisms. The most common ones that people hear about are *Lactobacillus acidophilus* (different strains of this organism live primarily in the small intestine) and *Bifidobacterium bifidum* (lives in the large intestine). All of the different strains have slightly different functions, including helping to break down and absorb different nutrients. In general, this normal flora makes significant amounts of B vitamins, makes short-chain fatty acids, improves digestion and absorption of nutrients by producing enzymes, increases the bioavailability of vitamins and minerals, biodegrades bacterial toxins, detoxifies carcinogens, metabolizes drugs and hormones, acts as natural antimicrobials (helping to prevent infections), helps reduce cholesterol, helps prevent colonization of parasites in the gut, decreases ammonia produced by bacteria in the gut, and strengthens the immune system.

Another beneficial organism is a yeast called *Saccharomyces boulardii.* This yeast helps digest carbohydrates and dairy products, fights several bacterial pathogens and *Candida albicans* (the yeast that causes many yeast infections), increases enzyme activity, and enhances the immune system. It is known to prevent antibiotic-associated diarrhea and is used commonly in Europe for this purpose.

An imbalance of the normal flora can cause Vitamin B deficiencies, indigestion, bloating, gas, and diarrhea. *Candida albicans* actually attaches to the mucosal wall of the intestine, causing inflammation and a breakdown of the immune barrier, weakening the barrier between the GI tract and the bloodstream. There is evidence to suggest that this plays a role in allergy response and autoimmune diseases.

If someone is taking an antibiotic, it will kill this "good gut bacteria." It is often recommended to take *Saccharomyces boulardii* during antibiotic therapy and an acidophilus product for two weeks following antibiotic therapy. It is best to take these on an empty stomach because the normal acid produced during digestion will kill most of these organisms on the way to the small intestine.

Table 1 Recommended Daily Allowances

The values given are mostly affected by the size of a person. A larger child would require a greater amount than recommended for children in general. There are other important nutrients required for the body, but no recommended daily allowances have been established.

	Infants	Children	Men	Women
Protein	13-14g	16-28g	45-63g	46-50g
Vitamin A (beta-carotene, retinol)	375mcg	400-700mcg	1,000mcg	800mcg
Vitamin D (cholecalciferol)	7.5-10mcg	10mcg	10mcg (5 mcg over 25 yrs old)	10mcg (5 mcg over 25 yrs old)
Vitamin E (tocopherol)	3-4mg (d-alpha tocopherol)	6-7mg (d-alpha tocopherol)	10mg (d-alpha tocopherol)	8mg (d-alpha tocopherol)
Vitamin K (phytonadione)	5-10mcg	15-30mcg	45-80mcg	45-65mcg
Vitamin C (ascorbic acid)	30-35mg	40-45mg	50-60mg	50-60mg
Thiamin (Vitamin B1)	0.3-0.4mg	0.07-1.0mg	1.3-1.5mg	1.1mg
Riboflavin (Vitamin B2)	0.4-0.5mg	0.8-1.2mg	1.5-1.8mg (teens need most)	1.3mg (1.2mg for seniors)
Niacin (Vitamin B3)	5-6mg NE *(1 NE = 1mg niacin or 60mg dietary tryptophan)*	9-13mg NE	15-20mg NE *(teens need most; seniors the least)*	15mg NE (13mg for seniors)
Vitamin B6 (pyridoxine pyridoxal, pyridoxamine)	0.3-0.6mg	1.0-1.4mg	1.7- 2.0mg	1.4-1.6mg
Folic Acid (Vitamin B9)	25-35mcg			
Vitamin B12 (cyanocobalmin)	0.3-0.5mcg	0.7-1.4mcg	2.0mcg	2.0mcg
Calcium (as calcium carbonate, $CACO_3$)	400-600mg	800mg	1,200mg (11-24 yr) 800mg (25+yr)	1,200mg (11-24 yr) 800mg (25+yr)
Phosphorus	300-500mg	800mg	1,200mg (11-24 yr) 800 (25+yr)	1,200mg (11-24 yr) 800 (25+ yr)
Magnesium	40-60mg	80-170mg	270-350mg	280-300mg
Iron	6-10mg	10mg	10-12mg	10-15mg
Zinc	5mg	10mg	15mg	12mg
Iodine	40-50mcg	70-120mcg	150mcg	150mcg
Selenium	10-15mcg	20-30mcg	40-70mcg	45-55mcg

Table 2 Drugs causing nutrient depletions[4,5]

Top 20 Drugs dispensed/categories	Depletion	Interactions	Nutritional support
Norvasc®, Procardia®, and Adalat® *Description: Types of calcium channel blockers drugs used for heart disease and blood pressure.*	Procardia® and Adalat® can cause potassium depletion (hypokalemia).	Ingestion of grapefruit or grapefruit juice has been shown to increase the blood levels of these drugs and may increase side effects.	Potassium (B12, B6, and folic acid lower homocysteine levels)
NSAIDs including Aleve®, aspirin, ibuprofen, Feldene®, Indocin®, Relafen®, Naprelan®, Naprosyn®, etc. *Description: Types of anti-inflammatory drugs.*	Iron, folic acid, zinc, Vitamin C, and possibly Vitamin B12.	High dosages of Vitamin E (>400 IU/day) can decrease platelet aggregation. This may result in additive blood thinning effects already present with NSAIDs.	Glucosamine sulfate, a high-potency daily multiple vitamin for women or men; omega-3 fatty acids as in fish and flax seed oil promote noninflammatory prostaglandin function
Premarin®, Prempro®, and other estrogen hormones *Description: Types of estrogen replacement used for menopause.*	Vitamin B6, folic acid, niacin, Vitamin C, and magnesium.	Red clover extracts and soy isoflavones may interfere with absorption. Vitamin D, calcium, zinc, magnesium, and ipriflavone may increase absorption.	A high potency, daily multiple vitamin; standardized black cohosh.
Prilosec® and other proton pump inhibitors *Description: Types of ulcer/gastroesophageal reflux medications (GERD).*	Vitamin B12, Thiamine Calcium, Magnesium	May decrease the absorption of calcium, magnesium, and other minerals by blocking the release of stomach acid.	Vitamin B12 and a high potency, daily multiple vitamin
Prozac®, Zoloft®, and other SSRIs *Description: Types of antidepressants.*	Melatonin	Low levels of B vitamins may reduce the effectiveness of these drugs. St. John's wort extract and 5-Hydroxytryptophan (5-HTP) should not be taken with any SSRI unless under a physician's supervision.	Melatonin and a complete daily multiple vitamin
Synthroid® and other thyroid hormone medications (Eltroxin®, Levo-T®, Levothroid®, Levoxyl®, Thyrolar®, etc.) *Description: Types of thyroid hormone replacement.*	Calcium	Iron supplements and soy products taken at the same time as Synthroid® may interfere with absorption.	Milk thistle extract standardized to contain 70% silymarin
Vasotec®, Capoten®, Prinivil®, Zestril® *Description: Types of ACE inhibitors used for high blood pressure.*	Zinc	These drugs may increase blood levels of potassium above normal or reduce potassium excretion in urine.	A high-potency, daily multiple vitamin for women or men

Table 2 Drugs causing nutrient depletions[4,5] (continued)

Top 20 Drugs dispensed/categories	Depletion	Interactions	Nutritional support
Proventil®, Ventolin® *Description: Types of bronchodilators used for asthma.*	Magnesium and calcium		A high-potency, daily multiple vitamin; magnesium
Amoxicillin preparations including Augmentin®, Amoxil®, Polymox®, Trimox®, and others *Description: Types of antibiotics.*	Vitamin K, all B vitamins, *Lactobacillus acidophilus* and *bifidobacterium.*[2]	The enzyme bromelain increases the absorption of amoxicillin and other antibiotics.	*Acidophilus* and bromelain, B complex
Claritin®, Claritin-D® *Description: Types of allergy medications.*	None known	None known	A high-potency, daily multiple vitamin
Coumadin® *Description: Types of anticoagulant (blood thinner) therapy used for heart disease.*	None known	Vitamin K may decrease the effect of Coumadin®. Ginkgo biloba extract, Vitamin E, and aspirin may increase the effect of Coumadin®.	A high-potency, standardized grape seed extract helps to maintain healthy blood vessels

When a person is taking prescription medications, the chance of nutrient deficiencies increases. Table 2 shows the Top 20 drugs that are prescribed and the nutrients that they deplete. It also shows interactions that may occur with nutrients, herbs, and prescription drugs. (Chapter 19 describes herbals in more detail.) For example, many anti-hypertensives deplete zinc. Note that the third largest category of drugs is the cholesterol-lowering drugs. These can easily deplete CoQ10 or ubiquinone, which is important for the cardiovascular system. CoQ10 is a vitamin-like substance that normally occurs in the body, though its production decreases with age. Also, Dilantin® (phenytoin) and Tegretol® (carbamazepine) interfere with absorption of biotin.

Conclusion

The body needs a host of nutrients to keep it functioning properly and optimally. Eating the right types of food enables a person to receive such nutrients. But there is the possibility of getting "too much of a good thing;" therefore, people need to be aware of the maximum levels of vitamins they can safely consume. Additionally, when people take prescription medications that rob the body of certain nutrients, care must be taken to offset the loss and restore optimal levels.

References

1. Bock, Kenneth, M.D., Sabin, Nellie, The Road to Immunity; How to Survive and Thrive in a Toxic World, Pocket Books, 1997.
2. Colgan, Michael Ph.D., CCN, Optimum Sports Nutrition, Advanced Research Press, NY, 1993.
3. Margen, Sheldon, M.D., The Wellness Nutrition Counter, Rebus, Inc., New York, NY, 1997.
4. Pelton, Ross, R.Ph., Ph.D., CCN, et al., Drug-Induced Nutrient Depletion Handbook, Lexi-Comp, Inc. and Natural Health Resources, 1999.
5. "Patients Taking Prescription Drugs Need to be Nutrition-Conscious," Natural Medicine Online, www.nat-med.com/feat.html, April 2000.

Bibiography

Griffith, H. Winter, M.D., Complete Guide to Vitamins, Minerals & Supplements, Fisher Books, Tucson, AZ, 1988.

About the authors

James "Mike" Sadler is a 1977 graduate of Ferris State University College of Pharmacy and has always worked in retail pharmacy. Since 1981 he has owned the Advanced Pharmacy and Nutrition Center located in North Branch, Michigan, a combination pharmacy and health food store. Sadler became a Certified Clinical Nutritionist in 1997. In addition to owning and operating his pharmacy, Sadler conducts individualized nutritional and natural medicine counseling.

Pamela M. Sadler is a 1977 graduate of Lincolnland Community College where she received her associate's degree in nursing. She received her Bachelor of Science in Nursing from the University of Michigan in 1989 and became a Certified Clinical Nutritionist in 1997. Her nursing expertise includes 15 years in obstetrics, as well as experience in intensive/coronary care, medical-surgical, and emergency room nursing. She has also experienced community nursing by working in public health for the Maternal Infant Support Services and Home Health Care. Currently, she runs the health food store part of the Advanced Pharmacy and Nutrition Center and does individual nutrition and natural medicine counseling.

Self-assessment questions

1. If a nutrient is classified as "essential," it means that:
   a. the body manufactures enough of the nutrient so additional consumption is not needed.
   b. the body needs the nutrient to maintain life.
   c. the body does not manufacture that nutrient, so it must be obtained from food.
   d. the nutrient is needed to digest food.
2. What is the only water-soluble vitamin stored in the body?
   a. Vitamin C
   b. Vitamin K
   c. Vitamin A
   d. Vitamin B12
3. A deficiency in what nutrient in pregnant women causes neural tube defects such as spina bifida in babies?
   a. Folic acid
   b. Vitamin B12
   c. Vitamin E
   d. Iron
4. The best supplement for someone suffering from osteoporosis includes what nutrients?
   a. Calcium only
   b. Calcium and magnesium
   c. Calcium, Magnesium, Boron, Vitamin D and Silica
   d. Magnesium, Vitamin D
5. The number one cause of childhood poisoning death is:
   a. iron supplements.
   b. cleaning products.
   c. rat poison.
   d. prescription medicine.
6. Signs of magnesium deficiency may include:
   a. heart abnormalities and muscle weakness.
   b. constipation and heart irregularities.
   c. drowsiness and confusion.
   d. diarrhea and nausea.
7. A probiotic should be recommended if someone is taking what kind of medication?
   a. Antibiotic
   b. Laxative
   c. Diuretic
   d. "Statin" drug
8. NSAIDs, including aspirin and ibuprofen, cause deficiencies in which nutrients?
   a. Vitamins E and B12
   b. CoQ10
   c. Glucosamine sulfate
   d. Iron, Folic Acid, Zinc, and Vitamin C
9. What herb has an additive effect with Coumadin?
   a. Gingko biloba
   b. Echinacea
   c. St. John's Wort
   d. Vitamin K
10. According to the 1988 Surgeon General's report, what percentage of deaths were associated with diet and nutrient imbalances?
    a. 0 percent
    b. 25 percent
    c. 50 percent
    d. 66 percent

Chapter 19

Herbals

Susan C. Smolinske, Pharm.D., BCPS, DABAT

Learning objectives

Upon completion of this chapter, the technician should be able to do the following:

- Define *dietary supplement.*
- Explain the labeling requirements for herbals and their place in medical therapy according to the Dietary Supplement Health and Education Act (DSHEA).
- Differentiate between homeopathic and herbal remedies.
- Identify methods to obtain patient history of dietary supplement use.
- Explain potential hazards of dietary supplement use, including contamination, adulteration, interactions with medications, and adverse reactions.
- Develop techniques to determine which patients using dietary supplements need counseling by a pharmacist.

Introduction

Herbal products have been regulated since 1994 under the Dietary Supplement Health and Education Act (DSHEA), which created a new category of foods, separate from food additives. The new category, dietary supplements, includes vitamins, minerals, herbs, botanicals, and amino acids, as well as concentrated extracts, individual constituents, and even metabolites of a naturally occurring compound. Only oral formulations can be considered to be a dietary supplement.[1] Definitions and examples of types of products are listed in Table 1.

Labeling requirements

As of March 23, 1999, dietary supplements must contain the common name or Latin botanical name, the part of the plant used, the amount, a box with "supplement facts," and the FDA disclaimer "These statements have not been evaluated by the FDA. This product is not intended to diagnose, treat, cure, or prevent any disease." Products may contain structure and function claims, but not disease claims. An acceptable example would be, "Glucosamine builds strong joints." The disease "arthritis" is not mentioned, only the part of the body and the effect of the supplement.

Homeopathic products

True homeopathic products are not considered dietary supplements under the DSHEA regulation. Homeopathic products are drugs regulated by the Food and Drug Administration (FDA) under the Food, Drug, and Cosmetic (FD&C) Act. Ingredients must be published in the Homeopathic Pharmacopoeia of the United States (HPUS) and can include minerals, plants, or animals. Labels must contain ingredients (usually a Latin zoological or botanical term),

Table 1 Types of dietary supplements

Product type	Definition	Examples
Herb	Flowering plant whose stem above ground does not become woody; valued for medicinal properties, flavor, or scent.	Valerian root, green tea
Botanical	An item pertaining to, made from, or containing plants.	Any plant
Concentrate	A substance that contains a higher percentage of ingredients than found in nature.	Ma Huang
Constituent	An individual chemical component of a plant.	5HTP derived from *Griffonia*
Metabolite	A product of metabolic action.	Androstenedione metabolized from DHEA in humans
Standardized extract	Preparation containing the active principles extracted from a plant; containing a consistent amount of one or more constituents in all batches.	*Gingko biloba* extract, St John's wort extract
Functional Food	Food product containing dietary supplement ingredients intended primarily as a nutritional source.	*Gingko biloba* potato chips, candy bars, or gum

usage instructions, at least one major therapeutic indication, and dilution. The major premises of homeopathy are contained in three "laws" or "tenets."

1. Law of Similars: If a large amount of a substance causes symptoms in a healthy person, a smaller amount of the same substance will treat similar symptoms in someone who is ill.
2. Law of Infinitesimals: A substance's strength and effectiveness increases the more it is diluted. Strength is achieved by vigorous shaking (succession) after each dilution, which releases the energy of the substance. With sufficient dilution, the material content of the substance disappears, and only its energy, imprint, or spirit-like substance remains.
3. Law of Single Remedy: Generally, only a single remedy is prescribed to cover all symptoms, but the use of multi-ingredient products is also a recognized practice.

The strength of a homeopathic formulation is described in terms of the extent of dilution. A 1X dilution represents a 1 in 10 dilution of the crude herbal material. Thus, a tablet weighing 100mg labeled as "atropa belladonna 1X" would contain 10mg of crude drug. Since the active constituent atropine is only present in the crude drug at a concentration of about 0.5 percent, the actual amount of atropine in this 1X product would be 0.05mg. A 2X product would represent two successive 1 in 10 dilutions, or a 1 in 100 dilution. The centesimal scale is also used, where 1C is equal to 2X. Because of this dilution, homeopathic drugs are generally extremely safe. They are, however, exempt from ethanol limits, and liquid formulations may contain very high concentrations of alcohol.[2]

Medication history

Dietary supplements and other alternative medicine therapies are being increasingly used. It is estimated that 60 million adult Americans have used herbs, generally as "complementary" medicine as a supplement to conventional medications. Less than 40 percent of herbal users inform their health-care providers spontaneously, but studies have shown that patients will provide this information if asked. There is a growing trend of pediatric herbal use, and several surveys have shown that up to 20 percent of children are given herbal products to promote health or enhance mental or physical performance. Therefore, it is very important to include use of dietary supplements as part of a complete medication history.[3]

Obtaining and maintaining a history of dietary supplement use can be challenging for many reasons. Many products contain multiple herbs in combination. Some multi-herb products may change the components of the combination frequently without changing the product name. It is not unusual for a patient to be using more than one dietary supplement product simultaneously or sequentially; therefore, pharmacy professionals need to persist in questioning until all supplements are described. Functional foods may not be perceived as herbal products by the patient. Dates and frequency of dosing should be obtained. Ideally, patients should bring in all products so that actual labels can be examined. Botanical names can be too complicated and confusing for patients to rely on his or her memory. Brand names will not be included in standard reference textbooks; therefore, obtaining ingredient information is difficult without looking at the label. The history may change frequently as patients try the latest advertised product. Questions about new supplements should be asked at frequent intervals. Finally, because some herbs contain caffeine or substances with additive toxicity to caffeine, a history of dietary caffeine intake should be obtained as part of the complete medication history. Include all sources, such as beverages, chocolate, over-the-counter (OTC) drugs, and dietary supplements.

Safety issues

Safety provisions for dietary supplements under DSHEA are markedly different than that for drugs. While drugs must undergo extensive safety testing in animals and humans prior to marketing, dietary supplements are marketed with the presumption that they are safe if used according to the labeled guidelines. Action can be taken only if a supplement is proven to present a significant or unreasonable risk of illness or injury under recommended conditions of use. Evidence of abuse or overdose cannot be used to assess risk. Safety provisions under the Food Additives Amendment of the FD&C Act that require premarketing testing for carcinogenicity also do not apply to dietary supplements. An example of effective action is the herbal ingredient *aristolochic acid,* which was recently shown to be associated with a high risk of urinary injury and cancer. The response from FDA was to declare herbs containing this ingredient to be adulterated.[4]

Adulteration of herbal products with drugs or other toxins continues to be a sporadic problem due to variations in good manufacturing practices among herbal companies. Most herbal products can be expected to contain variations in the amount of active ingredients as this is a natural phenomenon. Ranges of active ingredients for several herbs, including ginseng, feverfew, and St John's wort, were from zero to 20 times the labeled amount. However, heavy metals such as lead or arsenic, or drugs such as digoxin, corticosteroids, benzodiazepines, glyburide, and melatonin, have been found in some herbal products. These are either cases of mistaken identity between plants with similar appearance or deliberate contamination in the case of many products originating from Asia.[5]

Herbal products may contain constituents with potent pharmacologic activity. When prepared as a concentrated extract, the action in the body is that of a drug. Most drugs have side effects, and herbal concentrates are not an exception. The FDA maintains a website called the Special Nutritionals Adverse Event Monitoring System (http://vm.cfsan.fda.gov/~dms/aems.html), which contains 2,621 cases of adverse reactions to herbs and other nutritionals, including 184 deaths. In addition to dose-related side effects, many herbal side effects are allergic in nature and can be life-threatening, resulting in asthma, hives, or anaphylactic shock. Echinacea has recently been shown to be one of the more common causes of herbal allergy.[6]

Herbal products may interact with prescribed or OTC drugs, resulting in an adverse event. For most herbs, their potential for interaction is unknown. Interactions can result from predictable, additive pharmacologic effect; such is the case when Ma Huang, which contains ephedrine, is mixed with caffeine to cause additive stimulant effects. Interactions can also result from pharmacokinetic effects, when an herb prevents a drug from being metabolized in the liver, or when the herb increases the metabolism to render the drug less effective. For example, there is now good data to suggest that St. John's wort activates liver enzymes to increase metabolism and reduce effectiveness of many drugs, such as cyclosporine, indinavir, and theophylline.[7-9] While computerized databases are now available to screen for some interactions with herbs, new interactions are being reported with increased frequency, and the vast majority of interactions are unknown. Patients should always be referred to the pharmacist when taking both herbal and conventional medicines.

Perhaps the greatest danger from herbal medicines is when patients decide to discontinue conventional therapy in favor of herbal medicine. Major consequences, such as progression of cancer to an untreatable stage or extreme hypertension from discontinuation of blood pressure drugs, have been reported in patients seeking alternative therapies.[10]

Counseling techniques

The pharmacy technician should use the same care in referring patients using dietary supplements to the pharmacist as they do with any OTC medication. Consider referral for any of the following situations:

- Patient is pregnant or breast-feeding
- Patient is a child
- Patient has a history of allergies
- Patient has a history of high blood pressure or diabetes
- Patient is taking prescription medications
- Patient has discontinued a prescription medication
- Patient is using more than one herbal product
- Patient is self-treating a serious condition
- Patient is experiencing a side effect after taking the herbal product
- Patient has purchased an herb with significant side/adverse effect potential (see Table 2)

Table 2 Dietary supplements with significant side/adverse effect potential

Common name	Botanical or chemical name	Side/adverse effect
American mandrake, mayapple	*Podophyllum peltatum*	Extremely toxic to multiple organs
Borage	*Borago officinalis*	Severe liver disease
Calamus	*Acorus calamus*	Some varieties are carcinogenic
Chaparral	*Larrea tridentata*	Liver damage
Coltsfoot	*Tussilago farfara*	Severe liver disease
Comfrey	*Symphytum* species	Severe liver disease
Dong quai	*Angelica sinensis*	Skin rash when exposed to sun, carcinogen, stimulates uterus
Fang ji	*Aristolochia fangchi*	Chronic renal failure, carcinogen
Germander	*Teucrium chamaedris*	Liver damage
Germanium	not applicable	Kidney damage
Khat	*Catha edulis*	High blood pressure, high fever, stroke, heart attack, liver cirrhosis, eye nerve damage, birth defects, oral cancers
Ku shen	*Sophora flavescens*	Seizures
Lobelia	*Lobelia inflata*	Drooling, tearing, stomach upset, diarrhea, coma, rapid heart rate, liver damage
Ma Huang extract	*Ephedra* species	High blood pressure, heart attack, stroke, liver damage
Monkshood, Wolfsbane	*Aconitum* species	Abnormal heart rhythm, death, toxic at very small doses
Paraguay tea	*Ilex paraguayensis*	Liver damage, cancer of the esophagus
Passion flower	*Passiflora incarnata*	Abnormal heart rhythm
Pennyroyal	*Mentha pulegium*	Extremely toxic to multiple organs (liver, kidney, nerves)
Petasites	*Petasites hybridus*	Severe liver damage
Pokeweed	*Phytolacca americana*	Vomiting, diarrhea, low blood pressure
Rue	*Ruta graveolens*	Induces abortion, liver damage, kidney damage, skin blisters

Table 2 Dietary supplements with significant side/adverse effect potential (continued)

Common name	Botanical or chemical name	Side/adverse effect
Sassafras	*Sassafras albidum*	Carcinogen, liver damage, diarrhea
Scullcap	*Scutellaria lateriflora*	Liver damage
Senecio	*Senecio* species	Severe liver damage
White cohosh	*Actaea* species	Skin rash, bloody diarrhea, kidney damage
Wormwood	*Artemesia absinthium*	Hallucinogenic
Yohimbe	*Pausinystalia yohimbe*	Extremely high blood pressure, heart palpitations, hallucinations

Conclusion

Dietary supplements are popular, and they are increasingly being added to a host of common foods and beverages. However, the number of adverse events associated with these products is also increasing. The pharmacy technician who has a good working knowledge of herbal and homeopathic products can act as a true patient advocate by obtaining complete histories of a patient's consumption of such products, and referring patients who could be placing themselves at risk by taking dietary supplements.

References

1. Bass, I. S., Young, A. L., Dietary Supplement Health and Education Act: A Legislative History and Analysis, The Food and Drug Law Institute, Washington, D.C., 1996.
2. Stehlin, I., "Homeopathy: Real Medicine or Empty Promises?," *FDA Consumer*, pp. 15-19, December 1996.
3. U. S. Food and Drug Administration, Letter to Industry-FDA Concerned About Botanical Products, Including Dietary Supplements, Containing Aristolochic Acid, May 16, 2000. (http://vm.cfsan.fda.gov/~dms/ds-botl1.html)
4. Eisenberg, D.M., Davis, R.B., Ettner, S.L., et al., "Trends in alternative medicine use in the United States, 1990-1997," *Journal of the American Medical Association*, Vol. 280, pp. 1569-1575, 1998.
5. Miller, L.G., Hume, A., Harris, I.M., et al., "White Paper on Herbal Products," *Pharmacotherapy*, Vol. 20, No. 7, pp. 877-891, 2000.
6. Mullins, R., Abstract presented at American Academy of Allergy, Asthma, and Immunology, 56th Annual Meeting, 2000.
7. Ruschitzka, F., Meier, P.J., Turina, M., "Acute heart transplant rejection due to Saint John's wort," *The Lancet*, Vol. 355, No. 9203, pp. 548-549, 2000.
8. Piscitelli, S.C., Burstein, A.H., Chaitt, D., et al. "Indinavir concentrations and St. John's wort," *The Lancet*, Vol. 355, No. 9203, pp. 547-548, 2000.
9. Nebel, A., Schneider, B.J., Baker, R.K., "Potential metabolic interaction between St. John's wort and theophylline," *Annals of Pharmacotherapy*, Vol. 33, pp. 502, April 1999.
10. Rivera, J.O., Verma, K.M., "Hidden problems with herbal remedies," *Pharmacotherapy*, Vol. 20, No. 7, pp. 874-876, 2000.

About the author

Susan C. Smolinske received her bachelor's of science in pharmacy from the University of Florida in 1977 and her Doctor of Pharmacy degree from Idaho State University in 1993. She is certified by the Board of Pharmaceutical Specialties in pharmacotherapy and by the American Board of Applied Toxicology in clinical toxicology. Her career has included several years in retail pharmacy, two years at the Rocky Mountain Drug Information Center, and 10 years as an editor at Micromedex. For the past six years, she has been employed by Wayne State University. Dr. Smolinske is currently an assistant professor in the College of Medicine Department of Pediatrics. She is also currently Managing Director of the Children's Hospital of Michigan Regional Poison Control Center in Detroit, Michigan.

Self-assessment questions

1. Herbal medicines are regulated under which federal law?
   a. Food, Drug, and Cosmetic Act
   b. United States Pharmacopeial Convention Act
   c. Consumer Product Safety Act
   d. Dietary Supplement and Health Education Act

2. Which of the following would be an acceptable label for a dietary supplement?
   a. Gingko biloba prevents memory loss in Alzheimer's disease.
   b. St John's wort cures mild depression.
   c. Saw palmetto promotes good prostate health.
   d. Echinacea is effective treatment for the common cold.

3. Which of the following is clearly a homeopathic drug?
   a. Ma Huang standardized extract
   b. Atropa belladonna HPUS, 3X
   c. Goldenseal root capsule
   d. Green tea

4. Which is the best method to obtain a dietary supplement history?
   a. Question the patient over the phone while they are looking at labels.
   b. Have the patient bring containers to the pharmacy.
   c. Rely on the patient's memory about what they are taking.
   d. Ask the patient's physician about their supplements.

5. What food ingredient is most important to question when taking a dietary supplement history?
   a. Sugar
   b. Artificial sweeteners
   c. Caffeine
   d. Nicotine

6. Which scenario could prompt the Food and Drug Administration to prohibit marketing of an herbal product?
   a. The product commonly produces minor allergic reactions.
   b. The product causes immediate, life-threatening effects.
   c. The product is dangerous when taken in overdose.
   d. The product was not tested for safety prior to marketing.

7. Which is an example of a harmful drug-herb interaction?
   a. St John's wort caused failure of heart transplant in a patient taking cyclosporin.
   b. Echinacea caused hives in a patient with history of allergies.
   c. Ma Huang caused a heart attack in a patient who took more than the labeled amount.
   d. Gingko biloba caused bleeding in an elderly man not taking any medications.

8. Which of these patients should be referred to the pharmacist for counseling?
   a. Patient taking a multivitamin with herbs, not on any medications.
   b. Patient who discontinued blood pressure medication and is purchasing garlic pills.
   c. Patient taking goldenseal, with no history of allergies.
   d. Patient with borderline high cholesterol taking green tea.

9. Which of these products would be considered a functional food?
   a. Green tea
   b. Garlic capsules
   c. Candy bar with Gingko and Bacopa herbs
   d. Potato chips

10. Which herbal ingredient has been declared unsafe due to concerns over urinary cancer?
    a. Ma Huang
    b. Saw palmetto
    c. Echinacea
    d. Aristolochic acid

Chapter 20

Endocrine Disorders

Stephen Freed, R.Ph., CDE, FAADE

Learning objectives

Upon completion of this chapter, the technician should be able to do the following:

- ♦ Differentiate between type 1 and type 2 diabetes.
- ♦ Explain the criteria for the diagnosis of diabetes.
- ♦ Explain *insulin resistance.*
- ♦ Discuss the importance of monitoring blood sugars.
- ♦ Explain the purpose of the hemoglobin A_{1C} blood test.
- ♦ Differentiate between the five classes of oral medications for diabetes.
- ♦ Explain the role of insulin treatment in diabetes.
- ♦ Discuss the importance of controlling blood glucose.
- ♦ Explain the role of thyroid hormones in the body.
- ♦ Discuss estrogen replacement therapy.
- ♦ Explain the role of estrogen and progestin in oral contraceptives.

Introduction

The endocrine system is comprised of a group of organs and body tissues that produce, store and secrete hormones directly into the bloodstream. Among their functions, the organs of the endocrine system regulate metabolism, regulate the body's growth and development, and support reproductive functions. This chapter will focus on the pancreas, the thyroid gland, and the organs of the female reproductive system, which are part of the endocrine system.

The pancreas

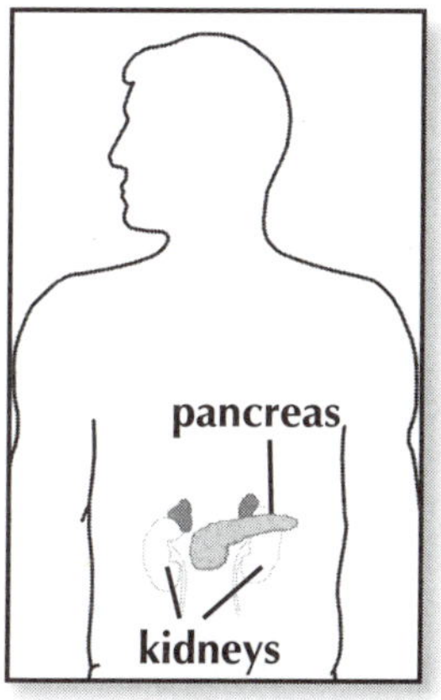

Diabetes

Diabetes—the complete name is *diabetes mellitus*—is one of the oldest diseases known. It was first described by the ancient Greeks as early as 100 AD. The word *diabetes* originates from the ancient Greek word for "flow through," since two of the most common symptoms are extreme thirst and a need to urinate frequently.

Scattered throughout the pancreas are cells called islets of Langerhans. Approximately 75 percent of these cells produce insulin, and about 20 percent of these cells produce glucagon. Insulin decreases blood glucose (sugar) and glucagon increases blood glucose. During normal food metabolism, insulin is released in response to blood glucose, to cause the uptake and storage of glucose (in the form of glycogen and fat). Without insulin, the body cannot use the glucose. Glucagon (from the pancreas) is released to oppose the actions of insulin.

An estimated 16 million people in the United States are known to have diabetes, with 40 percent not even knowing they have diabetes, and approximately 1 million of these being insulin dependent. Diabetes is a metabolic disorder that will progress over time to more serious problems unless it is managed properly.

In diabetes, the body cannot properly use the energy it gets from food. Normally, many foods we eat are broken down by digestion to *glucose,* which is a sugar. Glucose travels through the bloodstream to give the body's cells the energy they need. Glucose needs the help of *insulin,* a hormone produced by the pancreas, to get inside the cells, where the glucose is burned for energy or stored.

Although there is no cure for diabetes, it can be kept under control with proper care and attention. Monitoring blood sugar, establishing a proper diet and exercise routine, and making other lifestyle commitments can help keep diabetes under control. Checking blood sugar regularly and recording the readings are the best way to know whether a person is keeping his or her blood sugar levels under control. It is important to keep blood sugar levels within the boundaries set by the doctor throughout the course of the day and over time. This is the best way to avoid the long-term complications of diabetes, which can be serious. They can include heart and kidney problems, blindness, and nerve damage, possibly leading to toe or foot amputation.

The Diabetes Complications and Control Trials Study (DCCT), the largest study ever done on diabetics, showed that if a person can keep blood glucose levels as close to normal as possible, he or she can prevent the long-term complications of eye disease by almost 80 percent, kidney disease by more than 50 percent, and nerve disease by more than 60 percent.

In diabetes, there is a problem with insulin; either there is no insulin, hardly any insulin present, or the body has trouble using the insulin that is present. Without enough insulin, the glucose cannot be used by the body and it accumulates in the blood. This is called *hyperglycemia,* or too much sugar in the blood. Hyperglycemia is most common after meals, when sugar from digested food reaches the bloodstream. When there is too much sugar in the blood for a long period of time, complications such as heart disease can develop.

Symptoms of diabetes

Most of the symptoms of diabetes are similar for type 1 and type 2 diabetes. These symptoms include:

- Extreme thirst
- Need to urinate frequently
- Lack of energy
- Weight loss
- Nausea and vomiting
- Irritability
- Blurry vision
- Slow healing of cuts and bruises
- Frequent infections
- Mood changes

Type 1 diabetes

Type 1 diabetes used to be called *insulin-dependent diabetes mellitus* (IDDM) because the pancreas produces very little or no insulin. The cause of type 1 diabetes in unknown. It is believed to be an *autoimmune disease,* meaning that something causes the body's immune system to destroy normal insulin-producing cells. Another older term for type 1 diabetes is *juvenile-onset diabetes* because it is often diagnosed in children and young adults. People with type 1 diabetes need insulin injections to control their disease.

Type 2 diabetes

Type 2 diabetes used to be called *non-insulin-dependent diabetes mellitus* (NIDDM) because it sometimes can be managed without the need for insulin injections. However, some people with type 2 diabetes do have to use insulin. In type 2 diabetes, the pancreas makes some insulin, but it is not enough to manage the body's glucose. Or, the pancreas may make enough insulin, but the body can't use it properly to transport glucose into the cells. Another term formerly used for type 2 diabetes is *adult-onset diabetes,* because it typically affects people who are more than 40 years old, have a family history of diabetes, and are overweight.

Type 2 diabetes is much more common than type 1 diabetes. Approximately 90 percent of people with diabetes have type 2 diabetes. Also, about 80 percent of people who have type 2 diabetes are overweight. Being overweight is very strongly linked to the development of type 2 diabetes.

Many people with type 2 diabetes can successfully manage their disease with weight control. Proper diet and exercise can help achieve weight control. Those who cannot manage type 2 diabetes with weight control alone need oral medication or insulin, or a combination of both, to control their blood glucose.

Gestational diabetes

Diabetes that develops during pregnancy is called *gestational diabetes.* During pregnancy, certain hormones may cause glucose levels in the blood to rise. In some cases, the pancreas cannot keep up with the demand for extra insulin, and gestational diabetes develops. The symptoms of gestational diabetes usually disappear after the baby is born. But approximately one third of women who have gestational diabetes will develop type 2 diabetes later in life. This type of diabetes cannot be treated with oral drugs because of potential harm to the fetus, so only insulin injections can be used if diet and exercise are not sufficient in lowering blood glucose to normal levels.

Insulin resistance

Sometimes there is enough insulin in the body, but the body is unable to use it properly to reduce blood glucose. This is called *insulin resistance.* Usually, insulin resistance is due to problems in the cells that the insulin affects. Rarely, insulin resistance may be due to antibodies that bind to the insulin and prevent it from acting in the normal way. Either way, the result is that blood sugar levels may become too high.

People who are obese often have problems with insulin resistance. No one knows why, but in people who are very overweight, the insulin does not work properly. So being overweight may trigger diabetes in people with a family history of the disease. Insulin resistance is usually treated with diet and, if necessary, oral diabetes medications.

Who gets diabetes?

In the United States, nearly 16 million people have been diagnosed with diabetes, which means that approximately one of every 20 people has this disease. Many people have diabetes but do not know it yet. For example, approximately half of the people with type 2 diabetes have not yet been diagnosed. Diagnosing diabetes early is important so that weight control and, possibly, medication can be started as soon as possible to help avoid serious long-term complications.

Risk factors

Some reports have linked type 1 diabetes to viral infections and an impaired immune system. Other reports suggest toxins in the environment may damage the cells and affect insulin production in the pancreas. This can lead to type 1 diabetes. Family history may play a role in the development of type 1 diabetes. Other associations between risk factors and the development of type 1 diabetes are less clear. For example, there does not seem to be a link between race and the development of type 1 diabetes.

Type 2 diabetes has several well-established risk factors. The chances of developing type 2 diabetes increase with age. There is a very strong link between family history and the development of type 2 diabetes. People in several ethnic groups, including Native Americans, Mexican Americans, African Americans, and inhabitants of Pacific islands such as Polynesia and Samoa, have a high risk of type 2 diabetes. However the most significant risk factor for type 2 diabetes is being overweight. Researchers have discovered that it is not just the amount of body fat that is important, but where the fat is distributed on the body. People who have an increased amount of body fat at or above the waist are more at risk for developing type 2 diabetes than those who carry body fat below the waist. Inactivity also adds to diabetes risk. Exercise is important in preventing or delaying the onset of diabetes because it improves the body's use of glucose.

Diagnosing diabetes

Often there are few symptoms in the early stage of diabetes. It's important for patients to have regular check-ups so their physicians can check for diabetes. If diabetes is suspected, a doctor can make the diagnosis based on a complete medical history, physical examination, and blood and urine tests. Once diagnosed, treatment will be based on the type and severity of diabetes.

Table 1 Criteria for diagnosing diabetes

1. Symptoms of diabetes plus casual plasma glucose concentration ≥ 200mg/dl (11.1 mmol/l). Casual is defined as any time of day without regard to time elapsed since last meal. The classic symptoms of diabetes include polyuria (production of large volumes of pale, dilute urine), polydipsia (abnormal, intense thirst which leads to the drinking of large quantities of fluids), and unexplained weight loss.

OR

2. FPG (Fasting Plasma Glucose) ≥ 126mg/dl (7 mmol/l). Fasting is defined as no caloric intake for at least 8 hours.

OR

3. 2 hour PPG (Post-Prandial Glucose, meaning after meals) ≥ 200mg/dl (11.1 mmol/l) during an OGTT (Oral Glucose Tolerance Test). The test should be performed using a glucose load containing the equivalent of 75 grams anhydrous glucose dissolved in water.

In the absence of unequivocal hyperglycemia with acute metabolic decompensation, these criteria should be confirmed by repeat testing on a different day. The third measure (OGTT) is not recommended for routine clinical use.

Source: American Diabetes Association.

Glucose tolerance test

The *glucose tolerance test* is a very sensitive test, meaning it can firmly establish the presence or absence of diabetes. The test is given in the morning. After not eating since the night before, the patient will consume a drink containing glucose. The blood glucose level will be measured at least four or five times over the next two to three hours. The most important measurement is the one at two hours after drinking the glucose. (See Table 2.)

Table 2 Interpretation of glucose tolerance test*

Milligrams per deciliter (mg/dl)	Interpretation
80-140	normal
141-199	glucose intolerance
Over 200	diabetes

*These values do not apply to patients with gestational diabetes.

Fasting blood sugar

The *fasting blood sugar* (also called *fasting plasma glucose)* is a simple screening test for diabetes. It is not a very sensitive test, but is generally useful in identifying which patients should be followed closely for signs of diabetes. One must not eat anything beginning the night before the test. Then a blood sample will be drawn in the morning. Table 3 below shows the meaning of the test measurements.

Table 3 Fasting blood sugar measurements

Milligrams per deciliter (mg/dl)	Interpretation
Below 110	normal
111-125	impaired
Over 126	abnormal (you may have diabetes)

Urine sugar

When the level of sugar (glucose) in the blood gets too high for the kidneys to handle, some sugar "spills" into the urine. In most people, blood sugar levels have to be very high (approximately 250mg/dl) for sugar to get into the urine; therefore, blood sugar levels are now the standard measurements instead of urine tests.

Monitoring diabetes

Keeping track of blood sugar levels is the most important step in knowing that a patient's diabetes is under control. When the blood sugar levels are checked regularly, patients get an accurate record of the readings over time. This will help the patient, doctor, and diabetes educator to adjust diet, exercise, and medication as needed.

Finger stick blood sugar

Patients can easily test blood sugar with a simple finger stick device. A tiny blade will prick the finger to get a single drop of blood that is put on a test strip, pad, or sensor. The blood is automatically tested for its sugar level. The doctor or pharmacist can help to decide which type of device is best and help the patient learn how to use it.

When and how often to test blood sugar depends on many factors. When diabetes is first diagnosed, many people need to check their sugar three to four times each day. This will help determine if diet or medicine need to be adjusted. If diabetes is well controlled, blood sugar levels will not need to be checked as frequently.

Fasting and postprandial levels

The doctor and diabetes educator will also set up goals for fasting and *postprandial* (after eating a meal) blood sugar levels. Many doctors want fasting (more than eight hours after eating) levels of 80 to 120mg/dl and postprandial (less than two hours after eating) levels of less than 160mg/dl. These levels show tight control of blood sugar. However, these goals can vary for each patient.

Hemoglobin A_{1c} test

The hemoglobin (HbA_{1c}) test is a laboratory blood test that should be done by the doctor every three months to help patients keep tight control of diabetes. Keeping tight control is measured by long-term results and is the best way to avoid long-term complications.

Hemoglobin is a substance in blood that carries oxygen from the lungs to all parts of the body. A type of hemoglobin called *hemoglobin A_{1c}* forms when glucose attaches to hemoglobin. This happens only when blood glucose levels are high. The HbA_{1c} level can be used to measure a person's average blood sugar over the past two to three months. A normal HbA_{1c} value for a non-diabetic is approximately 4 percent to 6.2 percent. The American Diabetes Association recommends that it should be below 7 percent for diabetics to help prevent the complications from diabetes.

Treating and controlling diabetes

How diabetes is treated depends on the type and severity of the disease. The cornerstones of diabetes management are diet and exercise. If diet and exercise alone are not enough to control blood glucose levels, one or more oral medications, or perhaps even insulin, will need to be added.

Diet control

Diet control is the first step in the treatment of diabetes. Proper diet can help control the blood sugar level. In many cases of type 2 diabetes, proper diet, along with exercise, can control the disease without the need for oral medications.

Meal planning

The most important aspect of the diabetic diet is meal planning. A typical meal plan includes breakfast, lunch, dinner, and a nighttime snack. Some people also need to plan other between-meal snacks. Being consistent in a diet is the most important part of meal planning. It is advisable to eat the same number of calories, the same amounts of food, and the same types of food at the same times each day. It is also important to eat all of the meals on a regular schedule to help avoid sharp ups and downs in blood sugar.

Exercise

Exercise is important for the patient with diabetes. Exercise makes insulin work better in the blood and can help lower blood sugar levels. Exercising for just 20 to 30 minutes, three times per week, can lower the amount of medication needed for people with type 1 and type 2 diabetes. It can also improve overall health. People with diabetes have to be careful not to let the blood sugar get too low when exercising. The easiest to prevent low blood sugar is to eat within three hours before exercising. The doctor should be consulted before starting an exercise program.

Reducing stress

There is evidence linking stress with blood sugar levels. Stress has been shown to cause blood sugar to either rise or fall. Many people with diabetes notice that the stresses of daily living can affect their blood sugar levels. In some people, long-term stress can cause the onset of diabetes. Reducing stress is an important part of diabetes management.

Oral medications

Oral medications for diabetes are used when diet and exercise alone are not enough to control diabetes. Most people with type 2 diabetes can be helped by oral medications. Even if oral medications are used, it is still very important to follow a doctor's advice about diet and exercise.

Many medications are available for the treatment of diabetes. They all work by reducing blood sugar, but they work in different ways. None of these medications contains insulin. The oral medications available now all belong to one of five types:

- Sulfonylureas
- Biguanides
- Alpha-glucosidase inhibitors
- Thiazolidinediones
- Meglitinides

Sulfonylureas

This was the only class of oral diabetic medicine available from 1950 to 1995. The other four classes of medications did not become available until after 1995.

Sulfonylureas help the body release more insulin from the pancreas. They may also make it easier for the insulin to work. Sulfonylureas are usually taken before meals, although the exact time will vary according to the exact medication used. A sulfonylurea may be used alone, with another oral medication, or combined with insulin.

All sulfonylureas may cause the blood sugar to go too low (hypoglycemia). Symptoms of hypoglycemia can include nervousness, dizziness, sweating, weakness, and a pounding heart. This is more likely to happen if a meal is missed or when used in combination with other diabetic drugs, including insulin. When taking a sulfonylurea, it is important not to skip meals. The most common side effects with a majority of the sulfonylureas are gastrointestinal in nature, such as nausea or heartburn.

Biguanides

The biguanides are another class of oral diabetes medication. Sometimes biguanides are prescribed when people have been taking sulfonylureas for a long time and the sulfonylureas no longer lower the blood sugar enough. The biguanides cause the liver to release stored sugar into the blood more slowly, which makes it easier for insulin to work. They are taken several times a day, always with meals. A biguanide may be used alone or in combination with a sulfonylurea.

Biguanides alone usually don't cause low blood sugar, but it may occur when one is used in combination with a sulfonylurea. The most common side effects of biguanides are diarrhea, nausea, and vomiting.

Biguanides should not be taken by people with kidney disease. They also should not be taken if a patient is having a certain type of radiologic exam using a radiologic dye. There is a risk of a rare but life-threatening condition called lactic acidosis. The doctor may perform blood tests to monitor kidney and liver function to guard against this rare occurrence.

Alpha-glucosidase inhibitors

The alpha-glucosidase inhibitors are a type of medicine that works in a unique way. They slow down the digestion of carbohydrates after a meal. This means postprandial blood sugar levels do not rise so sharply. Alpha-glucosidase inhibitors must be taken with the first bite of each meal, three times a day. An alpha-glucosidase inhibitor may be taken alone or in combination with a sulfonylurea.

Alpha-glucosidase inhibitors themselves do not cause hypoglycemia or hyperinsulinemia (too much insulin in the blood), but it is still possible to develop hypoglycemia if the patient is taking an alpha-glucosidase inhibitor along with a sulfonylurea. If this happens, the patient needs to use a special sugar to raise his or her blood sugar level. This sugar is glucose (dextrose), which is different than sucrose (cane sugar) found in table sugar or candy. The patient should not use sucrose to treat hypoglycemia if taking an alpha-glucosidase inhibitor. Glucose is found in honey or bananas and lesser amounts in orange juice. Glucose (dextrose) tablets can be found in the pharmacy.

Alpha-glucosidase inhibitors should not be taken by patients with diabetic ketoacidosis (which is described later under "Complications of diabetes"), cirrhosis (hardening of the liver caused by the formation of connective tissue), or chronic intestinal disorders. The most common side effects are gas, diarrhea, and abdominal pain.

Thiazolidinediones

The thiazolidinediones are another type of oral diabetes medication. These medications are also referred to as insulin sensitizers. They are useful for patients already taking insulin and type 2 diabetics who are obese and insulin resistant, because they work by making the body's cells more responsive to insulin. Thiazolidinediones are taken only once per day, usually with breakfast, in the middle of the meal. They can also be used alone with another oral medication.

Hypoglycemia may occur when a thiazolidinedione is used in combination with insulin or another medication. It has not occurred when used alone. The most common side effects reported include increased risk of infection, headache, and pain.

Meglitinides

The meglitinides are another type of oral medicine that helps the body release more insulin from the pancreas. The medicine responds to the body's blood sugar level by signaling the pancreas to produce more insulin when the blood glucose level is high. Meglitinides may be used alone or with metformin. Meglitinides are taken before meals, usually three times a day, and only work if food is present.

Meglitinides can cause the blood sugar to go too low, but the risk of this is less than with the sulfonylureas.

People with diabetic ketoacidosis should not take meglitinides. Higher doses of meglitinides should be used carefully in patients with liver or kidney problems. The most common side effects reported include increased risk of infection, headache, diarrhea, and vomiting.

Combinations

Glucovance® is a combination of glyburide and metformin in three different dosage combinations.

Insulin

Initially all patients with type 1 diabetes and a few with type 2 diabetes need insulin. Many people with type 2 diabetes may eventually need insulin.

Types of insulin

So far, insulin is only available as an injection. There are several different types of insulin. These are:

- Ultra-short-acting insulin (an example is *Lysine-proline analog* insulin, also called Lispro® or Humalog® insulin). This insulin is only available with a prescription, where most of the other insulins are available without a prescription. Humalog® 75/25 is a mixture of NPH (75) and Humalog® (25) available only in a pen.
- Short-acting insulin (an example is Regular Insulin® or Humulin®R)
- Intermediate-acting insulin (examples are NPH and Lente® or Humulin® N insulin)
- Long-acting insulin (an example is Ultralente® insulin or Humulin® U)
- Mixed insulins (mixtures of NPH and Regular Insulin®; examples are 70/30 and 50/50)
- Buffered insulin (which is used in insulin pumps)

These types of insulin are not alike in terms of when and how long they act in the body. *Onset* is how long the insulin takes to begin working. *Peak* is the time after taking the insulin when it is working the most. *Duration* is how long the insulin keeps working. Onset, peak, and duration for each type of insulin are shown in Table 4.

The doctor will prescribe the type of insulin that is best for the patient based on how difficult it is to control the blood sugars and other factors. It should be noted that ultra-short-acting insulin is not approved for use during pregnancy.

Table 4 Activity of different types of insulin

	Example	Onset	Peak	Duration
Ultra-Short-Acting Insulin	Humalog®	5 min.	1 hour	2-4 hours
Short-Acting Insulin	Humulin®R	1/2 hour	2-4 hours	6-8 hours
Intermediate-Acting Insulin	Humulin® N	2-4 hours	6-12 hours	18-24 hours
Long-Acting Insulin	Humulin® U	4-8 hours	12-18 hours	24-36 hours
Long-Acting Insulin	Lantus® (glargine)	1-2 hours	Peakless	24 hours

How insulin is administered

Insulin shots can be administered by several techniques. The first is the traditional *syringe* and needle. The second is a special insulin *pen* in which a cartridge of insulin is put into a pen-like syringe and used multiple times. There are also pens with a single dose of insulin that are thrown away after use. The third is a *pump* the size of a pager that injects the right amount of insulin automatically into the bloodstream. The pump is used by people with brittle diabetes or those who want very tight control of their diabetes and more control over their lives.

Important considerations when using insulin

Self-administering insulin is not difficult to learn. Usually, a doctor, pharmacist, nurse, or diabetes educator can provide this training. Insulin comes in different strengths. Most manufacturers recommend that insulin be stored in the refrigerator *(not the freezer)* when not in use. Insulin should not be used after the expiration date shown on the package. It is also important to learn to recognize the normal appearance of insulin. Regular Insulin® should be clear. NPH®, Lente®, Lantus®, and Ultralente® insulin should be cloudy. No type of insulin should have any little specks (called *precipitates)* floating in it. If the insulin doesn't look right, it should not be used.

Most important is that the patient uses the insulin exactly as directed by the doctor. Insulin has a very strong effect on blood sugar. Taking the wrong type of insulin or the wrong dose of insulin can have serious results. Insulin should not be mixed unless the patient has been instructed to do so.

Complications of diabetes

Short-term complications

Short-term complications of diabetes (also called *acute complications)* occur because the blood sugar gets too high or too low and causes immediate symptoms. It is important to keep short-term complications under control so they don't lead to long-term problems. Short-term complications include:

Hypoglycemia (low blood sugar) symptoms	**Hyperglycemia (high blood sugar) symptoms**	**Ketoacidosis symptoms**
Nervousness	Thirst	Extreme thirst
Dizziness	Frequent urination	Loss of appetite
Sweating	Tiredness	Abdominal pain
Weakness		Nausea
Pounding heart		Vomiting
		Flushed skin
		Fever
		Frequent urination
		Drowsiness
		Alcohol breath
		Rapid breathing

Low blood sugar (also called hypoglycemia*)*. In hypoglycemia, the blood sugar becomes too low. This might happen if a person with diabetes misses a meal and still takes the normal dose of insulin. It might also happen during exercise if a person with diabetes has not eaten extra carbohydrates before exercising. Or, it might happen if a person with diabetes takes too much of some oral medications. Symptoms of hypoglycemia include nervousness, dizziness, sweating, weakness, and a pounding heart. However, there may be no symptoms at all.

Moderate hypoglycemia can usually be treated by taking some milk and crackers. If the blood sugar is extremely low, eating candy or drinking orange juice can help. If the blood sugar of a patient drops too low when he or she is taking an alpha-glucosidase inhibitor, the patient needs to use a special sugar (glucose/dextrose) to bring it back up; the sugar found in table sugar or candy will not work. If the symptoms do not improve after approximately 15 minutes, emergency help should be called for, since uncontrolled hypoglycemia is very dangerous. If low blood sugar continues to the point where the patient passes out and something cannot be given to them orally, then the alternative is to give the patient an injection of Glucagon®, which is available by prescription.

High blood sugar *(hyperglycemia).* It can occur if a patient has not taken oral medication or insulin, if he or she has eaten too much food, or hasn't exercised enough. Many times, there won't be symptoms during hyperglycemia. Other times, there may be thirst, frequent urination or tiredness. Hyperglycemia can be controlled by changing the diet or adjusting insulin or oral medications.

Ketoacidosis. Ketoacidosis (also called *diabetic ketoacidosis* or DKA) happens when there is no insulin in the blood and glucose can't be used by the body's cells. This occurs more commonly in people with type 1 diabetes. The body starts using stored fat for energy, and ketone (a simple sugar) bodies increase in the blood. Ketoacidosis starts slowly and builds up. The symptoms of ketoacidosis include extreme thirst, loss of appetite, abdominal pain, nausea, vomiting, flushed skin, fever, frequent urination, drowsiness, alcohol breath, and rapid breathing. It can cause dehydration, and if the person is not given fluids and insulin right away, ketoacidosis can lead to coma and even death.

Long-term complications

The long-term complications (also called *chronic complications)* of diabetes are those that typically occur after years of elevated blood sugar. Perhaps the most important reason for good blood sugar control in people with diabetes is that the longer the blood sugar remains elevated, the greater the chances of developing one or more of the complications of diabetes. Keeping blood sugar under control can actually reduce the chances of developing complications. If short-term complications can be controlled, then long-term complications are less likely to occur.

Blurry vision. This can occur if the blood sugar level is too high. Vision usually returns to normal when the blood sugar level returns to normal.

Retinopathy. Long-term diabetes can affect the retina of the eye, causing vision problems and, eventually, blindness. It is very important for people with diabetes to have regular eye examinations. Retinopathy from diabetes is the leading cause of blindness.

Nephropathy (kidney damage). A major job of the kidneys is to filter all of the waste products of the body out of the blood into the urine. When the small blood vessels in the kidneys become damaged, the kidneys cannot do this work as well. If this happens, a doctor can prescribe a blood pressure medication to help the kidneys work better. The doctor may also advise the patient to change the amount of protein and potassium in the patient's diet. Sometimes patients with diabetic nephropathy require *dialysis,* in which a machine does the filtering for them. Nephropathy from diabetes is the leading cause of kidney failure.

Neuropathy (nerve damage). Neuropathy can occur after years of poor blood sugar control because the small blood vessels feeding the nerves become blocked. *Peripheral neuropathy* is the most common type of diabetic neuropathy. Typically, patients with peripheral neuropathy feel numbness, tingling, or pain in the feet, legs, hands, and arms due to poor circulation caused by diabetes. This may even lead to foot amputation.

Macrovascular complications. Macrovascular complications are those affecting the large blood vessels (arteries and arterioles) of the body. Macrovascular complications include heart and blood-vessel disease and high blood pressure.

Heart and blood-vessel disease can develop because of poor circulation, caused by damage to the blood vessels. This can increase the chances of a heart attack or stroke. To help prevent heart disease and circulation problems, people with diabetes should eat a low-fat diet and exercise regularly.

High blood pressure can cause a strain on the kidneys, which may make it more likely for nephropathy to develop. High blood pressure can be controlled with changes in the diet and with medications.

Living with diabetes

The key to controlling diabetes is by educating and empowering patients to manage their own diabetes. With modern advancements in diabetes treatments and the availability of widespread support from doctors, pharmacists, nurses, diabetes educators, and organizations like the American Diabetes Association, American Association of Diabetes Educators, and the American Dietetic Association, it is possible now more than ever to successfully manage diabetes. Diabetes must be controlled by self-management, and in order to do that, patients need to become educated on their diabetes.

Table 5 Diabetes oral medications

Name of class	Examples	Mechanism of action	Unique factors	Major side effect or disadvantages of use	Primary site of action
Sulfonylureas	glyburide (Micronase®, DiaBeta®) micronized glyburide (Glynase®, Glynase PresTab®) glimepride (Amaryl®)	Increases the release of insulin from the pancreas.	Can be used in combination	Hypoglycemia, weight gain, beta cell depletion	Pancreas
Biguanides	metformin (Glucophage®) glucophage® XR	Reduces the production of glucose by the liver.	Can be used in combination	Abdominal distress	Liver
Alpha-glucosidase inhibitors	acarbose (Precose®) miglitol (Glyget®)	Delays the adsorption of carbohydrates in the intestinal tract.	Abdominal distress; can be used in combination	Abdominal distress	Intestines
Meglitinides	repaglinide (Prandin®)	Similar to sulfonylurea, except it is shorter acting and only works when glucose is present.	Taken with food. Not to be taken without food. Can be used in combination.	Short Duration — A mealtime drug	Pancreas
Thiazolidinediones	rosiglitazone (Avandia®) pioglitazone (Actos®)	Insulin sensitizer, allows for the more effective use of insulin.	Can be used in combination. Liver enzyme test must be performed at onset and every 2 months for 1 year.	Decreases the amount of insulin required, including a body's own insulin and injectable insulin.	Skeletal muscle

This chart is only a brief overview; for more information, review the information from computer printouts or drug inserts.

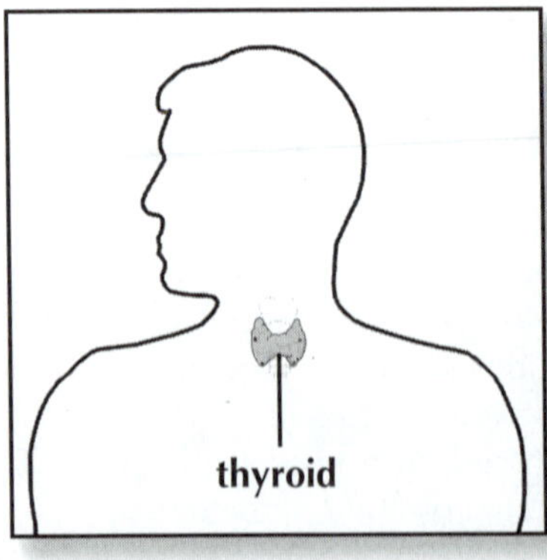

Drugs used to treat thyroid disorders[1]

The thyroid is an endocrine gland that releases thyroid hormones. The normal thyroid gland secretes (releases) sufficient amounts of the hormones triiodothyronine (T_3) and tetraiodothyronine (T_4 or thyroxine) to maintain normal body temperature, energy levels, growth, and development. These hormones contain 59 percent and 65 percent, respectively, of the iodine that comes from the daily food supply. The parafollicular cells of the thyroid gland also secrete calcitonin, which helps regulate body calcium.

As with most glandular systems, the thyroid is usually balanced, secreting just enough hormone to meet the body's need. However, if the thyroid gland does not respond to the signal to make and secrete T_3 and T_4 hormones, hypothyroidism will occur. Symptoms include lethargy, slowed speech and thought, swelling, puffy face, anemia, and weight gain. Replacement therapy is available as synthetic products (levothyroxine, liothyronine, liotrix) or those of animal origin (desiccated thyroid).

Table 6 Comparison of thyroid drugs

Drug	Content	Brand	Source
Thyroid desiccated	T_3 & T_4	Armour Thyroid®	Animal
Levothyroxine	T_4	Levothyroid®, Synthroid	Synthetic
Liotrix	T_3 & T_4	Euthyroid®, Thyrolar	Synthetic
Liothyronine	T_3	Cytomel®	Synthetic

Synthetic levothyroxine is the preparation of choice for thyroid replacement because of its stability, uniformity, low cost, easy measurement from blood levels, and once daily dosing. Some of this T_4 preparation converts to T_3 intracellularly so that both hormones are available. Generic levothyroxine provides comparable efficacy and is acceptable.

Estrogen, progestin, and oral contraceptives[1]

Estrogens produced by women include estradiol (E_2), estrone (E_1), and estriol (E_3). Estrogens are responsible for the development of the female reproductive system, the monthly buildup of the endometrium of the uterus during each reproductive cycle, and for the maintenance of pregnancy. Estrogens help to maintain healthy skin, blood vessels, heart, and bone. Estrogen increases blood coagulation and blood triglycerides (fat).

Post menopausal hormone therapy

Estrogen is replaced after menopause (when ovulatory function ceases) to reduce hot flashes, sweating, insomnia, and loss of genital tone. The goal of long-term replacement therapy is to retard the loss of bone (avoiding wrist, hip, and spine fractures) and to avoid lipid changes that lead to heart disease. Natural estrogens include conjugated estrogens (Premarin®), estradiol (Estrace®), and estradiol transdermal patch (Estraderm®, Climara®, Vivelle®). Synthetic estrogens that seem equally effective include estrified estrogens (Estratab®, Estratest®), and ethinyl estradiol (Estinyl®). Side effects of estrogen therapy include an increased risk of blood clots, endometrial cancer, breast cancer, and hypertension.

Progestin

Natural and synthetic progestin prepares the endometrium for pregnancy and breasts for milk production. Progestin is used in postmenopausal women, along with estrogens to oppose the risk of cancer from the estrogen and promote cyclic shedding (bleeding) to maintain a healthy uterus. Progestins include medroxyprogesterone (Provera®) and norethindrone acetate (Aygestin®). The single tablet combination of estrogen and progestin (Prempro®) is used for fixed-dose treatment or a cyclic therapy pack (Premphase®).

Oral contraceptives

Most contraceptives contain estrogen and progestin. Estrogen interferes with implantation of the fertilized ovum; progestin prevents sperm migration and promotes endometrial changes that make it unsuitable for ovum implantation. Monophasic therapy provides a fixed dose of estrogen and progestin for a 21-day cycle. Triphasic therapy provides a progestin dose that varies every seven days, and the estrogen dose may vary every seven days or remain fixed. This is intended to mimic normal hormone variation.

Oral contraceptives are used primarily to prevent pregnancy, but may be used to regulate menses characterized with extreme bleeding or pain. The most common side effects of oral contraceptives are nausea and areas of darkened skin color. The most severe effects include heart attack, hypertension, weight gain, blood clots, and possibly cervical cancer.

Table 7 Selected oral contraceptives

Monophasic combination tablets		Estrogen (mg)		Progestin (mg)	
Loestrin 1/20®		ethinyl estradiol	0.02	norethindrone acetate	1
Desogen®		ethinyl estradiol	0.03	desogestrel	0.15
Nordette®		ethinyl estradiol	0.03	L-norgestrel	0.15
Ortho-Novum 1/35® (Genora, Norinyl)		ethinyl estradiol	0.035	norethindrone	1
Ortho-Cyclen®		ethinyl estradiol	0.035	norgestimate	0.25
Ovcon 50®		ethinyl estradiol	0.05	norethindrone	1
Ortho-Novum 1/50® (Genora, Norinyl)		mestranol	0.05	norethindrone	1
Triphasic combination tablets		**Estrogen (mg)**		**Progestin (mg)**	
Triphasil®	Day 1-6	ethinyl estradiol	0.03	L-norgestrel	0.05
	Day 7-11	ethinyl estradiol	0.04	L-norgestrel	0.075
	Day 12-21	ethinyl estradiol	0.3	L-norgestrel	0.125
Ortho-Novum 7/7/7®	Day 1-7	ethinyl estradiol	0.035	norethindrone	0.5
	Day 8-14	ethinyl estradiol	0.035	norethindrone	0.75
	Day 15-21	ethinyl estradiol	0.035	norethindrone	1
Ortho-Tri-Cyclin®	Day 1-7	ethinyl estradiol	0.035	norgestimate	0.18
	Day 8-14	ethinyl estradiol	0.035	norgestimate	0.215
	Day 15-21	ethinyl estradiol	0.035	norgestimate	0.25

Conclusion

The medications used to treat diabetes and thyroid disorders and regulate the female reproductive system continue to appear on the list of Top 200 Prescriptions according to the number of prescriptions dispensed in the United States. Because of large numbers of patients taking such medications, pharmacy technicians need to understand how these medications work.

Reference

1. Pharmacy Certified Technician Training Manual, 7th edition, Michigan Pharmacists Association, Lansing, MI, 1997, pp. 153-155.

About the author

Stephen Freed, R.Ph., CDE, FAADE, received his pharmacy degree from the University of Illinois at Chicago and is the chief executive officer for Partners In Control, Inc., a diabetes education and management company based in Deerfield, Illinois. Freed started this company after spending 15 years as a successful independent pharmacy owner of four pharmacies. Shortly after starting Partners In Control, Freed became a Certified Diabetes Educator (CDE). After two years of success in having his own disease management company, Freed became a speaker for many pharmaceutical companies such as Eli Lilly, Parke Davis, and SmithKline Beecham, which enabled him to become a faculty member for the American Association of Diabetes Educators. Freed then took a clinical director position with The Gladstone Group, a disease management company that signs contracts with self-insured companies to provide disease management for employees with asthma, diabetes and cardiovascular disease.

Self-assessment questions

1. Which of the following is an accurate statement regarding type 1 and type 2 diabetes?
   a. Persons with type 1 diabetes can usually be treated with diet, exercise or, if needed, oral hypoglycemic drugs or in combination with insulin, and persons with type 2 diabetes require insulin injections to maintain their blood glucose in an acceptable range.
   b. Persons with type 1 diabetes require insulin injections to maintain their blood glucose in an acceptable range, and persons with type 2 diabetes can usually be treated with diet, exercise or, if needed, oral hypoglycemic drugs or in combination with insulin.
   c. Persons with type 1 and type 2 diabetes can only be treated with insulin.
   d. In persons with type 1 diabetes, their pancreas produces too much insulin, whereas the pancreas in persons with type 2 diabetes does not produce enough insulin.
2. Which of the following is ***not*** considered a criterion for the diagnosis of diabetes?
   a. Symptoms of diabetes plus casual plasma glucose concentration over 200mg/dl
   b. Fasting plasma glucose level greater than or equal to 126mg/dl
   c. A fasting plasma glucose level less than 126mg/dl and a post-prandial glucose level less than 200mg/dl
   d. A glucose level of 200mg/dl either after a meal or during an Oral Glucose Tolerance Test
3. Which of the following is ***not*** a class of diabetes oral medications?
   a. Thiazolidinediones
   b. Alpha-glucosidase inhibitors
   c. Glyburides
   d. Biquanides
4. If a patient has a hypoglycemic reaction while on Precose®, what would be the most effective product to take?
   a. Orange juice
   b. Snickers candy bar
   c. Sucrose
   d. Glucose tablets
5. How long does it take for Humulin R to begin working?
   a. 5 minutes
   b. 30 minutes
   c. 2-4 hours
   d. 4-8 hours
6. Which of the following is ***not*** a long-term complication from diabetes?
   a. Retinopathy
   b. Neuropathy
   c. Ketoacidosis
   d. Macrovascular
7. The hemaglobin A_{1c} or HbA_{1c} test:
   a. is a two- to three-month average of a person's blood sugar.
   b. has a normal range of 6 percent to 8 percent for a non-diabetic.
   c. is recommended once a year.
   d. can be done by the patient on a blood glucose monitor.
8. Which of the following is a possible symptom for hypoglycemia?
   a. nervousness
   b. thirst
   c. frequent urination
   d. tiredness
9. Which oral diabetes medication causes the liver to release stored sugar into the blood more slowly?
   a. Glucotrol®
   b. Prandin®
   c. Glucophage®
   d. Micronase®

10. Which oral diabetes medication requires that a liver enzyme test must be performed at onset and every two months for one year?
    a. Glucophage®
    b. Glyset®
    c. Avandia®
    d. Rezulin®

11. The statement, "Once a diabetic, always a diabetic," is:
    a. true for both type 1 and type 2 diabetics.
    b. false for both type 1 and type 2 diabetics.
    c. true only for type 1 diabetics.
    d. false only for type 2 diabetics.

12. Which of the following drugs is used for thyroid hormone replacement?
    a. Levothyroxine®
    b. Premarin®
    c. Prozac®
    d. Glucophage®

13. Benefits of estrogen replacement in postmenopausal women include all of the following *except*:
    a. it reduces the amount of hot flashes.
    b. it helps avoid lipid changes that lead to heart disease.
    c. it increases the loss of genital tone.
    d. it reduces insomnia.

14. Which of the following is a triphasic oral contraceptive?
    a. Loestrin®
    b. Nordette®
    c. Triphasil®
    d. Ovcon®

15. Which of the following statements regarding oral contraceptives is ***not*** true?
    a. They are used primarily to prevent pregnancy.
    b. They may be used to regulate menses.
    c. They may cause hypotension.
    d. They may cause blood clots.

CHAPTER 21

RESPIRATORY FUNCTION

Paul J. Munzenberger, Pharm.D., and Beverly P. Kershaw, Pharm.M.S.

Learning objectives

Upon completion of this chapter, the technician should be able to do the following:

- Explain the anatomy of the respiratory tract.
- Explain the characteristics of asthma.
- Explain the drug therapy of asthma.
- Explain the characteristics of chronic obstructive airway disease.
- Explain the drug therapy of chronic obstructive airway disease.
- Explain the actions of expectorants, antitussives, and decongestants.

Introduction

The respiratory system is a series of airways, starting with the nose and mouth, leading all the way to the smallest alveoli in the lung where gas exchange occurs. Air moves through the nose to the trachea that divides into two main bronchi (one for each lung). Each bronchus progressively divides into smaller airways (bronchioles) leading through the alveolar ducts to the alveoli (air sacs). Layers of smooth muscle wrap around the airway structures with progressively thinner amounts of muscle as it progresses toward the alveoli. These muscles help control the diameter of airways. If they constrict, the airway diameter becomes smaller. If they relax, the airway diameter is larger and air will flow more easily. The airways also contain mucus-producing glands. The mucus within the airway helps to humidify incoming air and trap pollutants, dust, and other unwanted substances. The walls of the structures get thinner so that at the level of the alveoli, there is only a thin layer of cells surrounded by the capillaries. This permits the gas exchange of oxygen into the capillary blood and the removal of carbon dioxide.

Normal lungs

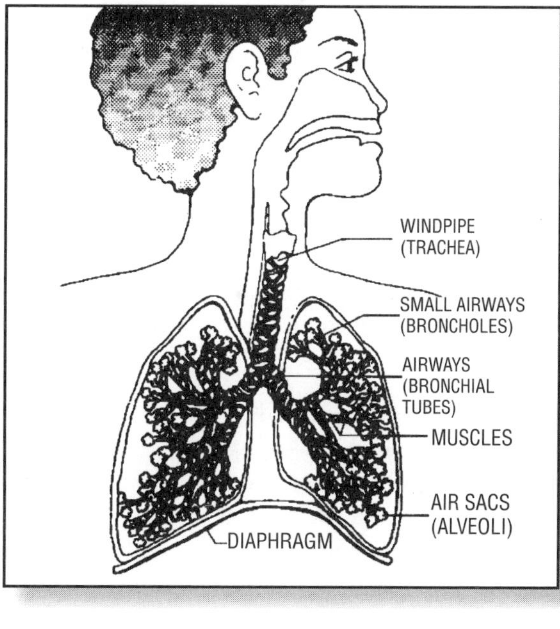

Characteristics of asthma

The national Asthma Education Program, Expert Panel Report defines asthma as a lung disease that is characterized by:

- airway obstruction that is reversible either by itself or with treatment
- airway inflammation
- increased airway responsiveness to various stimuli

In patients with asthma, the bronchi and smaller airways are more responsive to stimuli (i.e., cold, allergens, exercise) and become narrowed from muscle contraction, inflammation, swelling, and thick mucus. This results in the patient wheezing, coughing and being short of breath. Drug treatments include bronchodilators (beta agonists and theophylline), anti-inflammatory drugs (corticosteroids, antileukotrienes), and other preventative therapies (cromolyn, nedocromil).

Characteristics of chronic obstructive airway disease

Chronic obstructive airway disease (COAD) is usually a combination of chronic bronchitis (inflammation of the bronchi) and emphysema (enlarged and damaged alveoli making it hard for gas exchange to occur). While a number of risk factors are associated with the development of COAD, smoking is the main cause. Patients with COAD produce excessive amounts of mucus within the lungs. This results in coughing up large volumes of sputum (saliva mixed with mucus) and increased risk of infection. They also have increased smooth muscle around the airways, chronic airway inflammation, and destruction of the walls of the air sacs causing gas exchange to be reduced. COAD is a progressive disorder. Treatment is aimed at slowing the progression of the disease and providing symptomatic relief.

Beta agonists

Beta agonists stimulate the beta-2 receptors causing smooth muscle relaxation within the airways and increased ciliary activity to help clear mucus. Some of the inhaled drug is absorbed into the blood and may cause side effects of nervousness, tremor, and tachycardia (increased heart rate). Beta agonists are available in solutions for nebulizer treatments, metered-dose inhalers, tablets, and liquid. More side effects occur with the tablets and liquid.

Short-acting, quick-relief beta agonists are used in the treatment of asthma and COAD. Examples include albuterol (Proventil®, Ventolin®), bitolterol (Tornalate®), and pirbuterol (Maxair®). These are used primarily to treat asthma and COAD symptoms such as wheezing, shortness of breath, or coughing. They are also sometimes used before exercise or hard playing to prevent the symptoms of asthma. These drugs are most frequently used on an "as needed" basis. Rarely should short-acting beta agonists be used on a regular schedule in the treatment of asthma. These drugs generally become effective in 15 minutes (inhalers) to 30 minutes (oral medicines) and last about four to six hours in duration.

There are also long-acting beta agonists (e.g., salmeterol, sustained release albuterol tablets). These are used on a regular schedule for more persistent asthma or COAD. The long-acting inhaler, salmeterol (Serevent®), lasts 12 hours. This duration provides good control of nocturnal asthma symptoms. If breakthrough wheezing, shortness of breath, or other symptoms occur within the 12 hours, a shorter acting inhaler should be used. Additional doses of long-acting beta agonists should not be used.

Ipratropium bromide

Ipratropium bromide (Atrovent®) is an anticholinergic drug. (Anticholinergic activity was discussed in Chapter 11.) It blocks the airway constrictor effect of cholinergic stimulation to the smooth muscles around the airways. Because of this anticholinergic activity, airway dilation occurs. Ipratropium bromide is used primarily in patients with COAD. Occasionally it is used in combination to treat acute episodes of asthma. One advantage of this medication is the low risk of side effects or adverse reactions.

Theophylline

Related to caffeine, theophylline relaxes the smooth muscle that dilates the respiratory tract and relieves obstruction. The side effects seen are similar to those of caffeine and include nervousness, insomnia, stomach pain, muscle tremor, and tachycardia. Theophylline is available as an intravenous (IV) infusion or in oral sustained-release products (Theodur®, Slophyllin®) that provide continuous activity. Because this medication is maintained within a narrow range of acceptable blood concentrations, periodic blood tests are needed. The usual target range is 5mcg/mL to 15mcg/mL. There are many known interactions between theophylline and other drugs such as ciprofloxacin, cimetidine, erythromycin, clarithromycin, and others. Theophylline also interacts with certain diseases and conditions such as liver failure, pneumonia, and smoking. Such factors necessitate close monitoring and dosage adjustment.

Corticosteroids and antileukotrienes

In patients with asthma, corticosteroids are considered first-line drug therapy to reduce airway obstruction from inflammation and reduce airway hyperreactivity. Inhaled corticosteroids, including beclomethasone (Vanceril®), triamcinolone (Azmacort®), budesonide (Pulmicort®), flunisolide (AeroBid®),. and fluticasone (Flovent®), offer an effective delivery to the airways with minimal systemic absorption. Inhaled corticosteroids are not effective for acute wheezing and require continued use to reduce inflammation and airway hyperreactivity.

Short-term intravenous (IV) or oral corticosteroids (methylprednisolone, hydrocortisone, prednisone) are used to treat acute episodes of asthma and COAD. If given for short periods, systemic (IV or oral) corticosteroids cause few side effects. However, long-term use of oral corticosteroids cause many systemic side effects, such as cataract formation, electrolyte disorders, and "moon face." ("Moon face" is when the face of the patient swells to a round appearance, similar to the appearance of the moon.) The oral route is reserved for patients with severe asthma or COAD, and the dose is tapered to the lowest dose possible.

The antileukotrienes are also anti-inflammatory medications. They are not as potent as the corticosteroids. These products are only available for oral administration. Similar to the inhaled corticosteroids, they must be taken on a regular basis to be effective. Unlike the oral corticosteroids, their administration over a long period causes few side effects. Currently, three products are available. Montelukast (Singulair®) may be given once a day, while zafirlukast (Accolate®) is given twice a day. Zileuton (Zyflo®) has the disadvantage of requiring administration four times a day. These agents are used primarily in patients with asthma.

Cromolyn and nedocromil

Treatment with a cromolyn (Intal®) or nedocromil (Tilade®) inhaler is effective when used before an exposure to an asthma-causing trigger (i.e., cold air, exercise, allergens such as hay fever). They prevent mast cells (a large cell in connective tissue) from releasing histamine and other inflammatory substances and avoid the inflammatory process from the start. Like inhaled corticosteroids and antileukotrienes, these drugs should be inhaled routinely.

Asthma treatment

The treatment selected will depend on the severity of asthma. Severity is determined from the frequency of symptoms, needed visits to the doctor or hospital, and measurements of respiratory function (pulmonary function tests). Categories of asthma severity include mild intermittent, mild persistent, moderate persistent, and severe persistent. In patients with asthma, severity may change over time. They may improve, requiring less medication, or worsen, with the need of more aggressive treatment.

Table 1 represents a summary of the treatment of asthma based on the 1998 Global Strategy For Asthma Management And Prevention NHLBI/WHO Workshop Report.

Table 1 Treatment of adults & children over 5 years old

	Long-term preventive	**Quick-relief**
Severe Persistent	• **Inhaled corticosteroid** (high dose) and • Either **long-acting inhaled beta agonist**, and/or sustained-release theophylline, and/or long-acting beta agonist tablets and • Oral corticosteroids long term	• Short-acting **inhaled beta agonist**
Moderate Persistent	• **Inhaled corticosteroid** (medium dose) and, if needed, • **Long-acting inhaled beta agonist**, sustained-release theophylline, long acting beta agonist tablets, antileukotriene	• Short-acting **inhaled beta agonist**
Mild Persistent	• Either **inhaled corticosteroid** (low dose) or cromolyn, nedocromil, antileukotriene, sustained-release theophylline	• Short-acting **inhaled beta agonist**
Intermittent	• None Needed	• Short-acting **inhaled beta agonist**

Asthma monitoring

Monitoring patient response to treatment is an essential part of pharmaceutical care. Indicators of patient response include:

- frequency of asthma symptoms
- frequency of asthma symptoms that awaken the patient from sleep (nocturnal symptoms)
- frequency of short-acting beta agonist use
- limitations on physical activity
- frequency of symptomatic doctor office and emergency room visits
- frequency of hospitalizations
- pulmonary function tests

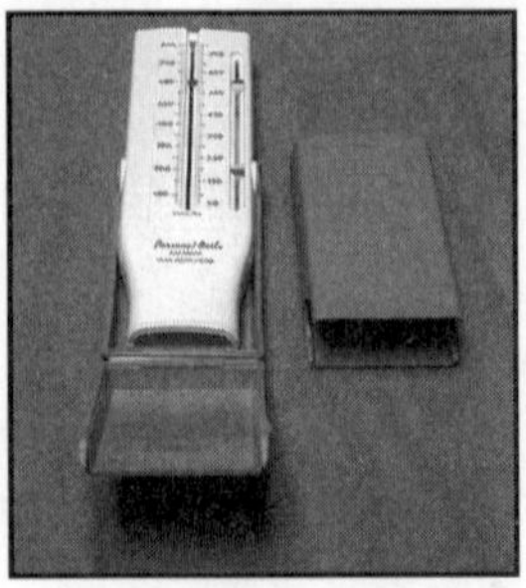

Example of a peak flow meter

Pulmonary function tests are done at the doctor's office with a spirometer or peak flow meter. Peak flow meters, a simple device available from many community pharmacies, are frequently used for home monitoring of peak expiratory flow rate (PEFR). The patient exhales forcefully and evaluates the PEFR value against a three-zone system of asthma management on a color coded scheme that uses a traffic light analogy (Table 2).

Table 2 Three-zone system of asthma management

Zone	Percent of personal best	Action
Green	>80% of patient personal best	Go! continue present activity and medication.
Yellow	50 - 80% of patient's personal best	Caution! may need additional medication. Take quick-relief medication and repeat PEFR in 15 minutes.
Red	<50% of patient's personal best	Stop! Take quick-relief medication and contact your doctor.

Chronic obstructive airway disease (COAD) treatment

The drug treatment for COAD depends on the severity. The more severe, the more aggressive the treatment. COAD severity is classified as episodic symptomatic, chronic mild, moderate, or severe. Patient severity is determined by symptom frequency, severity, and resistance to treatment, pulmonary function tests, activity limitations, and frequency and severity of acute episodes. The necessity for hospitalization during acute episodes is also considered. These same characteristics are used as long-term monitoring parameters. Table 3 is a summary of COAD treatment.

Table 3 Treatment of COAD

Disease severity	Drug treatment
Episodic Symptomatic	• Short-acting inhaled beta agonist as needed for symptoms
Chronic Mild	• Ipratropium bromide MDI, 3-6 puffs four times a day, and, • short-acting inhaled beta agonist as needed for symptoms
Chronic Moderate	• Ipratropium bromide MDI, 3-6 puffs four times a day; and, • Beta agonist on a regular schedule; and/or, • Sustained release theophylline; and, • short-acting inhaled beta agonist as needed for symptoms
Chronic Severe	• Ipratropium bromide MDI, 3-6 puffs four times a day; and, • Beta agonist on a regular schedule; and/or, • Sustained-release theophylline; and/or • Oral corticosteroids; and, • short-acting inhaled beta agonist as needed for symptoms

Drugs used to treat the common cold

Coughs and colds account for more time lost from work and school than all other diseases combined. A significant amount of money is spent annually on nonprescription cough and cold products. Colds are usually self-limiting viral infections causing inflammation of the upper respiratory tract. The inflammatory symptoms may involve the nose (rhinitis), throat (pharyngitis), larynx (laryngitis), or bronchi (bronchitis). Medicines are used according to the specific symptoms or patient complaints.

Respiratory system

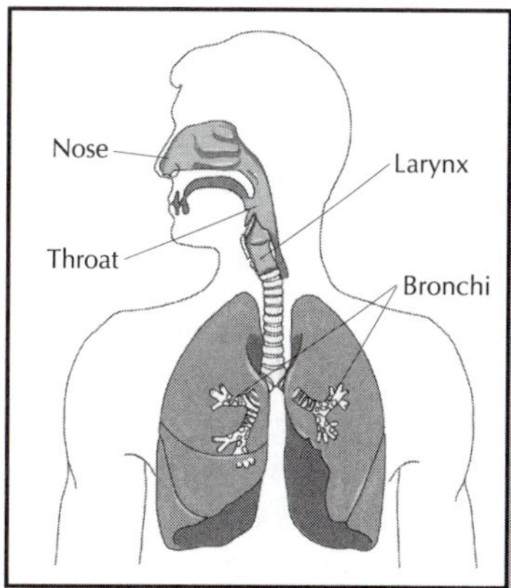

The surface of the nasal passages extending into the bronchi, are coated with a thin layer of mucus and lined with fine, hair-like cilia. The cilia constantly beat to sweep the mucus (along with any trapped particles) to the pharynx, moving mucus and debris downward from the nose and upward from the lungs to be expectorated (spit out) or swallowed.

Expectorants

Muco-ciliary clearance is one of the body's defenses against bacteria and viruses. Expectorants help in the removal of mucus by increasing the volume and decreasing the viscosity (thickness) of bronchial mucus. Guaifenesin (Robitussin®), available in a number of products, acts by irritating the gastric mucosa causing a reflex increase in respiratory tract secretions. The dose is variable, ranging from a maximum 600mg per day in children 2 to 6 years of age to 2,400mg per day in adults. Extra fluid intake (several glassfuls daily) is recommended to assist in better expectoration of mucus and debris.

Antitussives

Antitussive cough suppressants are used to reduce dry, hacking, nonproductive coughs. Antitussives are not used in productive (mucus being expectorated) or congested coughs. Three cough suppressants have FDA approval for this use: codeine, dextromethorphan (often referred to as DM in name brands), and diphenhydramine.

Codeine (Cheracol Syrup®, Robitussin AC Syrup®) is the standard against which other cough suppressants are measured. It works by depressing the cough center in the central nervous system, reducing the coughing reflex. The usual adult dose is 10mg to 20mg (less than the pain relieving dose of 30mg), not to exceed 120mg per day in adults. Antitussive action begins in about 30 minutes and lasts for three to eight hours. Codeine, as a narcotic drug, causes side effects of drowsiness, stomach pain, and constipation.

Dextromethorphan (Benylin Pediatric Syrup®), like codeine, works by depressing the cough center in the central nervous system, thereby reducing the coughing reflex. Dextromethorphan is found in many over-the-counter and prescription products. The usual dose is from 10mg to 30mg, not to exceed 120mg per day. Dextromethorphan does not have the side effects that are seen with narcotics. Dextromethorphan interacts with a group of drugs known as monoamine oxidase inhibitors (MAOI), resulting in an extreme rise in blood pressure. MAOIs include phenelzine (Nardil®), tranylcypromine (Parnate®), and selegiline (Eldepryl®).

Diphenhydramine has both antitussive action on the cough center of the central nervous system and antihistamine activity. A dose of 25mg to 50mg of diphenhydramine is equal to 15mg of codeine. Side effects include sedation and overdrying of the nose and mouth. The sedation is so pronounced that patients should be warned not to drive or operate hazardous machines while taking diphenhydramine.

Decongestants

Decongestants are used to treat the swelling or nasal stuffiness frequently associated with a cold. They act by causing vasoconstriction in the mucous membranes. Orally administered decongestants may cause side effects of increased blood pressure, heart arrhythmia, and increased blood glucose. These drugs must be used cautiously in patients with known hypertension, hyperthyroidism, diabetes or heart disease. Names of cold products often use the letter "D" to indicate that a decongestant is included. The two commonly used oral decongestants are pseudoephedrine (Sudafed®, Drixoral®) and phenylpropanolamine (Dimetapp®, Contac 12-Hour Cold Capsules®). However, in November 2000, the FDA issued a public health advisory on phenylpropanolamine concerning the risk of hemorrhagic stroke (bleeding into the brain) that has been associated with use of that medication. Shortly after issuing the advisory, the FDA began taking steps to remove phenylpropanolamine from all drug products and requested that all drug companies discontinue marketing products containing that drug.

Topical decongestants decrease the diameter of blood vessels and reduce nasal stuffiness. Available as drops, sprays, inhalers and gels, they act rapidly on the mucous membrane with only small amounts swallowed and absorbed systemically. While few systemic side effects occur with topical decongestants, congestion may rebound with prolonged use. This means that after several days of use, the vasoconstrictor effect subsides, causing an even more severe congestion or swelling. Topical decongestants should not be used for more than four days to avoid rebound. Some common decongestants include oxymetazoline (Neo-Synephrine 12-Hour Spray®), xylometazoline (Otrivin®), and naphazoline (Privine®).

Antihistamines

Histamine is a potent chemical found in body tissue. Histamine is stored in mast cells and basophils (white blood cells that are capable of ingesting foreign particles) located in the skin, respiratory tract, and GI tract. It is activated when it is released by tissue injury, infection, or allergic reaction. In colds, histamine causes a local inflammatory response from the cells injured by the invasion of virus particles. The released histamine causes blood vessels to dilate (congestion) and an increase in vascular permeability resulting in a "leakage" of fluid. In addition to congestion, the patient frequently complains of a runny nose due, in part, to the action of histamine. Antihistamines are useful in allergic rhinitis. Although they are present in many cold preparations, their efficacy has been questioned.

Table 4 Drugs used in respiratory diseases

Anticholinergic drugs
ipratropium (Atrovent®)

Beta adrenergic agonist
albuterol (Proventil®, Ventolin®)
bitolterol (Tornalate®)
pirbuterol (Maxair®)
salmeterol (Serevent®)

Bronchodilators
theophylline (TheoDur®, SloBID®, Slophyllin®)

Anti-inflammatory drugs

Corticosteroids
beclomethasone (Vanceril® inhaler)
budesonide (Pulmicort® inhaler)
flunisolide (AeroBid® inhaler)
fluticasone (Flovent® inhaler)
hydrocortisone [Solu-Cortef® (IV)]
methylprednisolone [Solu-Medrol® (IV)]
prednisone (Deltasone®)
triamcinolone (Azmacort® inhaler)

Antileukotrienes
montelukast (Singulair®)
zafirlukast (Accolate®)
zileuton (Zyflo®)

Other preventative therapy for asthma
cromolyn (Intal®)
nedocromil (Tilade® inhaler)

Expectorants
guaifenesin (Robitussin®)

Antitussives
codeine (Cheracol Syrup®, Robitussin® AC)
dextromethorphan ("DM," Robitussin® DM)
diphenhydramine (Benylin® Cough)

Decongestants
naphazoline (Privine® Nasal Spray)
oxymetazoline (Neo-Synephrine® 12-Hour Spray)
pseudoephedrine (Sudafed®, Drixoral®)
xylometazoline (Otrivin® Nasal Spray)

Antihistamines
cetirizine (Zyrtec®)
diphenhydramine (Benadryl®)
fexofenadine (Allegra®)
loratadine (Claritin®)

Conclusion

The severity of asthma and COAD will determine how a patient is treated for those diseases. Asthma patients need to be monitored to ensure the highest quality of life for persons living with that condition. Even though the common cold is self-limiting, adequately treating colds can reduce the number of school and work days lost due to this ailment.

About the authors

Paul J. Munzenberger received his bachelor's degree, master's degree and Doctor of Pharmacy degree from Wayne State University College of Pharmacy & Allied Health Professions in 1968, 1970, and 1971, respectively. Dr. Munzenberger is an Associate Professor of Pharmacy Practice at Wayne State University. His research has focused on pediatric pulmonary disease, including asthma and cystic fibrosis. Most recently, he has pursued the relationship of these diseases, treatments, and patient quality of life. Dr. Munzenberger has published a number of articles in medical and pharmacy journals. Currently, he serves as a referrer for several journals. Dr. Munzenberger has practiced at Children's Hospital of Michigan in Detroit for a number of years. He provides pharmaceutical care to patients with asthma and other pulmonary diseases. He is also a preceptor for an inpatient and outpatient pediatric experience. Dr. Munzenberger is responsible for the Pharm.D. students and pharmacy residents in these clinical sites. Dr. Munzenberger is a member of the American Pharmaceutical Association, Michigan Pharmacists Association, American Society of Health-System Pharmacists, and American College of Clinical Pharmacy. He is a board member of the American Lung Association of Michigan and the Detroit Asthma Coalition.

Beverly P. Kershaw is the assistant director of pharmacy at William Beaumont Hospital in Royal Oak, Michigan. Kershaw received both her bachelor's and master's degrees in pharmacy from Wayne State University in Detroit, Michigan. She has served as an officer and board member the Michigan Society of Health-System Pharmacists (MSHP), the Southeastern Michigan Society of Health-System Pharmacists, and the Macomb County Pharmacists Association, as well as on numerous professional committees. As a member of the American Society of Health-System Pharmacists, Kershaw served on the Council for Educational Affairs from 1999 through 2001.

Self assessment questions

1. The exchange of oxygen into the capillary blood occurs at the:
   a. trachea.
   b. bronchus.
   c. alveolar ducts.
   d. alveoli.

2. Which of the following is ***not*** a characteristic of asthma as defined by the Asthma Education Program, Expert Panel Report?
   a. Airway obstruction that is reversible either by itself or with treatment
   b. Airway inflammation
   c. Decreased airway responsiveness to various stimuli
   d. Increased airway responsiveness to various stimuli

3. First-line drug therapy to reduce airway obstruction due to inflammation in patients with asthma includes:
   a. beta agonists.
   b. theophylline.
   c. corticosteroids.
   d. antihistamines.

4. Which of the following is ***not*** a beta agonist?
   a. Albuterol
   b. Bitolterol
   c. Pirbuterol
   d. Zafirlukast

5. Which of the following drugs preserve mast cell function and prevent the inflammatory process from starting?
   a. Pirbuterol
   b. Cromolyn
   c. Zafirlukast
   d. Theophylline

6. A measurement of lung function which can be performed by patients at home is:
   a. Peak Expiratory Flow Rate.
   b. Peak Expiratory Filter Rate.
   c. Post Expiratory Force Rate.
   d. Positional Expiratory Flow Rate.

7. A drug which aids in the removal of mucus is called a(n):
   a. antitussive.
   b. expectorant.
   c. decongestant.
   d. corticosteroid.

8. Pseudoephedrine is classified as a(n):
   a. expectorant.
   b. antitussive.
   c. antihistamine.
   d. decongestant.

9. Which of the following may be a side effect of prolonged use of a topical decongestant?
   a. Sedation
   b. Rebound congestion
   c. Blurred vision
   d. Headaches

10. Drugs that are used to reduce dry, hacking, nonproductive coughs are called:
    a. antitussives.
    b. expectorants.
    c. decongestants.
    d. antihistamines.

CHAPTER

22

CANCER

Kathy Diener, Pharm.D.

Learning objectives

Upon completion of this chapter, the technician should be able to do the following:

- Define the word *cancer*.
- Identify the seven warning signs of cancer.
- Discuss proper technique and precautions that should be used in preparing and dispensing chemotherapy.
- Discuss the most common side effects associated with chemotherapy and discuss why these side effects occur.
- Discuss agents typically used in bone marrow transplantation and note the dosing implications of these agents.
- Identify chemotherapy agents that are typically given with an antidote.

Introduction

Cancer is perhaps the most-feared disease in the world because, after years of research and billions of dollars spent, a cure for many common cancers still eludes us. Cancer has been defined as a large group of diseases characterized by uncontrolled, rapid growth and the spread of abnormal cells. Finding a cure is complicated by the fact that there are more than 100 distinct types of cancer. Cancer cells are essentially our own body cells multiplying, growing, and using nutritional sources without heed to normal growth-controlling mechanisms. Because those cells are our own, the body does not set out to destroy them, even though they could be considered foreign and should be destroyed by the body's normal protective mechanisms.

Cancer can be treated by surgery, radiation, hormones, biologic therapy, and chemotherapy. We typically think first of chemotherapy, partly because of the fear of the many side effects seen with the administration of these agents. Most chemotherapy agents target rapidly dividing cells that can be either normal or malignant. This accounts for their activity against cancer, but also explains many of the side effects which involve normal cells that rapidly divide. These side effects include mouth sores, hair loss (alopecia), sterility, impotence, anemia, bleeding (due to decreased numbers of platelets), and infections (due to decreased numbers of white blood cells). The effects on the red and white blood cells and platelets is termed bone marrow depression. Side effects from chemotherapy can also be related to how the drug is cleared from the body. Thus patients receiving certain medications that are cleared by the kidney or metabolized in the liver should be closely monitored for damage to those organ systems. Other side effects commonly associated with chemotherapy include rash, fatigue, nausea, vomiting, diarrhea, weight loss, and anorexia (loss or lack of appetite). Research continues to find new drugs and techniques that can better differentiate between the cells, thereby enhancing the killing of cancer cells without harming normal cells. Antidotes for other commonly encountered side effects are also taking away some of the concerns of receiving cancer treatment.

Warning signs of cancer

Seven specific warning signs of cancer have been recognized. Even though a person may have one or more of these signs, it does not mean that they have cancer, but they should seek medical attention to rule out cancer. The word "caution" is the acronym for the seven warning signs. They are as follows:

C hange in bowel or bladder habits (greater than two weeks duration).
A sore that does not heal.
U nusual bleeding or discharge.
T hickening or lump in breast or other tissue.
I ndigestion or difficulty in swallowing.
O bvious change in a wart or mole.
N agging cough or hoarseness.

Alkylating agents

Alkylating agents (alkylators) bond to the parts of the cell that contain genetic material preventing the cell from further dividing. Because of the cancer cell's faster growth rate, these agents have a greater effect on cancer cells than normal cells. Once again, however, side effects commonly associated with chemotherapy administration occur with administration of alkylators because of the cytotoxic effects of these drugs on normal cells. Thus, alopecia, anemia, bleeding, and infections can occur. Other side effects common to many chemotherapy agents are also seen with alkylators, such as nausea, vomiting, diarrhea, nephrotoxicity, and hepatotoxicity. Side effects unique to alkylators include hearing loss associated with cisplatin (Platinol®), seizures associated with busulfan (Myleran®), lung damage associated with long-term busulfan use, hemorrhagic cystitis (bleeding from the bladder) associated with ifosfamide (Ifex®), confusion progressing to coma associated with ifosfamide, and cardiac toxicity associated with high-dose cyclophosphamide (Cytoxan®). These drugs are teratogenic, meaning they can cause cancers themselves.

Alkylating agents are a part of almost every chemotherapy regimen. They are used to treat various types of leukemia, multiple myeloma, non-Hodgkin's lymphomas, Hodgkin's disease, and testicular, ovarian, breast, and bladder cancer. Alkylating agents are often seen given in high-dose regimens prior to bone marrow transplantation. For example, a typical dose of busulfan for the treatment of chronic myelogenous leukemia is 4 to 6mg/m^2/day, which would result in a dose of 6.8-10.2mg for an average-sized patient, while the busulfan dose given prior to bone marrow transplantation is 4mg/*kg*/day, which would equal a dose of 280mg for that same patient. However, it is important to question any dose outside conventional limits or not documented to be correct.

Antimetabolites

All cells, cancer or normal, need nutrients to survive and reproduce. Certain cancer drugs may mimic a necessary nutrient or block a reaction which synthesizes a necessary nutrient. Drugs that do this are called antimetabolite drugs. Antimetabolites are utilized by both normal and cancerous cells. Since cancer cells generally have a faster growth rate, multiplying faster and taking up more nutrients than normal cells, the antimetabolite drug is more effective on the cancerous cells. However, the nutrient disruption to the normal cells is enough to cause severe side effects which can limit treatment. Other side effects seen with antimetabolites can include severe hepatotoxicity and nephrotoxicity. Damage to the kidneys is due to the drug crystallizing in the kidney. To keep crystals from forming, large quantities of intravenous fluids are given.

Methotrexate (Rheumatrex®) is often given directly into the central nervous system (intrathecally). Side effects associated with intrathecal methotrexate can include anything from headaches to infections to seizures or coma. Intrathecal methotrexate should always be prepared with preservative-free diluents and the dose should be carefully checked. Overdoses of intrathecal methotrexate are common and the damage is typically irreversible. Vincristine (Oncovin®), a mitotic inhibitor (this class of drugs is discussed later in this chapter), is often given to children with leukemia on the same day they receive intrathecal methotrexate. These two drugs are both dispensed in syringes and could be mistaken for each other. Vincristine given intrathecally is always fatal. Thus, the syringes containing the drugs should never be dispensed together and labels should always be double-checked.

Certain chemotherapy protocols call for the use of massive amounts of antimetabolite drugs to be given over a short period of time in hopes of killing off the cancer cells, with an antidote drug given immediately thereafter to try to spare the body's normal cells. An example of this is the use of high dose methotrexate with a rescue "antidote" of leucovorin calcium (Wellcorvin®).

Hormone therapy

Hormone therapy, or endocrine therapy, may be used to treat hormone-dependent cancers. In other words, this type of therapy can be used to counteract the effect of the body's own hormones which may make a certain cancer grow. For example, tamoxifen (Nolvadex®) works in breast cancer by blocking the effect of estrogen, which can make certain breast cancers grow.

Side effects of these agents are often associated with the effect a certain hormone would normally have on the body, or the side effects may be similar to what would happen if certain hormones were taken away. For example, some drugs used to treat prostate cancer result in the body no longer being able to produce testosterone. Thus, a man who is receiving treatment for his prostate cancer with such a drug may experience hot flashes, impotence, loss of sex drive (libido), and breast enlargement (gynecomastia). Other side effects may include nausea, vomiting, diarrhea, alopecia, headache, weight gain or loss, rash, irregular menses, thrombophlebitis (inflammation of the wall of a vein that is associated with blood clots), and fluid retention.

Antibiotic type

Antibiotic type agents are capable of disrupting cellular functions. Although antibiotic types have different mechanisms of action, they primarily interfere with the cell DNA replication.

In addition to side effects commonly seen with chemotherapy such as nausea, vomiting, alopecia, and bone marrow depression, antibiotic type agents have some unique and important side effects. The most deadly and debilitating is toxicity to the heart (cardiac toxicity) that can occur with doxorubicin (Rubex®). Chances of cardiac toxicity occurring are greater when increased drug dosages are given. For example, a person who has received 600mg/m^2 of doxorubicin has a greater chance of developing cardiac toxicity than a person who has received only 300mg/m^2. Other risk factors for developing cardiac toxicity include a patient's present cardiac status, the age of the patient, and the length of the infusion (longer infusions, less toxicity). Another toxicity associated with these agents is the severe skin reaction if the drug is infused outside the vein (extravasation) by accident. A harmless side effect may occur when the drugs are cleared from the body by the kidney—the urine changes color. For example, doxorubicin and daunorubicin can change the urine red to orange in color, and mitoxantrone (Mutamycin®) can change the urine to a dark blue color.

Mitotic inhibitors

Mitotic inhibitors have an effect on cancer cells by arresting a step in the cell cycle. Thus, they "freeze" the cell at a certain point of division.

In addition to common side effects seen with all chemotherapy such as bone marrow depression, these agents also have an effect on different parts of the nervous system. They can cause constipation by affecting nerves which act on the gastrointestinal system, and they may cause numbness and tingling of the hands and feet by affecting those nerves. One of the most common side effects associated with newer mitotic inhibitors such as paclitaxel (Taxol®) is severe allergic reactions which are prevented by giving such drugs as diphenhydramine (Benadryl®), dexamethasone (Decadron®), and cimetidine (Tagamet®). Paclitaxel can also cause cardiac arrhythmias (irregular heart beats). These arrhythmias are usually not noticed by the patient (asymptomatic), but once documented, the patient typically is not given the drug again.

Topoisomerase inhibitors

Topoisomerase inhibitors kill cancer cells by causing a break in DNA, thus stopping DNA copying for new cells. One new agent in this category is irinotecan (Camptosar®), which is used in the treatment of colon cancer. The primary side effect seen with this agent is severe diarrhea. Other side effects commonly seen with chemotherapy administration are often seen with these agents.

Radiopharmaceuticals

Radiopharmaceuticals destroy cancerous cells directly by emitting radiation on exposed tissue. Only specialized, nuclear pharmacies would dispense radiopharmaceuticals.

Side effects which have been associated with radiopharmaceuticals might include bone pain, bone marrow depression, anemia, radiation sickness (nausea and vomiting), rash, hives, itching, temporary hair thinning, and abdominal cramping.

Miscellaneous antineoplastics

There are other cancer agents that cannot be classified in one of the above categories. Their mechanisms of action are unique from other agents. Common side effects of these agents are similar to other chemotherapeutic drugs and might include nausea, vomiting, alopecia, diarrhea, abdominal cramping, etc.

Antineoplastic adjuncts

Some drugs are used in conjunction with chemotherapeutic agents to minimize the toxic effects they can exert upon normal cell tissue. These agents include mesna (Mesnex®), which is used with ifosfamide to treat hemorragic cystitis (inflammation of the bladder); amifostine (Ethyol®), which is used with cisplatin to treat renal toxicity; and dexrazoxane (Zinecard®), which is used with doxorubicin to prevent cardiomyopathy (a chronic disorder of the heart).

Precautions surrounding cancer medications

Special precautions should be used in the preparation of any cancer medication. Intravenous cancer medications should be prepared in a vertical laminar flow hood using proper technique and precautions, such as wearing chemoprotective gowns and gloves. (See Chapter 27 for further discussion of how to prepare chemotherapy treatments.) Oral agents should not be handled without gloves. Cancer medications dispensed for use outside the hospital should be packaged in child-proof containers. Directions for administration should be followed exactly. All medications, but especially cancer medications, should be taken only by the individual for whom they are prescribed and should be kept out of children's reach.

Table 1 Drugs used to treat cancer

Alkylating agents (alkylators)
busulfan (Myleran®)
carboplatin (Paraplatin®)
carmustine (BiCNU®)
chlorambucil (Leukeran®)
cisplatin (Platinol®)
cyclophosphamide (Cytoxan®, Neosar®)
estramustine (Emcyt®)
ifosfamide (IFEX®)
lomustine (CeeNu®)
mechlorethamine, also called nitrogen mustard (Mustargen®)
melphalan (Alkeran®)
streptozocin (Zanosar®)
thiotepa (Thioplex®)
uracil mustard (Uracil Mustard®)

Antimetabolites
cytarabine also commonly called ARA-C (Cytarabine®, Cytosar-U®)
floxuridine (Floxuridine®, FUDR®)
5-Fluorouracil also commonly called 5-FU (Fluorouracil®, Adrucil®)
fludarabine (Fludara®)
hydroxyurea (Hydrea®)
mercaptopurine (Purinethol®)
methotrexate (Methotrexate®, Rheumatrex®, Folex®)
pentostatin (Nipent®)
thioguanine (Thioguanine®)

Hormones
aminoglutethimide
anastrozole (Arimidex®)
bicalutamide (Casodex®)
diethylstilbestrol (Stilphostrol®)
flutamide (Eulexin®)
goserelin (Zoladex®)
irinotecan (Camptosar®)
leuprolide (Lupron®)
medroxyprogesterone (Depo-Provera®)
megestrol (Megestrol®, Megace®)
mitotane (Lysodren®)
nilutamide (Nilandron®, Anandron®)
polyestradiol (Estradurin®)
tamoxifen (Nolvadex®)
testolactone (Teslac®)
topotecan (Hycamtin®)

Antibiotic type
bleomycin (Blenoxane®)
dactinomycin (Cosmegen®)
daunorubicin (DaunoXome®)
doxorubicin (Doxorubicin®, Rubex®, Adriamycin®, Doxil®)
idarubicin (Idamycin®)
mitomycin (Mutamycin®)
mitoxantrone (Novantrone®)
plicamycin (Mithracin®)

Mitotic inhibitors
docetaxel (Taxotere®)
paclitaxel (Taxol®)
teniposide (Vumon®)
vinorelbine (Navelbine®)
vincristine (Vincristine®, Oncovin®, Vincasar PFS®)
vinblastine (Vinblastine®, Velban®)

Radiopharmaceuticals
chromic phosphate P 32 (Phosphocol P 32®)
sodium iodide I 131 (Sodium Iodide I 131®, Iodotope®)
sodium phosphate P 32 (Sodium Phosphate P 32®)
strontium-89 chloride (Metastron®)

Topoisomerase inhibitors
etoposide, also commonly called VP-16 (VePesid®)
irinotecan (Camptosar®)
topotecan (Hycamtin®)

Miscellaneous antineoplastics
aldesleukin, also commonly called interleukin-2 (Proleukin®)
altretamine (Hexalen®)
asparaginase (Elspar®)
cladribine (Leustatin®)
dacarbazine (DTIC-Dome®)
gemcitabine (Gemzar®)
hydroxyurea (Hydrea®)
interferon ALFA-2a (Roferon-A®)
interferon ALFA-2b (Intron A®)
interferon ALFA-n3 (Alferon N®)
levamisole (Ergamisol®)
mitotane (Lysodren®)
pegaspargase (Oncaspar®)
porfimer sodium (Photofrin®)
procarbazine (Matulane®)
tretinoin (Vesanoid®)

Antineoplastic adjuncts
amifostine (Ethyol®)
dexrazoxane (Zinecard®)
mesna (MESNEX®)

Conclusion

While cancer is a very common disease, there are numerous ways it can be treated. Treatment is more successful when the cancer is detected early; therefore, knowing the warning signs of cancer is important. Medications used to treat cancer can prevent cancer cells from dividing, stop the cells while they are dividing, kill the cancer cells, or have other unique mechanisms of action. Proper handling of cancer medications can ensure the safety for the technician and the patient.

Acknowledgment

The author and publisher wish to acknowledge Beverly P. Kershaw, Pharm.M.S., for her extensive contributions to this chapter in the previous edition of this manual.

Bibliography

Perry, M.C., The Chemotherapy Source Book, 2nd edition, Williams & Wilkins, Baltimore, MD, 1997.

Pharmacy Certified Technician Training Manual, 7th edition, Michigan Pharmacists Association, Lansing, MI, 1997, pp. 197-210.

About the author

Kathy Diener received both her bachelor's of science degree in pharmacy and her Doctor of Pharmacy degree from Ferris State University College of Pharmacy in Big Rapids, Michigan. After obtaining her Pharm.D., she completed a specialty residency in hematology/oncology at the University of Texas M.D. Anderson Cancer Center. Dr. Diener is currently employed as a Clinical Scientist in Oncology for Pfizer Global Research and Development, and holds Adjunct Faculty Appointments at Ferris State University, the University of Michigan, and Wayne State University colleges of pharmacy. Prior to this position, she was a clinical pharmacist/clinical assistant professor at the University of Michigan Hospitals and College of Pharmacy, specializing in adult oncology. Dr. Diener has also held a position as a specialist in bone marrow transplantation at Harper Hospital in Detroit, Michigan. She has authored several articles and continuing education modules dealing with oncology practice and has delivered multiple lectures related to oncology to various professional and non-professional groups.

Self-assessment questions

1. Which of the following is true of cancer?
   a. Cancer is a disease characterized by uncontrolled growth and spread of abnormal cells.
   b. Cancer cannot be treated by surgery.
   c. All cancers have a cure.
   d. Cancer has five specific warning signs.

2. All of the following are warning signs of cancer *except*:
   a. unusual bleeding or discharge.
   b. obvious changes in a wart or mole.
   c. nagging or persistent headache.
   d. thickening or lump in breast or other tissue.

3. Chemotherapy given intravenously should be prepared in a:
   a. horizontal laminar air flow hood, wearing special protective gear, such as gowns and gloves.
   b. vertical laminar flow hood, wearing chemoprotective gowns and gloves.
   c horizontal laminar air flow hood reserved for chemotherapy preparation, and the individual preparing the chemotherapy should wear gloves.
   d. patient's room, at the bedside to ensure stability of the compound.

4. All of the following are side effects of chemotherapy *except*:
   a. weight loss.
   b. nausea.
   c. constipation.
   d. hair growth.

5. You notice that a patient who has just been admitted to the hospital is to start receiving oral busulfan 70mg every 6 hours, starting tomorrow at 6 a.m. You also note that oral busulfan is only supplied in 2mg tablets, leading you to:
   a. assume this is a bone marrow transplantation patient, since this is such a high dose, and proceed to fill the prescription as it was written.
   b. conclude this is an error and ask the pharmacist to contact the physician writing the order.
   c. check the patient profile and other orders to verify this is a bone marrow transplant patient, and once this is verified, dispense the medication.
   d. assume the physician had meant to write for intravenous busulfan, and ask the pharmacist to make the change in the formulation.

6. Which of the following medications bonds to the parts of the cell that contain genetic material, which prevents the cell from further dividing?
   a. Myleran®
   b. Tamoxifen®
   c. Taxol®
   d. Rubex®

7. The appropriate antidote for ifosamide is:
   a. eucovorin
   b. amifostine
   c. dexrazoxane
   d. mesna

8. The appropriate antidote for methotrexate is:
   a. leucovorin
   b. amifostine
   c. dexrazoxane
   d. mesna

9. The appropriate antidote for cisplatin is:
   a. leucovorin
   b. amifostine
   c. dexrazoxane
   d. mesna

10. The appropriate antidote for doxorubicin is:
   a. leucovorin
   b. amifostine
   c. dexrazoxane
   d. mesna

CHAPTER
23

INFECTIONS

Mark Weiss, Pharm.D.

Learning objectives

Upon completion of this chapter, the technician should be able to do the following:

- Define *infection, microorganisms,* and *anti-infective agents.*
- Explain how aminoglycoside dosage is adjusted.
- Explain the generation classification for cephalosporins.
- Compare the benefits of azithromycin to erythromycin.
- Explain the various classifications of penicillins.
- Explain common indications for sulfonamides and tetracyclines.
- Explain the place of fluoroquinolones in contemporary antibiotic therapy.
- Explain the advantages and disadvantages of vancomycin therapy.
- Discuss the carbapenems.
- Explain common indications for fluconazole and amphotericin B.
- Discuss the antiviral medications acyclovir and valacyclovir.

Introduction

Infections result when microorganisms in body tissues or fluids begin to damage the body, produce symptoms, and evoke an immune response from the host.[1] Microorganisms that cause infections include bacteria, mycobacteria, fungi, protozoa, and viruses. Some microorganisms are present in our environment but do not infect humans. Other microorganisms are normal inhabitants of our bodies, or may be residing within the body without causing any harm (colonization). When the microorganism begins to do damage and an immune response is triggered, an infection results and the organism is called a pathogen or has become pathogenic. The microorganism causing an infection may be identified microscopically with the aid of stains (the gram stain being most common) and by growing colonies of the organism in laboratory cultures. Then, a variety of drugs are tested against the organism in the culture (sensitivity testing) to find effective agents that will eradicate the microorganism. Antibiotics may be started empirically (before the pathogen is identified), based on clinical experience suggesting that a drug will be effective.

Drugs to prevent or treat infections

Anti-infective drugs from natural substances are called antibiotics and those from synthetic substances are called antimicrobials. These terms are often used interchangeably. They work by suppressing the growth (bacteriostatic) or by killing (bacteriocidal) the bacteria. These drugs vary in effectiveness against bacteria, and their spectrum of activity refers to the group of bacteria that is vulnerable (susceptible) to the drugs. Broad-spectrum drugs affect a wide variety of bacteria, and narrow-spectrum affect only a few.

A combination of anti-infectives may be used when there is synergy (two agents more effective together than either alone) between the agents, when there are multiple pathogens present, or to treat a highly resistant pathogen (poor sensitivity to any one drug). The patient may be assessed for response to the anti-infective by monitoring for a reduction in fever, white blood cell count (WBC), reduction in pain and inflammation, or improvement in x-ray findings. Anti-infectives used to treat bacterial infections include aminoglycosides, cephalosporins, erythromycins, penicillins, sulfonamides, tetracyclines, fluorquinolones, vancomycin, and carbapenems. Antifungal agents include fluconazole and amphotericin B. The most common antiviral agents are acylovir and valacyclovir.

Aminoglycosides

Aminoglycoside antibiotics are bacteriocidal (they kill bacteria) and are most effective against gram-negative bacteria (identified by the gram staining process), causing infection of the blood (sepsis), lung (pneumonia), brain (meningitis), abdomen (peritonitis), or urinary tract. The aminoglycosides include streptomycin, amikacin, gentamicin, and tobramycin. Streptomycin is sometimes used in treating tuberculosis,[2] while the other aminoglycosides are commonly used in hospitals. They are primarily given by intravenous (IV) administration and pharmacists may provide assistance in calculating the right dose for the individual patient. The dose is calculated based on the patient's height, weight, age, kidney function, and seriousness of the infection. Further dose adjustments are based on blood levels immediately after drug infusion (peak level) and just before the next dose (trough level). Adjusting the dose is important not only to achieve an effective dose, but also to avoid loss of hearing (ototoxicity) or damage to the kidneys (nephrotoxicity). Aminoglycosides are often combined with other antibiotics to expand the spectrum of microorganism coverage and/or to achieve a synergistic effect against those microorganisms.

Cephalosporins

These agents are often called beta-lactam antibiotics because their chemical structure includes a beta-lactam ring (a characteristic molecular feature of penicillins and cephalosporins). Some bacteria have learned to resist these agents by producing an enzyme (beta-lactamase) which destroys the beta-lactam ring of the molecule. Cephalosporins are used for infections of the respiratory tract, skin, bones, joints, and urinary tract. Cephalosporins are bacteriocidal and are classified into four generations based on their spectrum of activity. First-generation cephalosporins are most active against gram-positive bacteria (streptococcal or staphylococcal) and may be alternatives to penicillin in penicillin-allergic patients. However, a few patients allergic to penicillins will also be allergic to the cephalosporins. Second-generation cephalosporins are active against bacteria covered by first-generation agents with added gram-negative coverage. The second-generation cephalosporins are ideal for infections caused by multiple organisms (polymicrobic) such as foot ulcers, some pneumonias, and pelvic and intra-abdominal infections. Third-generation cephalosporins have an even wider spectrum of activity and are effective for some cases of meningitis, pneumonia, and other severe infections. A fourth-generation cephalosporin (cefepime) features enhanced activity (vs. the third-generation drugs) against certain gram-negative organisms and the gram-positive organisms.[3]

Cephalosporins are very safe, available for both oral and IV administration, widely prescribed, and have a high dollar cost. Cephalosporins cause few adverse effects, but they can cause diarrhea, vomiting, oral thrush or kidney toxicity. Patients who have had only mild skin reactions to penicillin may be cautiously given cephalosporins.[4]

Erythromycins (macrolides)

Erythromycins are bacteriocidal or bacteriostatic against many gram positive microbes, as well as *Mycoplasma* and *Legionella* (in legionnaires' disease). Oral products include erythromycin (Emycin®, Ery-Tab®), erythromycin ethylsuccinate (EES®, Pediamycin®), and erythromycin stearate (Erythrocin®).

The IV products are erythromycin gluceptate or lactobionate. The erythromycins are good alternatives to penicillin in penicillin-allergic patients. While serious adverse effects are rare, nausea, vomiting, and abdominal cramping can be bothersome with all forms. Transient hearing loss has occurred with prolonged, high dosages. Erythromycins interact with other drugs, causing toxic concentrations of the target drug (e.g., theophylline, felodipine, nicardipine, nifedipine, cyclosporin, and simvastatin).

Clarithromycin (Biaxin®) and azithromycin (Zithromax®), although similar in antimicrobial spectrum to erythromycin, are effective against some organisms not covered by erythromycin. They are generally better tolerated (little nausea/vomiting/cramping) and cost more than erythromycin. Clarithromycin often causes a bad taste sensation. It is taken for 10 days, the same as erythromycin. Azithromycin is unique in its dosing. It is taken (on an empty stomach) twice daily on the first day of treatment and then once daily for the next four days, for a total of five days of treatment. Azithromycin concentrates in tissue and is effective for approximately 10 days.

Penicillins

Penicillins are bacteriocidal and have a beta-lactam ring in their structure like cephalosporins. Penicillins are either naturally occurring or semisynthetic. Penicillins are classified based on spectrum of activity. Natural penicillin (Penicillin G) is available for IV, IM, and oral use, although the semisynthetic Penicillin V is more often used orally. They are highly effective for pharyngitis, sinusitis, otitis (ear infection), syphilis, and soft tissue and respiratory infections. Many bacteria have become resistant to natural penicillin by producing an enzyme, penicillinase or beta-lactamase, to destroy it.

A group of penicillins is not destroyed by penicillinase, which includes nafcillin, dicloxacillin, and others. These enzyme-resistant drugs may be used for staphylococcal infections when natural penicillin is not effective. While less potent than natural penicillin, they are bacteriocidal and fast-acting in susceptible bacteria.

Aminopenicillins are semisynthetic drugs and have a wider spectrum than natural penicillins. These are often used for upper respiratory infections, urinary tract infections and otitis media. Amoxicillin is more popular than ampicillin because it causes less diarrhea, and is normally given two or three times a day instead of every six hours. The spectrum of activity is enhanced when a beta-lactamase inhibitor like clavulanic acid is added to amoxicillin (Augmentin®) or sulbactam is added to ampicillin (Unasyn®).

Extended-spectrum penicillins (e.g., piperacillin) are further modified to enhance effectiveness against very pathogenic bacteria such as *Pseudomonas,* which is often a hospital-acquired infection. These are given by IV administration for serious infections such as sepsis and pneumonia.

Sulfonamides

These were the first drugs that successfully cured bacterial infections in humans. Sulfonamides are bacteriostatic. Sulfamethoxazole is most often prescribed in a combination with trimethoprim, commonly called TMP-SMZ. There is renewed interest in this combination to treat and prevent *pneumocystis carinii* pneumonia (associated with acquired immunodeficiency syndrome [AIDS]) and for other infections where the bacteria have again become sensitive to sulfonamides. The trimethoprim-sulfamethoxazole combination is used to treat upper respiratory tract infections, urinary tract infections, pneumonia, prostatitis, and otitis media. It is available for IV or oral administration. Sulfonamides are known to interact with other drugs, causing increased concentrations of warfarin or phenytoin, and may result in severe sunburn if the patient uses a sunlamp or gets too much sunlight. Sulfonamides are well tolerated, but skin rashes are common. TMP-SMZ is available generically and is quite low in cost.

Tetracyclines

The broad-spectrum tetracyclines are bacteriostatic and are among the most commonly prescribed antibacterials in the world, although they are rarely considered the drugs of choice for common infections. Tetracycline HCl (Achromycin®, Sumycin®), although popular some years ago, is seldom prescribed today. The most commonly used tetracyclines are doxycycline (Vibramycin®) and minocycline (Minocin®). These agents are used for upper respiratory tract infections, skin conditions, and certain sexually transmitted diseases. They are well tolerated with few adverse reactions or interactions. Absorption of tetracyclines is drastically reduced by intake of dairy products, iron preparations, and antacids, so these products should be avoided. Tetracyclines are not recommended for children under eight years of age or for pregnant patients. Patients should be cautioned to avoid unnecessary exposure to sunlight. Another tetracycline derivative, demeclocycline (Declomycin®), is not commonly used as an antibiotic but is used in a fluid imbalance condition called "Syndrome of Inappropriate Antidiuretic Hormone Secretion" (SIADH).

Fluoroquinolones

The fluroquinolones are highly active, bacteriocidal agents used against a wide variety of pathogens. They are not recommended in children less than 18 years of age. Norfloxacin (Noroxin®) is used for urinary tract infections. Ciprofloxacin (Cipro®), ofloxacin (Floxin®), and levofloxacin (Levaquin®) are used for prostatitis, urinary tract infections, traveler's diarrhea, bone and joint infections, respiratory tract infections, skin and soft tissue infections, and to prevent infections in patients with dangerously low white blood counts. These agents are well absorbed, resulting in similar blood concentrations with oral or IV administration. Patients should be advised to avoid taking these agents within four hours of antacids, iron preparations, or multivitamins containing iron or zinc because the fluoroquinolones will bind with those medications and, therefore, the body will be unable to absorb those medications. The most recently introduced fluoroquinolones, gatifloxacin (Tequin®) and moxifloxacin (Avelox®), may offer better coverage of certain gram-positive and anaerobic (don't require oxygen to grow) organisms.[5,6]

Vancomycin

Vancomycin (Vancocin®) is very poorly absorbed, and if it is given orally, it is intended to treat diarrhea-causing bacteria in the gastrointestinal tract. The dose is small, 125mg given every six hours. Vancomycin is given intravenously to treat systemic infections in higher doses such as 1,000mg every 12 hours. The dose of vancomycin needs to be adjusted for renal dysfunction, and as with aminoglycosides, pharmacists may assist in determining the appropriate dose. Vancomycin works slowly to damage the cell wall of the bacteria, which allows the body's natural defenses to attack and eradicate the bacteria.

Vancomycin is widely used even though bacteriocidal agents would work faster. It works well with aminoglycosides, is well tolerated, is a good alternative to penicillin in penicillin-allergic patients, and is effective against organisms like certain *Staphylococcus* species that have become resistant to penicillins and cephalosporins. Because some bacteria (e.g., *Enterococcus*) are now becoming resistant to vancomycin, the U.S. Centers for Disease Control and Prevention (CDC) in Atlanta, Georgia, has issued guidelines to reduce the use of vancomycin to retain its effectiveness. Many hospital pharmacists are evaluating patients to help determine if another agent could be used in place of vancomycin.

While some patients are truly allergic to vancomycin, there is a common symptom complex (Red Man Syndrome) that may occur when vancomycin is too concentrated or is infused intravenously too fast. The patient may experience flushing which gives the appearance of a red neck, sensation of heat, and scalp itching, all of which subside by slowing the rate of infusion or treating with diphenhydramine (Benadryl®).

Carbapenems

Imipenem-cilastin (Primaxin®) and meropenem (Merrem®) are very broad-spectrum antibiotics, effective against gram-positive, gram-negative, and anaerobic organisms. They contain a beta-lactam ring structure (like penicillins and cephalosporins) and are given by the IV route. These agents are used primarily for complex infections in hospitalized patients. Cilastin is given with imipenem to prevent enzyme inactivation of imipenem. Imipenem has been associated with nausea, vomiting, tremors and even seizures with high doses or in patients with renal dysfunction. Meropenem may have less seizure potential and is indicated for certain types of meningitis in pediatric patients. Patients who are allergic to penicillin or cephalosporins may be allergic to the carbapenems as well.

Table 1 Selected anti-infective agents

Aminoglycosides
amikacin (Amikin®)
gentamicin (Garamycin®)
tobramycin (Nebcin®)

Cephalosporins

First generation
cefadroxil (Duricef®)*
cephalexin (Keflex®)*
cefazolin (Ancef®, Kefzol®)

Second generation
cefaclor (Ceclor®)*
cefprozil (Cefzil®)*
cefuroxime axetil (Ceftin®)*
cefuroxime (Zinacef®)
cefpodoxime (Vantin®)*
loracarbef (Lorabid®)*

Third generation
cefixime (Suprax®)*
cefotetan (Cefotan®)
cefotaxime (Claforan®)
ceftazidime (Fortaz®)
ceftizoxime (Cefizox®)

Macrolides
axithromycin (Zithromax)
clarithromycin (Biaxin)
erythromycin (Emycin, Ery-Tab)
erythromycin ethylsuccinate (EES, Pediamycin)
erythromycin stearate (Eythrocin)

Penicillins

Natural penicillins
penicillin G potassium
penicillin V potassium (PenVeeK®)*

Penicillins (continued)

Penicillinase-resistant
cloxacillin (Tegopen®)*
dicloxacillin (Dynapen®)*
oxacillin (Prostaphlin®)*
nafcillin (Nafcil®)*

Aminopenicillins
amoxicillin* (Amoxil®, Trimox®)
ampicillin*(Principen®, Omnipen®)

Extended spectrum penicillins
piperacillin (Pipracil®)
piperacillin/tazobactam (Zosyn®)
ticarcillin (Ticar®)
ticarcillin clavulanate (Timentin®)

Sulfonamides
TMP-SMZ (Bactrim®, Septra®)
sulfisoxazole/erythromycin (Pediazole®)*

Tetracyclines
doxycycline (Vibramycin®)*
minocycline (Minocin®)*
tetracycline HCl (Achromycin®, Sumycin®)*

Fluoroquinolones
ciprofloxacin (Cipro®)*
gatifloxacin (Tequin®)*
levofloxacin (Levaquin®)*
moxifloxacin (Avelox®)*
norfloxacin (Noroxin®)*
ofloxacin (Floxin®)*

Miscellaneous antibiotics
imipenem-cilastin (Primaxin®)
meropenem (Merrem®)
vancomycin (Vancocin)*

*Available as oral dose form

Antifungals

The pathogenic fungi comprise a wide array of microorganisms, commonly classified as either yeasts or molds. Systemic fungal infections occur much more commonly in immunocompromised patients or those on long-term antibiotic therapy. Localized fungal infections, such as of the skin or vaginal mucosa, are quite common.

For the treatment of serious, life-threatening systemic fungal infections, amphotericin B (Amphocin®) remains the agent of choice. It is administered by the IV route. The use of amphotericin B is limited by its broad range of serious toxicities including electrolyte imbalances, renal toxicity, anemia, anorexia, and a flu-like syndrome consisting of fever, chills, headache, and generalized malaise (a feeling of not being in good health). In an attempt to reduce these toxicities, several formulations of amphotericin B in association with a lipid (fat) phase have been developed.

The "azole" antifungals, such as fluconazole (Diflucan®), are effective, well tolerated and much safer than amphotericin B. For these reasons, many clinicians now choose fluconazole when a localized or systemic fungal infection is suspected. Fluconazole is well absorbed and may be given orally or by the IV route. The most common adverse effects are headache, rash, nausea, vomiting, and diarrhea. Fluconazole may decrease the effectiveness of oral contraceptives; alternative contraceptive measures are advised while taking fluconazole. Fluconazole may increase the effect of other drugs such as warfarin, phenytoin, and theophylline. Fluconazole is approved for the treatment of vaginal candidiasis (a localized fungal infection) as a single, 150mg oral dose.

Antivirals

Viruses are microorganisms incapable of replicating independently; they must harness the cellular machinery of a host, instructing the host cells to produce more virus particles. Numerous viruses are capable of causing infections. Some of the more common and well known are the varicella group (chicken pox, shingles), herpes group (genital herpes), and the retroviruses (human immunodeficiency virus [HIV]). Viruses, unlike bacteria or fungi, are often not eradicated by drug therapy. Their replication and ability to cause disease, however, can be controlled by antiviral agents.

Acyclovir (Zovirax®) and valacyclovir (Valtrex®) are antiviral agents commonly encountered in pharmacy practice. Valacyclovir is absorbed orally to a much greater extent than acyclovir, and is almost immediately converted to acyclovir in the body. It is available only as an oral tablet. Acyclovir is available for IV, oral, or topical use. Both agents are used to treat infections caused by the herpes group, while acyclovir may be used to treat varicella zoster (chicken pox) in older children and adults, as well as life-threatening viral infections such as herpes simplex encephalitis. Although quite well tolerated, some of the more common adverse effects of these agents include headache, rash, dizziness, and nausea.

Conclusion

Technicians should know the classifications and the benefits of therapy with anti-infective agents. Having a good understanding of the various types of anti-infective agents will allow the pharmacy technician to aid in the distributive process, as well as in the identification of potential allergies in patients.

Acknowledgment

The author and publisher with to acknowledge Beverly P. Kershaw, Pharm.M.S., for her extensive contributions to this chapter in the previous edition of this manual.

References

1. Rybak, M.J., Aeschlimann, J.R., Laboratory Tests to Direct Antimicrobial Pharmacotherapy, Pharmacotherapy, Stamford, CT, Appleton and Lange, 1999, p. 1598.

2. American Thoracic Society, Treatment of Tuberculosis and Tuberculosis Infection in Adults and Children, *American Journal of Respiratory Critical Care Medicine*, 1994, pp. 1623-33.
3. Gilbert, D.N., Moellering Jr., R.C., Sande, M.A., editors, Features of 1st, 2nd, 3rd, 4th Generation Cephalosporins, The Sanford Guide to Antimicrobial Therapy, 1999, p. 55.
4. Dipiro, J.T., Schlesselman, L.S., Allergic and Pseudoallergic Drug Reactions, Pharmacotherapy, Stamford, CT, Appleton and Lange, 1999, pp. 1398-99.
5. Anonymous, AHFS firstFAX-gatifloxacin, *American Journal of Health-System Pharmacy*, Vol. 57, pp. 1125-26, 2000.
6. Anonymous, AHFS firstFAX-moxifloxacin, *American Journal of Health-System Pharmacy*, Vol. 57, pp. 1126-27, 2000.

Bibliography

Dipiro, J.T., et al., Pharmacotherapy, Stamford, CT, Appleton and Lange, 1999.

Gilbert, D.N., Moellering Jr., R.C., Sande, M.A., The Sanford Guide to Antimicrobial Therapy, Antimicrobial Therapy Inc., Hyde Park, VT, 1999.

Lacy, C.F., Armstrong, L.L., Goldman, M.P., Lance, L.L., Drug Information Handbook, 7th edition, Lexi-Comp Inc., Hudson, OH, 1999.

Pharmacy Certified Technician Training Manual, 7th edition, Michigan Pharmacists Association, Lansing, MI, 1997, pp. 191-196.

About the author

Mark Weiss received his bachelor's of science in pharmacy from the University of Michigan College of Pharmacy in 1978 and his Doctor of Pharmacy from the University of Illinois at Chicago in 1997. Dr. Weiss is a clinical pharmacist at Sparrow Health System in Lansing, Michigan. His responsibilities include clinical support for surgery/anesthesia, critical care, and the pharmacokinetic dosing service, as well as drug information. He has practiced in the institutional pharmacy environment for his entire career, most recently as a clinical pharmacist at W.A. Foote Memorial Hospital in Jackson, Michigan. He has also worked as a pharmacy manager, staff pharmacist, pharmacy technician, and pharmacy clerk (early in his career). Dr. Weiss' position as a pharmacy clerk has made him particularly sensitive to the needs of and demands placed on pharmacy technicians.

Self-assessment questions

1. An infection occurs when:
   a. a microorganism is found in the body.
   b. a microorganism begins to damage the body and causes an immune response.
   c. the patient has a fever.
   d. signs of inflammation are present.

2. An anti-infective that kills microorganisms is:
   a. bacteriostatic.
   b. bacteriocidal.
   c. broad spectrum.
   d. narrow spectrum.

3. Which of the following is a first-generation cephalosporin?
   a. Cefaclor
   b. Cefprozil
   c. Cefuroxime
   d. Cephalexin

4. Which of the following anti-infectives is usually administered once a day for five days?
   a. Erythromycin
   b. Azithromycin
   c. Clarithromycin
   d. Streptomycin

5. Fluconazole is an antimicrobial agent used to treat infections caused by:
   a. gram-negative bacteria.
   b. anaerobic bacteria.
   c. viruses.
   d. fungi.

6. Dosing adjustment for the aminoglycosides is based on:
   a. white blood cell count.
   b. blood levels of the anti-infective.
   c. bacteriocidal concentration.
   d. bacteriostatic concentration.

7. Which of the following is effective against *Pneumocystis carinii* pneumonia?
   a. Penicillin
   b. Cephalosporin
   c. Tetracycline
   d. Sulfamethoxazole-trimethoprim

8. Which of the following may reduce the absorption of tetracyclines when administered concomitantly?
   a. Laxatives
   b. Penicillin
   c. Antacids
   d. Aspirin

9. The U.S. Centers for Disease Control has issued guidelines to reduce the use of vancomycin because of:
   a. increased drug costs.
   b. increased side effects.
   c. emergence of resistant bacteria.
   d. inability of the manufacturer to meet demand.

10. Which of the following may cross react in a patient with a penicillin allergy?
    a. Erythromycin
    b. Aminoglycoside
    c. Fluoroquinolone
    d. Carbapenem

CHAPTER 24

HUMAN IMMUNODEFICIENCY VIRUS (HIV)

Betty J. Abate, Pharm.D., BCPS

Learning objectives

Upon completion of this chapter, the technician should be able to do the following:

- ♦ Recognize FDA-approved antiretroviral agents in the following classes: nucleoside reverse transcriptase inhibitors (NRTIs), protease inhibitors (PIs), and non-nucleoside reverse transcriptase inhibitors (NNRTIs).
- ♦ Identify the major adverse drug reactions, drug interactions, and special storage instructions associated with antiretroviral agents (both as a class and individually).
- ♦ Briefly describe the procedure for administering prophylaxis for HIV following a significant occupational exposure.
- ♦ Recognize the drugs used for prophylaxis *of Pneumocystis carinii* pneumonia (PCP) and *Mycobacterium avium complex* (MAC).
- ♦ Identify the major adverse drug reactions associated with the drugs used to treat PCP and MAC.

Introduction

HIV infection can be transmitted in one of three modes: parenteral (e.g., blood-transfusions, sharing of needles, needle sticks), sexual, or perinatal (through the birth canal). Sexual contact is the most common route of infection in adults, whereas perinatal transmission is the most common route in infants and children. HIV infection is diagnosed using a screening test called an Enzyme-Linked Immunosorbent Assay (ELISA) and confirmed by the Western Blot test.

Once HIV is acquired, it adheres to CD4 receptors or "CD4 cells." CD4 receptors are proteins on the surface of many cells of the immune system, including T-helper lymphocytes, monocytes, macrophages, and dendritic cells. These cells are responsible for stimulating other cells in the immune response. The body cannot mount an appropriate immune response when CD4 cells are greatly decreased. Thus, the patient with HIV infection becomes susceptible to a variety of serious bacterial, viral, and fungal infections.

Drugs used to treat any infectious agent must target biological features or processes unique to the infecting organism to prevent adverse effects to the host. The life cycle of HIV is quite complicated; however, several unique processes have been identified for therapeutic intervention.[1]

HIV initially adheres to a CD4 cell and is then absorbed into the cell to prepare for replication (making copies of itself). The genetic information of HIV is contained on single strand RNA and must be transcribed onto DNA for replication. (Transcription for human cell replication occurs in the reverse direction—DNA to RNA.) HIV possesses a unique enzyme for this process called *reverse transcriptase*. This enzyme is a prime target for therapeutic intervention.

Once the genetic information of HIV is replicated, large proteins must be "cut" into functional pieces to produce a complete virus. This is accomplished with another unique enzyme called *protease*. Without the enzyme protease, the virus is immature and incapable of infecting cells. Thus, inhibiting protease is another major drug target. If HIV is allowed to replicate and produce complete viruses, the body's CD4 cells are eventually destroyed, which leads to the development of acquired immune deficiency syndrome (AIDS).

Drugs used to treat HIV[2-4]

FDA-approved drugs to treat HIV infection are included in Table 1. All of the antiretrovirals are administered as tablets or capsules. Agents which are available in additional dosage forms are so noted at the end of the paragraph for that specific drug.

Table 1 FDA-approved antiretroviral agents

Nucleoside reverse transcriptase inhibitors (NRTIs)
abacavir (Ziagen®, ABC)
didanosine (Videx®, ddI)
lamivudine (Epivir®, 3TC)
stavudine (Zerit®, d4T)
zalcitabine (HIVID®, ddC)
zidovudine (Retrovir®, AZT)
zidovudine 300mg + lamivudine 150mg (Combivir®)

Protease inhibitors (PIs)
amprenavir (Agenerase®)
indinavir (Crixivan®)
nelfinavir (Viracept®)
saquinavir (Invirase® [hard-gel, original], Fortovase® [soft-gel, improved formulation])
ritonavir (Norvir®)

Non-nucleoside reverse transcriptase inhibitors (NNRTIs)
delavirdine (Rescriptor®)
efavirenz (Sustiva®)
nevirapine (Viramune®)

Nucleoside reverse transcriptase inhibitors (NRTIs)

NRTIs inhibit the enzyme reverse transcriptase preventing viral DNA replication. Adverse effects reported with NRTIs include lactic acidosis (a buildup of lactic acid in the bloodstream at a faster rate than the body can eliminate it) with hepatomegaly (enlargement of the liver) and hepatic steatosis (fatty degeneration of the liver). This effect is rare but is potentially life-threatening. Risk factors for developing these side effects include obesity, liver disease, and prolonged nucleoside exposure.

Zidovudine (Retrovir®) was the first antiretroviral agent to be used clinically. Side effects associated with zidovudine can be divided into "early" and "late" effects. Early effects occur usually within the first four weeks of therapy and include gastrointestinal (GI) intolerance (e.g., nausea and vomiting), fatigue, headache, fever, and rash. Late effects generally occur after four weeks and include anemia (decreased number of red blood cells), neutropenia (decreased number of white blood cells), neuropathy (nerve pain), and myopathy (muscular pain). Zidovudine is administered to help prevent pregnant women with HIV from passing the virus to their babies during birth.[5] Zidovudine is also available in oral forms and an injection.

Lamivudine (Epivir®) is the best tolerated NRTI. It is very common for doctors to prescribe lamivudine and zidovudine together, and they are manufactured as a combination product (Combivir®) to increase patient compliance. Lamivudine is also available as an oral solution.

Didanosine (Videx®) is associated with pancreatitis (15 percent of patients), and individuals with a history of pancreatitis or alcohol abuse should not use this drug. Signs and symptoms of pancreatitis include severe pain in the upper abdomen and back. Alcohol should be avoided while taking didanosine. Didanosine is best absorbed when taken on an empty stomach. Due to drug interactions, didanosine should not be administered at the same time as dapsone, ketoconazole (Nizoral®), itraconazole (Sporanox®), ciprofloxacin (Cipro®), indinavir (Crixivan®), or delavirdine (Resciptor®). Separate these drugs by one hour before or two hours after taking didanosine.

Painful peripheral neuropathy is associated with both zalcitabine (HIVID®) (17 percent to 31 percent of patients) and stavudine (up to 31 percent of patients). Peripheral neuropathy is a nerve disease causing weakness or numbness. This side effect is dose related; therefore, the patient should be advised to take this medication **exactly** as prescribed. Symptoms of peripheral neuropathy include tingling, burning, pain or numbness of hands or feet.

Abacavir (Ziagen®) is the newest NRTI to be approved by the FDA. The most serious side effect is a hypersensitivity reaction occurring in up to 3 percent of patients that can be life threatening. The reaction generally occurs during the first six weeks of therapy and symptoms include fever, skin rash, fatigue, and GI intolerance. A warning card must be dispensed with each prescription to be carried with the patient at all times. The reaction usually resolves within two days of discontinuing the drug. Patients who experience these symptoms should never receive the drug again. Abacavir is also available as an oral solution.

Protease inhibitors (PIs)

As described earlier, protease inhibitors act by inhibiting the enzyme protease, resulting in a newly replicated immature virus incapable of infecting new CD4 cells. All of the protease inhibitors are metabolized by the liver which has major implications for drug interactions. **The package insert must be consulted whenever beginning any protease inhibitor therapy and every time a new drug is prescribed for the patient to avoid serious drug interactions.** Patients should be advised to strictly adhere to their dosing schedule when taking PIs to prevent the development of resistance.

Common adverse effects reported with PIs include hyperglycemia, diabetes mellitus, increased bleeding episodes in hemophiliac patients, and fat redistribution with or without lipid abnormalities.

Saquinavir (Invirase®, soft-gel formulation) was the first FDA-approved protease inhibitor. Due to significant problems with bioavailability, a hard-gel formulation was developed (Fortovase®). Most patients have been transferred to the hard-gel formulation. Fortovase® is well tolerated by patients and should be stored in the refrigerator. Once brought to room temperature, Fortovase® must be used within three months.

Indinavir is associated with the development of kidney stones (6 percent to 8 percent of patients); therefore, patients must drink 48 ounces of fluids every day while taking indinavir. Occasional nausea and GI discomfort may occur. Two significant drug interactions that require dose adjustments include concomitant use of rifabutin (Mycobutin®) and concomitant use of ketoconazole. Indinavir capsules are very sensitive to moisture. For optimal absorption, patients should be advised to take indinavir one hour before or two hours after a meal. The drug must be stored in the original container that includes a desiccant (drying agent). The drug is stable for three days out of the original container.

Ritonavir (Norvir®) has the most side effects and drug interactions of all the PIs. The most frequent side effects include weakness, GI intolerance, diarrhea, anorexia, abdominal pain, change in sense of taste, numbness in the lips, and paresthesia (tingling sensations). The package insert must be consulted with every new prescribed drug to avoid drug interactions. Ritonavir should be taken with meals and one hour after antacids. The capsule form should be stored in the refrigerator, while the oral solution should be stored at room temperature. The taste of ritonavir oral solution may be improved by mixing it with chocolate milk, Ensure® or Advera® within one hour of dosing.

Nelfinavir (Viracept®)is associated with mild to moderate diarrhea, which may be relieved with the over-the-counter drug loperamide (Imodium®). Nelfinavir is best absorbed with a small meal. It is also available as an oral powder.

Amprenavir (Agenerase®) is the newest FDA-approved PI. Rash, diarrhea, and nausea are the most common side effects.

Non-nucleoside reverse transcriptase inhibitors (NNRTIs)

These agents exert their antiretroviral effects as non-competitive inhibitors of reverse transcriptase. Common adverse effects include the development of a rash and an increase in transaminase (an enzyme) levels.

Nevirapine (Viramune®) was the first FDA-approved NNRTI. The most common side effect of nevirapine is rash (15 percent to 44 percent of patients). The rash usually occurs between seven and 28 days of initiation of therapy, but it may be seen up to eight weeks after initiation of therapy. Gradually increasing the dose may decrease the incidence of rash. Other symptoms associated with the rash include fever, mucosal ulcerations of the mouth or conjunctivae (lining of the inner surface of the eyelids), or hepatitis. Some risk factors for developing the rash have been identified as concomitant use of trimethoprim-sulfamethoxazole (TMP-SMZ) (Bactrim®, Septra®) or amoxicillin-clavulanate (Augmentin®), CD4 count <50 cells/mm^3, or the dose given as single daily dose versus divided doses. Nevirapine is an inducer of hepatic enzymes, which results in many drug interactions.

Delavirdine is also associated with rash. It is a hepatic enzyme inhibitor which results in many drug interactions. A notable difference of delavirdine and nevirapine is dosing frequency; nevirapine requires once- or twice-daily dosing, and delavirdine is administered three times daily. Delavirdine tablets can be dispersed in water to make consumption easier.

Efavirenz (Sustiva®) is the newest NNRTI. It is associated with rash, dizziness, and insomnia. It is a hepatic enzyme inducer causing many drug interactions.

Combination treatment[3]

The decision to treat an HIV patient is based upon his or her clinical symptoms, CD4 cell count, and HIV RNA plasma level. The ultimate goal of HIV treatment is maximal suppression of viral replication to help preserve immune function, prolong health and life, and decrease the risk of drug resistance. Specific drug regimens are based upon many individual patient factors including, but not limited to, degree of infection, previous drug treatment, adverse drug reaction profiles, and patient compliance factors. Consult current literature for updated recommendations. The drugs discussed in this chapter are presented for teaching purposes only and no product should be construed as endorsed by the author or editors.

Monotherapy is no longer recommended for HIV treatment. As of this writing, the preferred combination of antiretroviral agents is a three-drug regimen consisting of one PI with two NRTIs such as 1) indinavir or ritonavir, plus 2) zidovudine, plus 3) didanosine, lamivudine or zalcitabine. Guidelines from the Centers for Disease Control and Prevention (CDC) should be consulted for more details and other possible regimens.[3]

Occupational exposure to HIV

Healthcare workers are at risk of contracting HIV from significant mucous membrane or skin exposures. The CDC has published guidelines for postexposure prophylaxis (PEP) of HIV infection.[6] It is recommended to administer **within one to two hours of exposure** a combination of zidovudine and lamivudine (usually as Combivir®), plus or minus nelfinavir. If the exposure is deemed significant, therapy is continued for four weeks.

Opportunistic infection prophylaxis regimens[7]

Drugs used as prophylaxis against *Pneumocystis carinii* pneumonia (PCP) and *Mycobacterium avium complex* (MAC) are listed in Table 2.

Table 2 Drugs used for prophylaxis of *Pneumocystis carinii* pneumonia (PCP) and *Mycobacterium avium complex* (MAC)

Drugs used as prophylaxis for PCP
trimethoprim-sulfamethoxazole (TMP-SMZ) (Bactrim®, Septra®)
dapsone (DDS)
pentamidine (Pentam®)
Drugs used as prophylaxis for MAC
azithromycin (Zithromax®)
clarithromycin (Biaxin®)
rifabutin (Mycobutin®)

Pneumocystis carinii pneumonia (PCP)

Pneumonia caused by *Pneumocystis carinii* is the most common life-threatening infection in HIV patients. *Pneumocystis carinii* is widespread in the environment and up to 80 percent of the population has been exposed. Infection does not occur unless a patient has a suppressed immune system.

HIV patients with CD4 counts less than 200 cells/mm^3 or who have had previous PCP should receive prophylaxis for PCP. TMP-SMZ is the current drug of choice. Side effects include rash, nausea, and abdominal pain. For patients who cannot tolerate TMP-SMZ, dapsone is an alternative. Side effects of TMP-SMZ include rash, nausea and hemolytic anemia. Both TMP-SMZ and dapsone regimens may provide additional prophylaxis against the disease toxoplasmosis. Pentamidine by nebulization (administration of a fine spray) once a month is another option. This treatment can be associated with bronchospasm.

Mycobacterium avium complex (MAC) infection

Mycobacterium avium complex is a nontuberculosis organism commonly found in water and soil. Systemic MAC infection is considered an end-stage AIDS complication consisting of high fevers, diarrhea, night sweats, malaise, weight loss, anemia, and neutropenia. Patients with CD4 counts less than 50 cells/mm^3 should receive prophylaxis for MAC. Azithromycin once weekly or clarithromycin daily are the current drugs of choice. Side effects are minimal. Patients unable to tolerate azithromycin or clarithromycin can be prescribed rifabutin. Side effects of rifabutin include rash, GI intolerance, uveitis (inflammation of the iris, ciliary body or the layer of blood vessels and connective tissue between the white of the eye and the retina of the eye), hepatitis, and orange-brown coloring of bodily secretions (tears, sweat, sputum, skin, urine, or feces). Patients should be warned that soft contacts may be permanently stained if worn while taking rifabutin.

Conclusion

Treatment of the HIV-infected patient is challenging; however, new drugs are continually-being-developed. Clinicians are optimistic that HIV infection may someday be compared to diabetes—a manageable condition not necessarily associated with early mortality. Pharmacy technicians can be an HIV-infected patient's advocate and resource. Pharmacy technicians providing either inpatient or outpatient services for HIV-infected patients must remain constantly updated on therapy recommendations, drug interactions, adverse reaction profiles, and administration techniques to help patients obtain the best benefit from their therapy.

References

1. Stanley S.K., Fauci A., Immunology of AIDS and HIV Infection, Principles and Practice of Infectious Diseases, New York, NY, pp. 1203-1217, 1995.
2. Fletcher C.V., Kakuda T. N., Collier A.C., Human Immunodeficiency Virus Infection, Pharmacotherapy: A Pathophysiologic Approach, Stamford, CT, 1999, pp. 1930-1956.
3. Medscape, http://hiv.medscape.com/govmt/DHHS/guidelines/HIV/pnt-HIV.html, December 8, 1999.
4. Medscape, http://hiv.medscape.com/updates/quickguide, December 8, 1999.
5. Anonymous, "Recommendations of U.S. Public Health Service Task Force on the Use of Zidovudine to Reduce the Perinatal Transmission of HIV," *Morbidity and Mortality Weekly Report*, Atlanta, GA, Vol. 43 (RR-11), pp. 1-20, May 8, 1994.
6. Anonymous, "Public Health Service Guidelines for the Management of Health-care Worker Exposure to HIV and Recommendations for Postexposure Prophylaxis," *Morbidity and Mortality Weekly Report*, Atlanta, GA, Vol. 47 (RR-07), pp. 1-28, May 15, 1998.
7. Anonymous, "1999 USPHS/IDSA Guidelines for Prevention of Opportunistic Infections in Persons Infected with HIV," *Morbidity and Mortality Weekly Report*, Atlanta, GA, Vol. 48 (RR-10), pp. 1-59, August 20, 1999.

About the author

Betty J. Abate earned her bachelor's of science in pharmacy from the Albany College of Pharmacy in Albany, New York, in 1987 and completed a one-year residency in hospital pharmacy at Rhode Island Hospital in Providence. She earned her Doctor of Pharmacy degree at the University of Rhode Island in Kingston in 1991 and completed a two-year fellowship in infectious diseases at Wayne State University/Detroit Receiving Hospital in Detroit, Michigan, from 1991-1993. Her primary focus of research was in-vitro modeling of drug treatment for *Pseudomonas aeruginosa* and the development of an in-vitro endocarditis model of infection. Dr. Abate taught infectious diseases at the University of Georgia College of Pharmacy in Augusta from 1993-1994. In 1994, she returned to the Detroit Medical Center/Grace Hospital in Detroit, Michigan, where she spent five years as a clinical pharmacist specialist in infectious diseases with teaching appointments at Wayne State University and the University of Michigan in Ann Arbor. She has worked extensively with HIV/AIDS patients.

Self-assessment questions

1. Which antiretroviral agent is administered to prevent perinatal transmission of HIV?
   a. Indinavir
   b. Lamivudine
   c. Nevirapine
   d. Zidovudine

2. Combivir® is a combination of the two antiretroviral drugs zidovudine and:
   a. didanosine.
   b. lamivudine.
   c. stavudine.
   d. zalcitabine.

3. Healthcare workers significantly exposed to HIV should receive antiretroviral prophylaxis within:
   a. 1 hour.
   b. 1day.
   c. 1 week.
   d. 1 month.

4. Which antiretroviral is sensitive to moisture and must be stored in its original container?
   a. Amprenavir
   b. Indinavir
   c. Ritonavir
   d. Saquinavir

5. Which NRTI must be dispensed with a patient information card warning of a life-threatening hypersensitivity reaction?
   a. Abacavir
   b. Didanosine
   c. Zalcitabine
   d. Zidovudine

6. Which of the following applies to Fortovase®?
   a. It belongs to the antiretroviral class NRTI.
   b. It should be refrigerated.
   c. It is a soft-gel formulation of saquinavir.
   d. It has very low bioavailability.

7. Diarrhea associated with nelfinavir can be treated with:
   a. azithromycin.
   b. bactrim.
   c. clarithromycin.
   d. loperamide.

8. The common adverse effect associated with NNRTIs is:
   a. hepatitis.
   b. kidney stones.
   c. bone marrow toxicity.
   d. rash.

9. Bactrim® can be used to prevent:
   a. HIV infection.
   b. MAC infection.
   c. PCP.
   d. tuberculosis.

10. Which of the following drugs can cause orange-brown secretions?
    a. Azithromycin
    b. Clarithromycin
    c. Loperamide
    d. Rifabutin

CHAPTER 25

POISONINGS

Susan C. Smolinske, Pharm.D., BCPS, DABAT

Learning objectives

Upon completion of this chapter, the technician should be able to do the following:

- Explain the general measures taken for the treatment of drug poisonings.
- Describe the symptoms of digoxin poisoning and discuss the drugs used for treatment.
- Describe the symptoms of narcotic poisoning and discuss the drugs for treatment.
- Describe the symptoms of benzodiazepine poisoning and discuss the drugs used for treatment.
- Explain the effects of hyperkalemia and identify an antidote for treatment.
- Explain the effects of acetaminophen poisoning and identify an antidote for treatment.

Introduction

Each year more than 2.5 million human poisoning cases are reported to poison control centers. Approximately 53 percent of victims are children less than 6 years of age. The most common drug products involved in accidental poisoning in children are pain relievers and cough/cold preparations. Drugs most likely to result in death after an overdose include pain relievers, antidepressants, and cardiac medications. Dispensing drugs in child-resistant closures is instrumental in preventing childhood poisoning. Parents should also be cautioned to keep all medications out of reach, since 20 percent of children are able to open these closures. Medications kept in food storage areas, such as liquid antibiotics, are often involved in pediatric poisoning.

When medications have been taken in an overdose, the patient is evaluated for symptoms and supportive measures are begun. Stabilization of an unconscious patient often includes protection of the airway (intubation) and administration of oxygen, glucose IV, naloxone IV, and thiamine IV.

Gastric decontamination

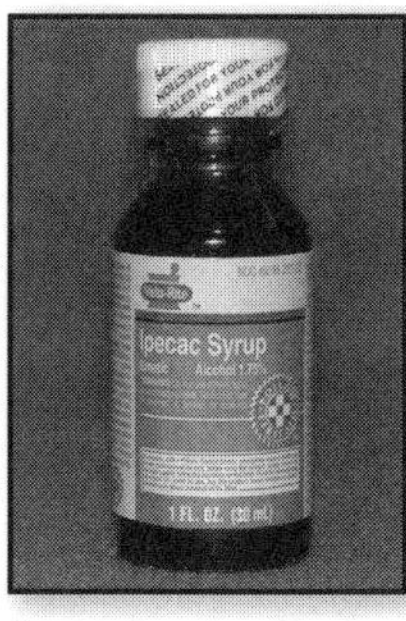

Ipecac syrup

To reduce the absorption of toxic drugs, ipecac syrup may be used to induce vomiting (only in a fully conscious patient) or the patient can undergo gastric lavage (pumping the stomach). Removal methods are most effective if used quickly (within one hour) after an overdose, and on average they remove approximately 30 percent of the substance. The poison control center should always be called prior to recommending home use of ipecac syrup since vomiting may increase the hazards of some substances. Activated charcoal may be used to bind the toxin and prevent further absorption, or to enhance removal of some drugs even after absorption has occurred. To promote passage of the charcoal-drug combination through the gastrointestinal tract, cathartics such as magnesium citrate or sorbitol 70% may be included in the charcoal mixture. Activated charcoal does not bind to certain drugs, such as iron and lithium. For these agents, rapid flushing of tablets through the gastrointestinal tract may be accomplished by administration of a polyethylene glycol/electrolyte solution. This is termed "whole bowel irrigation." When possible, a specific antidote is used to reverse or prevent the toxic effects, but there is not an antidote for every poison. Some poisons and antidotes are listed in Table 1.

Table 1 Poison with corresponding antidote

Poison	Antidote
acetaminophen (Tylenol®)	N-acetylcysteine (Mucomyst®)
digoxin (Lanoxin®)	digoxin immune Fab (Digibind®)
theophylline (Theodur®, Slophyllin®)	esmolol
benzodiazepines (Xanax®, Ativan®, Valium®)	flumazenil (Romazicon®)
iron salts (various vitamins)	deferoxamine (Desferal®)
narcotic drugs (opium derivatives, Demeral®, Percocet®)	naloxone (Narcan®)
methanol/ethylene glycol	fomepizole (Antizol®)
anticoagulants (rat poisons, Coumadin®)	phytonadione (Vitamin K1)
isoniazid (Laniazid®)	pyridoxine (Vitamin B6)

Digoxin poisoning[1]

Digoxin (Lanoxin®) is used in the treatment of certain heart arrhythmias and congestive heart failure. The therapeutic concentration of digoxin in the blood is usually less than two nanograms per milliliter (mg/ml). Increased blood concentration causing toxicity can occur due to advanced age, worsening of heart disease, poor kidney function, or a drug interaction. Evidence of digoxin toxicity (vomiting, diarrhea, headache, and visual changes) requires temporarily stopping digoxin therapy. Very high concentrations or severe symptoms, such as heart arrhythmias and hyperkalemia, are treated with the antidote digoxin immune Fab (Digibind®). It irreversibly binds with digoxin, rendering it inactive in the body. The amount of digoxin in the body is estimated and the number of vials of digoxin immune Fab is calculated and administered intravenously. Each 40mg vial of digoxin immune Fab will bind 0.6mg of digoxin. In patients with chronic digoxin intoxication who require digoxin for control of heart rate, a dose of digoxin immune Fab may be calculated that will bring the digoxin serum level down to a therapeutic range rather than inactivating the entire body stores.

Narcotic poisoning[1]

Narcotic pain relievers are classified according to their potential for addiction and abuse. (See Chapter 30.) In pain-relieving doses, these drugs cause few adverse effects. When the dose exceeds the pain-relief dosage, or in cases of a deliberate overdose, there is a dose-related progression of toxic symptoms. The symptoms include nausea, hypotension, sleepiness, coma, reduced respirations, and death. Narcotic toxicity is quickly reversed with a naloxone (Narcan®) injection. The naloxone dose may need repeating because the duration of action is two to three hours and may wear off before the body concentration of narcotic has diminished. A longer duration, reversal agent is nalmephene (Revex®) that lasts for several hours, but is more expensive. For long-acting narcotics, a continuous infusion of naloxone is commonly used. Naloxone is extremely safe, but may produce side effects in two settings: 1) administration of the full dose of naloxone (0.4mg to 2mg) may produce uncomfortable withdrawal symptoms in a patient who is addicted to narcotics, and 2) administration of naloxone to a patient taking tramadol, a synthetic narcotic, may produce seizures.

Benzodiazepine toxicity[1]

Benzodiazepine drugs such as diazepam (Valium®), lorazepam (Ativan®), alprazolam (Xanax®), and others, are used for treatment of anxiety, sleep disorders, and panic attacks, and for sedation. When the effect of these drugs becomes toxic due to an overdose, the symptoms include disinhibition, sleepiness, stupor and coma. Muscle tone decreases and breathing can become impaired. The benzodiazepine antidote is flumazenil (Romazicon®), given by IV route. Because the flumazenil binds with the benzodiazepine receptor, the benzodiazepine no longer has an effect, leaving some people at risk for seizure. Seizures may occur in patients who are benzodiazepine dependant, those who have taken a tricyclic antidepressant overdose, and those who are predisposed to seizures. While zolpidem (Ambien®) is not structurally a benzodiazepine, it acts like a benzodiazepine and is used for sleep. Flumazenil is also an effective reversal agent for a zolpidem overdose.

Hyperkalemia[1]

A high concentration of potassium in the blood, called hyperkalemia, is usually treated if the potassium level exceeds six milliequivalents (mEq) per liter. Sodium polystyrene sulfonate (Kayexalate®) is a cation-exchange resin that absorbs potassium in exchange for sodium in the GI tract. This is a slow process over several hours and, if the hyperkalemia is life-threatening, other measures should also be taken. The sodium polystyrene sulfonate is given orally or by enema. The high amount of sodium exchanged may worsen heart failure in some patients.

Acetaminophen

Acetaminophen (Tylenol®) is partly metabolized by cytochrome P450 to a compound that binds to liver cells and destroys them. After therapeutic doses of acetaminophen, the small amount of metabolite formed is scavenged easily by body stores of glutathione (a peptide that contains three amino acids) and no damage occurs. In patients who have depleted stores of glutathione, such as alcoholics or AIDS patients, even usual doses of acetaminophen can produce liver toxicity. Chronic overdose may occur in patients with chronic pain syndromes or in children who are given multiple sources of acetaminophen or treated with adult formulations. Overdose of acetaminophen usually causes no immediate symptoms, but it results in liver failure within two to three days. The antidote N-acetylcysteine binds to the toxic metabolite and prevents liver damage in nearly 100 percent of patients who receive it within the first eight hours after the overdose. N-acetylcysteine is given orally, generally for a three-day period of time. The major side effect is vomiting, which may require treatment with anti-emetic medications such as metoclopramide (Reglan®) or ondansetron (Zofran®).

Conclusion

The goals of treating poisonings and drug overdoses include removing the drug from the patient's body, administering an antidote that will bind to the toxic substance and make it ineffective, and stabilizing the patient. Not every drug has a specific antidote. A poison control center should be consulted before recommending gastric decontamination in the home.

Acknowledgment

The author and publisher wish to acknowledge Beverly P. Kershaw, Pharm.M.S., for her extensive contributions to this chapter in the previous edition of this manual.

Reference

1. Pharmacy Certified Technician Training Manual, 7th edition, Michigan Pharmacists Association, Lansing, MI, 1997, p. 178.

Bibliography

Litovitz, T.L., et al, "1998 Annual report of the American Association of Poison Control Centers Toxic Exposure Surveillance System," *American Journal of Emergency Medicine*, Vol. 17, No. 5, pp. 435-443, September 1999.

Olson, K.R., Poisoning & Drug Overdose, 3rd Edition, Appleton & Lange, Stamford, CT, 1999.

About the author

Susan C. Smolinske received her bachelor's of science in pharmacy from the University of Florida in 1977 and her Doctor of Pharmacy degree from Idaho State University in 1993. She is certified by the Board of Pharmaceutical Specialties in pharmacotherapy and by the American Board of Applied Toxicology in clinical toxicology. Her career has included several years in retail pharmacy, two years at the Rocky Mountain Drug Information Center in Denver, Colorado, and 10 years as an editor at Micromedex. For the past six years, she has been employed by Wayne State University in Detroit, Michigan. Dr. Smolinske is currently an assistant professor in the College of Medicine Department of Pediatrics. She is also currently Managing Director of the Children's Hospital of Michigan Regional Poison Control Center in Detroit.

Self-assessment questions

1. The best method to lessen absorption of lithium after an overdose is:
   a. activated charcoal.
   b. sorbitol.
   c. whole bowel irrigation.
   d. ipecac syrup.

2. What drug may be given to induce vomiting?
   a. Ipecac syrup
   b. Sorbitol
   c. Activated charcoal
   d. Naloxone

3. An antidote for acetaminophen toxicity is:
   a. ipecac syrup.
   b. sorbitol.
   c. activated charcoal.
   d. N-acetylcysteine.

4. The antidote for narcotic toxicity is:
   a. ipecac syrup.
   b. sorbitol.
   c. activated charcoal.
   d. naloxone.

5. Flumazenil is used to reverse the effects of:
   a. acetaminophen.
   b. benzodiazepines.
   c. theophylline.
   d. digoxin.

6. Kayexalate® is used to treat:
   a. hyerpcalcemia.
   b. hypermagnesemia.
   c. hyperkalemia.
   d. digoxin toxicity.

7. Death from respiratory depression may result from toxicity of which drug/class of drugs?
   a. Narcotics
   b. Acetaminophen
   c. Theophylline
   d. Digoxin

8. Death from liver toxicity may result from toxicity of which drug/class of drugs?
   a. Narcotics
   b. Acetaminophen
   c. Theophylline
   d. Digoxin

9. Flumazenil would be most useful as an antidote in which setting?
   a. Accidental diazepam overdose in a child
   b. Chronic diazepam overuse in an adult
   c. Suicidal overdose of diazepam in a patient taking amitriptyline, a tricyclic antidepressant
   d. Accidental diazepam overdose in a adult with epilepsy

10. What is the most common side effect of N-acetylcysteine?
    a. Liver damage
    b. Vomiting
    c. Kidney dysfunction
    d. Diarrhea

Part IV:
Medication Distribution and Control Measures

CHAPTER 26

QUALITY IMPROVEMENT

Judith Fedchenko, R.Ph, M.S.

Learning objectives

Upon completion of this chapter, the technician should be able to do the following:

- List healthcare organizations that incorporate a quality agenda.
- List JCAHO requirements that directly effect a pharmacy technician.
- List three reasons that JCAHO accreditation is important to a hospital.
- List at least five of the Deming management theory principles.
- State three reasons that TQM principles have been difficult to incorporate in hospitals.
- Define an *adverse drug reaction (ADR).*
- Differentiate between Type A and Type B ADRs.
- Define the *Drug Utilization Evaluation (DUE) process.*
- List the criteria used to select medications for DUE reporting.
- Explain the reasons for the Food and Drug Administration (FDA) MedWatch Program.

Introduction

Unfortunately, the drug distribution process is not perfect all of the time. It is important to identify processes that lead to errors or less-than-ideal delivery of medications. Improving the quality of a pharmacy's service is an ongoing process and involves every member of the healthcare team.

Joint Commission on Accreditation of Healthcare Organizations[1]

For healthcare facilities, an organization by the name of the "Joint Commission on Accreditation of Healthcare Organizations" (JCAHO) has set standards for hospitals in the United States. This non-profit organization accredits almost 20,000 healthcare organizations and programs in the United States. The corporate members are:

1. The American Society of Internal Medicine
2. The American College of Surgeons
3. The American Hospital Association (AHA)
4. The American Medical Association (AMA)
5. The American Dental Association (ADA)

A healthcare facility that wants accreditation requests a review by JCAHO. JCAHO charges a fee for this service, based on the size and services offered by the organization. The maximum accreditation period is three years.

While JCAHO is not a governmental agency, having their accreditation is very important. To participate in the Medicare program, a healthcare facility must be accredited by JCAHO or undergo a yearly Medicare survey. JCAHO accreditation is also sought by organizations for many of the following reasons:

- Improves the ability to recruit quality clinical staff.
- May fulfill licensing requirements.
- Improves the ability to attract patients to the facility.
- May reduce liability insurance premiums.
- Provides a tool for staff education.
- Helps organizations improve their quality of care.
- May provide financial incentives, such as bond ratings, a managed care contract, etc.

During a JCAHO survey, the accrediting team looks for many things, some of which have a direct impact on a pharmacy technician. JCAHO reviewers look to see that a healthcare facility:

1. complies with legal requirements;
2. meets safety requirements for both patients and employees;
3. follows its own policies and procedures;
4. employs competent staff; and
5. has a "Process Improvement" plan in place (a JCAHO term for a quality improvement plan).

In the past, the JCAHO survey team spent a lot of their time reviewing the facility's policy and procedure manuals and questioning the facility's administrators concerning the interpretation of those policies. More recently, it has become the practice of the survey team to question individual employees to determine if they know the hospital's policies and procedures and follow them. A pharmacy employee could expect to be questioned by a JCAHO surveyor on anything from where the fire extinguishers are located to the appropriate expiration dating to be applied to a specific compounded intravenous fluid.

Technicians working in a health facility pharmacy will have their competency checked at regular intervals in a number of areas of responsibility. Some of these areas might include: hazardous material handling, sterile technique, emergency code procedures, chemotherapy preparation, and confidentiality. If the technician is required to interact with patients, competency may be accessed for dealing with various age groups.

Incident reporting

Healthcare organizations reviewed by JCAHO are expected to have programs addressing any form of adverse incident that occurs. Pharmacies, of course, are particularly interested in incidents involving medications (also referred to as "drug misadventures"). The data helps determine deficiencies in the current systems and creates improvements to prevent future incidents. When the correction is identified, the monitoring process will determine whether the change is effective. If not, a new method for improvement is developed and the monitoring process continues.

If an incident involves the death or serious physical or psychological injury, a "sentinel event" has occurred. JCAHO requires that the healthcare organization notify them of such an occurrence and that a special review occurs in order to prevent a recurrence. The organization's leaders must be involved in identifying the problem, ensuring that an analysis occurs to determine how the error occurred (referred to as a "root cause analysis"), identifying mechanisms to prevent the recurrence, and monitoring the facility to determine if the new measures were effective.

JCAHO requires hospitals to develop and use an adverse drug reaction (ADR) reporting system and use the data obtained to improve the patient's quality of care. ADRs encompass what are referred to as "side effect" and allergic reactions. Some of these reactions are mild, and some of them may be life threatening. This topic will be discussed further along in the chapter.

Drug use evaluations (DUE) and ADRs are quality improvement mechanisms used to improve drug therapy outcomes for patients. Other areas of drug administration need constant evaluation to reduce the inherent risks associated with the use of medication, known as drug related problems (DRP). The problems range from those related to the individual healthcare worker (e.g., illegible handwriting, failure to follow policy and procedures); system problems (e.g., lack of or poor quality unit-dose distribution); or manufacturers' issues (e.g., different drug products with similar names, confusing labels, or packages that fail to prevent dangerous administration methods).

There are other organizations involved with quality improvement in health care that have shown major interest in the medication delivery system. Some of the organizations are described below.

Institute for Safe Medication Practices, Inc. (ISMP)[2]

The founders of ISMP have collected data for many years from pharmacists, technicians, and other practitioners on a voluntary basis. The ISMP and the United States Pharmacopeial (USP) Convention provide a 24-hour-a-day telephone and facsimile (FAX) reporting system to record and monitor errors involving prescribing, dispensing, and administering medication. The institute presents educational programs on preventing medication errors, incorporating data on the most common errors, and suggesting methods for "minimizing the consequences of errors and reducing the incidence of critical errors."[8] They also publish the "ISMP Medication Safety Alert" every two weeks that includes descriptions of errors that have occurred, suggestions for preventing that type of error, and other news pertinent to the topic of medication errors.

National Committee for Quality Assurance (NCQA)[3]

The NCQA is an accreditation agency that deals with managed care organizations (MCOs). Since hospitals and pharmacies are part of many MCOs, they have standards that apply to these areas. Some of the standards, which have particular application to the pharmacy, include:

- prohibiting health plans from using financial incentives to encourage utilization review staff to limit or deny care.
- requiring health plans to have a process for approving exceptions to restricted drug formularies.
- requiring plans to take extra steps to protect the confidentiality of medical information.

If an MCO restricts its formulary, it must have a method to deal with medications for an individual patient's need for drugs not on the formulary.

Health Plan Employer Data and Information Set (HEDIS)[3]

HEDIS workgroups set up measures for specified patient populations that have certain disease states. These measures indicate if the patient is receiving the proper care and management of their condition. NCQA monitors the HEDIS results to ensure that the data is correct. HEDIS data that is pertinent to pharmacy includes such items as ensuring that the influenza vaccine is administered to older adults, that beta blocker drugs are administered to patients who have had a heart attack (if not contraindicated for some other reason), that patients are being advised to quit smoking, and that personnel with whom the patient interacts are courteous and helpful.

National Coordinating Council for Medication Error Reporting and Prevention (NCC MERP)[4]

This organization was developed in 1995 and is led by the USP Convention. Representatives of many large healthcare associations joined with the USP to develop a nationwide campaign to improve medication error reporting and develop prevention methods that will be used nationally. This group developed the following definition of a medication error:

> *A medication error is any preventable event that may cause or lead to inappropriate medication use or patient harm while the medication is in the control of the healthcare professional, patient, or consumer. Such events may be related to professional practice, healthcare products, procedures, and systems, including prescribing; order communication; product*

labeling, packaging, and nomenclature; compounding; dispensing; distribution; administration; education; monitoring; and use.

USP provides a USP Medication Errors Reporting Program form to self-report errors that occur in the workplace or are identified by working with a problem (see Figure 1).

Figure 1 USP Medication Errors Reporting Program form

MEDICATION ERRORS REPORTING PROGRAM

USP MEDICATION ERRORS REPORTING PROGRAM

Presented in cooperation with the Institute for Safe Medication Practices

The USP Practitioners' Reporting Network℠ is an FDA MEDWATCH partner

❑ ACTUAL ERROR ❑ POTENTIAL ERROR

Please describe the error. Include sequence of events, personnel involved, and work environment (e.g., code situation, change of shift, short staffing, no 24-hr. pharmacy, floor stock). If more space is needed, please attach separate page.

Was the medication administered to or used by the patient? ❑ No ❑ Yes Date and time of event: ____

What type of staff or health care practitioner made the initial error? ____

Describe outcome (e.g., death, type of injury, adverse reaction). ____

If the medication did not reach the patient, describe the intervention. ____

Who discovered the error? ____

When and how was error discovered? ____

Where did the error occur (e.g., hospital, outpatient or retail pharmacy, nursing home, patient's home)? ____

Was another practitioner involved in the error ? ❑ No ❑ Yes If yes, what type of practitioner? ____

Was patient counseling provided? ❑ No ❑ Yes If yes, before or after error was discovered? ____

If a product was involved, please complete the following:

	Product #1	Product #2
Brand name of product involved		
Generic name		
Manufacturer		
Labeler (if different from mfr.)		
Dosage form		
Strength/concentration		
Type and size of container		
NDC number		

If available, please provide relevant patient information (age, gender, diagnosis, etc.). Patient identification not required.

Reports are most useful when relevant materials such as product label, copy of prescription/order, etc. can be reviewed.
Can these materials be provided? ❑ No ❑ Yes If yes, please specify. ____

Suggest any recommendations you have to prevent recurrence of this error or describe policies or procedures you have instituted to prevent future similar errors.

A copy of this report is routinely sent to the Institute for Safe Medication Practices (ISMP), to the manufacturer/labeler, and to the Food and Drug Administration (FDA). **USP may release my identity to: (check boxes that apply)**

❑ ISMP ❑ The manufacturer and/or labeler as listed above ❑ FDA ❑ Other persons requesting a copy of this report ❑ Anonymous to all

Your name and title

Telephone number (include area code)

Your facility name, address, and ZIP

Signature

Date

Return to the attention of:
Diane D. Cousins, R.Ph.
USP PRN
12601 Twinbrook Parkway
Rockville, MD 20852-1790

Call Toll Free: **800-23-ERROR** (800-233-7767)
or FAX 301-816-8532
USP home page: http://www.usp.org/prn
Electronic reporting forms are available. Please call for additional information and/or your free diskette.

Date Received by USP:

File Access Number:

C-194

Additional forms can be found in the *USP DI Vol. I* and *Vol. III* and in all monthly *Updates*.

Institute of Medicine (IOM)[5]

The IOM in a November 1999 report, entitled "To Err Is Human: Building A Safer Health System," stated that as many as 40,000 to 100,000 deaths occur in hospitals each year due to medical errors. This means that errors are the eighth leading cause of death in the Unites States. This report focused attention on issues that have been brought up previously but had failed to receive the national support needed to create major change in the healthcare delivery system. While there are many kinds of medical errors, many people associate them with medications. If medications are the focus by a majority of the public, it means pharmacy must step to the forefront with methods to reduce those errors.

Drug use evaluation[6]

Drug use evaluation (DUE) is a process that sets standards within the healthcare organization to assure that medications are used safely, effectively, and appropriately. This type of process is applied in many ambulatory (outpatient) settings and by agencies, such as state Medicaid programs, health maintenance organizations (HMO), health insurance companies, etc. JCAHO requires DUE in healthcare organizations subject to their accreditation. The data must be used to make improvements in patient care and to credential the medical staff. Since evaluating all drugs used is nearly impossible, the American Society of Health-System Pharmacists (ASHP) suggests the following criteria for choosing drugs for evaluation:

1. The medication is known or suspected to cause adverse reactions or it interacts with another medication, food, or diagnostic procedure in a way that presents a significant health risk.
2. The medication is used in the treatment of patients who may be at high risk for adverse reactions.
3. The medication-use process affects a large number of patients or the medication is frequently prescribed.
4. The medication or medication-use process is a critical component of care for a specific disease, condition, or procedure.
5. The medication is potentially toxic or causes discomfort at normal doses.
6. The medication is most effective when used in a specific way.
7. The medication is under consideration for formulary retention, addition, or deletion.
8. The medication or medication-use process is one for which suboptimal use would have a negative effect on patient outcomes or system costs.
9. The use of the medication is expensive.

The criteria for a DUE usually represent the judgment of the medical staff, are based on solid scientific knowledge, and should ensure that the medications are used appropriately, safely, and effectively. The criteria are compared with the actual drugs in the study. The pharmacy department review, either in an institution or ambulatory pharmacy, is done with the approval of the health system or pharmacy management.

Once the medication use is evaluated, the resulting information must be distributed to the appropriate committees and individuals. If the criteria were not met, action is taken to correct the medication program and the evaluation is repeated to learn if the problems were corrected satisfactory. The frequency of review of the drug(s) evaluated must be determined to identify that the criteria are still being met. The reviews continue until the drug is in one of these stages: no longer problem-prone, high volume, or high risk; lower priority; problems increase and require more frequent monitoring; or a consensus shows that the medication is used appropriately and the frequency of monitoring can be decreased.

Utilization of pharmacy technicians in drug use evaluation

Technicians have a valuable role in collecting data for DUE. The criteria require that laboratory tests and their subsequent results fall within certain parameters. The data can be collected and documented for a pharmacist's review. As with ADR, the technician can review individual patient medication charts, computer screens, or computer-generated reports. Technicians are used to prepare DUE reports on the findings for hospital committees, physicians' requests, and for meeting the objectives of a pharmacy department.

Adverse drug reactions[7]

ADRs are among the leading causes of people being admitted to a hospital each year. Adverse reactions may range from discomfort to permanent damage or death. In 1995, a study was published in the *Journal of the American Medical Association* (*JAMA*), entitled "Incidence of Adverse Drug Events and Potential Adverse Drug Events." The authors reviewed more than 4,000 adult admissions to hospitals. Adverse drug events were detected through self-reporting by nurses and pharmacists and by continuous review of charts by investigators. By extrapolating the number of incidents that happened to the patients in the study to the total number of patients hospitalized in the United States, more than 1 million patients are injured in hospitals each year and approximately 180,000 die each year.[8] Other articles printed in 1998 in both *JAMA* and *Lancet* reported death rates as very high due to drug related errors and/or adverse drug reactions. Although these studies did not use the same definition of problem areas, the numbers reported remain alarming.[9] Many ADRs are preventable through the proper education of the patient and medical personnel. To obtain the knowledge necessary to prevent an ADR, reporting every suspected ADR is necessary. Pharmacists evaluate the potential for the reaction to have been caused by a specific medication. A definition of an ADR is necessary to obtain consistent reports. The ASHP states that when developing a definition of an ADR, the following criteria are essential: "Any undesirable or unexpected event that required stopping a drug, modifying the dose, prolonging hospitalization, or providing supporting treatment." An example of an internal hospital ADR reporting form is shown in Figure 2.

Classification of adverse drug reactions[10]

ADRs are defined as Type A and Type B. Type A ADRs are those that could be expected from the known properties of the medication and are responsible for most ADR events (many people refer to these reactions as drug side effects). These reactions, though frequent, are unlikely to be life threatening, but they may cause considerable discomfort to the patient. Type B ADRs are infrequent and are not predictable. Type B includes allergic and immunological reactions and may cause cancer and birth defects. Type B reactions are often more serious and may be life threatening. How the drugs induce these effects is usually unknown.

The FDA is particularly interested in the more serious of either Type A or Type B ADRs. Premarketing studies required by the FDA are usually tested on 3,000 to 5,000 patients before the drug is released and are designed to learn if the medication's benefits outweigh the risks of side effects or adverse drug reactions. The premarketing studies are not able to detect ADRs that may occur after long-term use or in special populations (e.g., children, elderly, patients having multiple diseases, patients taking multiple medications, or certain ethnic groups).

Utilization of pharmacy technicians in ADR reporting

The Food and Drug Administration (FDA) developed the MedWatch program to standardize reporting ADRs. The FDA uses a definition of an ADR that is broader in scope; it includes adverse events associated with drug overdose, drug abuse, and drug withdrawal. The FDA focuses on problems related to product quality performance or safety. The MedWatch forms are used for suspected contamination, questionable stability, defective components, and poor packaging or labeling.

Figure 2 Internal hospital ADR form example

SAINT JOSEPH MERCY HEALTH SYSTEM
A Member of Mercy Health Services

ST. JOSEPH MERCY HOSPITAL
5301 East Huron River Drive, P.O. Box 995, Ann Arbor, Michigan 48106-0995

Adverse Drug Reaction Probability Scale
(For Pharmacist Use)

7071-016 R 1/98 (PC) D

Date Notified of ADR: ____________________

Patient Registration Number: ____________________

Attending MD: ____________ Service ________

Prescribing MD: ____________________

Admitting Diagnosis: ____________________

Gender: M F Age/Birthdate: ____________

Height (cm): ______ Weight (kg): ______ SCr (mg %): ______

LOS: ________ (if applicable)

In your opinion,, was the reaction (Check one):

❒ mild ❒ moderate ❒ severe

Pharmacist Name (Print) /Pager# ____________________

Date mailed to attending MD: ____________________

Allergy History: ____________________

Allergies Noted in Medical Records ❒ Yes ❒ No

Date of Admission: ____________________

Date of Reaction: ____________________

Suspected Medication(s): ____________________

Dates of Administration: ____________________

List of Significant Concurrent Medications:

Description of Reaction/Sequence of Events:

Pertinent Laboratory Data:

Action Taken:

Comments:

Patient Outcome (check one): ❒ **Recovered** ❒ **Recovered with Sequelae** ❒ **Not Yet Recovered**

To assess the adverse drug reaction, please circle the answer on the following questionnaire to give the pertinent score:

		YES	NO	UNKNOWN
1.	Are there previous conclusive (literature) reports on this reaction?	+1	0	0
2.	Did the adverse event appear after the suspected drug was administered?	+2	-1	0
3.	Did the adverse reaction improve when the drug was discontinued or a specific antagonist was administered? List antagonist:	+1	0	0
4.	Did the adverse reaction appear when the drug was readministered?	+2	-1	0
5.	Are there alternative causes (other than the drug) that could on their own have caused the reaction in this patient? List:	-1	+2	0
6.	Did the reaction reappear when a placebo was given?	-1	+1	0
7.	Was the drug detected in the blood (or other fluids) in concentrations known to be toxic?	+1	0	0
8.	Was the reaction more severe when the dose was increased, or less severe when the dose was decreased?	+1	0	0
9.	Did the patient have a similar reaction to the same or similar drugs in any previous exposure? List/when:	+1	0	0
10.	Was the adverse event confirmed by any objective evidence (other than serum drug concentration)?	+1	0	0

"This is a confidential professional/peer review and quality Improvement document of St. Joseph Mercy Hospital, Ann Arbor, MI. It is protected from disclosure pursuant to the provisions of MCL 33.20175. MCL 333.21515. MCL 331.51. MCL 331.533 and other state and federal laws. Unauthorized disclosure or duplication is prohibited."

TOTAL SCORE: ____________

Score: **≥ 9 DEFINITE** **5-8 PROBABLE** **1-4 POSSIBLE** **0 DOUBTFUL**

Naranjo CA, Busto U, Sellers EM et al. A method for estimating the probability of adverse drug reactions. *Clin Pharmacol Ther* 1981;30:239-45.

Pharmacy personnel, including technicians, are an important link in reporting any ADR to the FDA. A technician may be involved in the process of identifying, documenting, analyzing, and reporting of ADRs in many ways. Technicians are trained to participate in the original screening of patient medication pharmacy orders by looking for *target drugs* (e.g., Benadryl® IM STAT to treat an allergic reaction) used to treat the ADR. The technician may do this screening through manual review of written orders or by screening computer reports of patients receiving target drugs. Additionally, the technician may review laboratory results for abnormally high blood or serum levels of drugs or other body chemicals that show an ADR occurred. Some pharmacists develop a training program for specialized technicians that will allow them to do the initial patient chart reviews based on well-defined criteria. This is particularly valuable in hospitals that use post-discharge computer reporting. Technicians can maintain the computer database of the ADR reports received and can complete the FDA MedWatch forms (see Figure 3).

Figure 3 MedWatch form

MEDWATCH
THE FDA MEDICAL PRODUCTS REPORTING PROGRAM

For VOLUNTARY reporting by health professionals of adverse events and product problems

Page ___ of ___

Form Approved: OMB No. 0910-0291 Expires:12/31/94
See OMB statement on reverse

FDA Use Only
Triage unit sequence #

A. Patient information

1. Patient identifier — In confidence
2. Age at time of event: ___ or Date of birth:
3. Sex ☐ female ☐ male
4. Weight ___ lbs or ___ kgs

B. Adverse event or product problem

1. ☐ Adverse event and/or ☐ Product problem (e.g., defects/malfunctions)
2. Outcomes attributed to adverse event (check all that apply)
   ☐ death ___ (mo/day/yr)
   ☐ life-threatening
   ☐ hospitalization – initial or prolonged
   ☐ disability
   ☐ congenital anomaly
   ☐ required intervention to prevent permanent impairment/damage
   ☐ other: ___
3. Date of event (mo/day/yr)
4. Date of this report (mo/day/yr)
5. Describe event or problem
6. Relevant tests/laboratory data, including dates
7. Other relevant history, including preexisting medical conditions (e.g., allergies, race, pregnancy, smoking and alcohol use, hepatic/renal dysfunction, etc.)

C. Suspect medication(s)

1. Name (give labeled strength & mfr/labeler, if known) #1 #2
2. Dose, frequency & route used #1 #2
3. Therapy dates (if unknown, give duration) from/to (or best estimate) #1 #2
4. Diagnosis for use (indication) #1 #2
5. Event abated after use stopped or dose reduced
   #1 ☐ yes ☐ no ☐ doesn't apply
   #2 ☐ yes ☐ no ☐ doesn't apply
6. Lot # (if known) #1 #2
7. Exp. date (if known) #1 #2
8. Event reappeared after reintroduction
   #1 ☐ yes ☐ no ☐ doesn't apply
   #2 ☐ yes ☐ no ☐ doesn't apply
9. NDC # (for product problems only) – –
10. Concomitant medical products and therapy dates (exclude treatment of event)

D. Suspect medical device

1. Brand name
2. Type of device
3. Manufacturer name & address
4. Operator of device
   ☐ health professional
   ☐ lay user/patient
   ☐ other: ___
5. Expiration date (mo/day/yr)
6. model # ___ catalog # ___ serial # ___ lot # ___ other # ___
7. If implanted, give date (mo/day/yr)
8. If explanted, give date (mo/day/yr)
9. Device available for evaluation? (Do not send to FDA)
   ☐ yes ☐ no ☐ returned to manufacturer on ___ (mo/day/yr)
10. Concomitant medical products and therapy dates (exclude treatment of event)

E. Reporter (see confidentiality section on back)

1. Name, address & phone #
2. Health professional? ☐ yes ☐ no
3. Occupation
4. Also reported to
   ☐ manufacturer
   ☐ user facility
   ☐ distributor
5. If you do NOT want your identity disclosed to the manufacturer, place an " X " in this box. ☐

FDA

Mail to: MEDWATCH
5600 Fishers Lane
Rockville, MD 20852-9787

or FAX to:
1-800-FDA-0178

FDA Form 3500 (6/93)

Submission of a report does not constitute an admission that medical personnel or the product caused or contributed to the event.

Medication incident reporting

Most medical facilities have a mechanism for collecting data concerning medication errors. The data collected usually incorporates the type of error, where the breakdown in the system occurred that allowed the error to take place, the drug involved, and personnel involved. (See Figure 4.) It is important to document errors that never reached the patient (near misses), as well as those that do. It may take the occurrence of a number of similar incidents to be able to determine the actual source of the problem.

Figure 4 Medication incident reporting form example

SAINT JOSEPH MERCY HEALTH SYSTEM
A Member of Mercy Health Services

❐ ST. JOSEPH MERCY HOSPITAL, ANN ARBOR
❐ SALINE COMMUNITY HOSPITAL, SALINE

Medication Incident Report
(Not part of the medical record)

For Occurrence:
Date: ________ Time: ________ Location: (Rm.) ____________
Medication as Ordered (Drug, dose, route, schedule):
____
Medication as given (Drug, dose, route, schedule):
____

WHEN WAS ERROR DETECTED
- Greater than 24 hours ❐
- Same shift ❐
- Within 24 hours ❐
- Office/Clinic Visit #1-3 ❐
- Office/Clinic Visit #4 or more ❐

CATEGORIZE ERROR
- Allergic to drug ❐
- Charting related ❐
- DC'd drug given ❐
- Drug mislabeled ❐
- Drug omitted ❐
- Extra dose ❐
- Order related ❐
- Wrong dose/rate ❐
- Wrong drug ❐
- Wrong patient ❐
- Wrong route ❐
- Wrong schedule ❐
- Wrong time ❐

DISCREPANCIES**
(Please describe under "Other."
No other sections apply.)
- Narcotic/Controlled Substance ❐
- Non-narcotic ❐
- Pyxis ❐
- Non-Pyxis ❐

RATE POTENTIAL PROBLEMS*
(Consider drug and condition of patient)
- Patient never received ❐
- No reaction expected ❐
- Minimal intervention ❐
- Complex intervention ❐
- Extensive intervention ❐

RATE ACTUAL PATIENT OUTCOME*
- No apparent ADE ❐
- Minimal intervention ❐
- Complex intervention ❐
- Extensive intervention ❐

ADDITIONAL COST INCURRED*
Check all that apply)
- No apparent cost ❐
- Pharmacy ❐
- Lab or other testing ❐
- Additional hospitalization or ❐
- outpatient visit ❐
- ICU stay ❐

*See Instructions/Definitions on reverse side.

REASONS FOR ERROR
(MARK ALL THAT APPLY)
ORDER PROCESS/VERIFICATION
- Charting Discrepancy ❐
- Correct Drug/Dose not available ❐
- Drug given but not charted ❐
- Changed order overlooked ❐
- Communication between providers ❐
- Forgot to give medication ❐
- Incorrect dose calculated ❐
- Incorrect drug/dose ❐
- Med order correlation at D/C ❐
- New order overlooked ❐
- No order ❐
- Order transcription error ❐
- Outpatient prescription issues ❐
- Patient compliance-explain** ❐
- Pyxis downtime ❐
- Verbal/Telephone order ❐
- Written order confusing/ incomplete/illegible ❐
- Other** ❐

PCIS-RELATED PROBLEMS
- PCIS downtime ❐
- Wrong dose selected ❐
- Wrong drug selected ❐
- Wrong patient selected ❐
- Wrong route selected ❐

PHARMACY ERROR
- Drug label incorrect ❐
- Drug not available ❐
- Order entry error ❐
- Wrong drug sent ❐
- Other ** ❐

MAR ERROR
- Admin. drug not charted ❐
- Charted incorrectly ❐
- Given after drug DC'd ❐
- Held drug given ❐
- MAR check not completed/ accurate ❐
- Other** ❐

This is a confidential professional/peer review and quality improvement document of St. Joseph Mercy and Saline Community Hospitals. It is protected from disclosure pursuant to the provisions of MCL 333,20175, MCL 33.21515, MCL 331.531, CML 331.533 and other state and federal laws. Unauthorized disclosure or duplication is absolutely prohibited.

IV PUMP ISSUES (RETAIN ALL DISPOSABLE)
(See directions on reverse)
- Found IV pump off ❐
- Incorrect rate setting ❐
- Tubing not clamped ❐
- Other** ❐

PCA Infuser Issues
- Epidural Pump # ________ (Hospital Tag #) ❐
- Pump # ________ (Hospital Tag #) ❐
- Other** ❐

****Other** (Describe error); use back if needed:
____

DEPT./DISCIPLINE INVOLVED
(Name if known)
Nurse ____________
Pharmacist ____________
Pharm Tech ____________
MD ____________
PA ____________
Student:
Nurse ____________
MD ____________
Other ____________
Clerk ____________
Other ____________

FOR PERSONNEL INVOLVED
- Error self-reported ❐
- Error reported by other ❐

MD NOTIFIED OF INCIDENT?
❐ No
❐ Yes (name): ____________

Signature of person preparing report: ____________
Date: ____________

Supervisor/Manager Follow-up or Action:
(If more space needed, use back of pertinent copy)
____
Signature: ____________
Date: ____________

09046 R 10/97 (PC) White Copy - Risk Management • Yellow - Pharmacy • Pink - CNM/Dept. Dir.

After the incident reports are collected, the data is usually organized in a manner that ranks the severity of the errors, determines the drug class (e.g., antibiotics, controlled substances, cardiovascular agents, anticoagulants, etc.), and the type of error. This allows staff (usually an interdisciplinary committee) to analyze the data and make recommendations to changes in policies and procedures where necessary.[11,12]

To increase medication incident reporting, national organizations, including ISMP, are encouraging the elimination of a disciplinary response to an incident.

> *"While we must still hold individuals responsible for high standards of performance, we now recognize that most errors result from faulty systems, not faulty people. To identify systems' failures, we need to know about the errors they cause. We need to make it safe for all healthcare workers to report errors."*
>
> — Lucian L. Leape, "Board of registration in nursing action is misguided and harmful" *Boston Globe*, Jan. 12, 1999.

"[F]ear of making a mistake that could harm a patient, damage one's reputation or relationships at work, and ruin one's career or livelihood."[13] This fear prevents staff members from reporting medication errors that could lead to system corrections. Driving fear out of the workplace has not occurred in many institutions, but work continues on this part of incident reporting.

Utilization of pharmacy technicians in medication incident reporting

All technicians should utilize their organization's reporting mechanisms to report a medication incident they observe or in which they participate. These incidents should be reported even if the medication never reached the patient or did not even leave the pharmacy. Such reports, along with others, will allow the system to be evaluated and corrected to prevent further errors.

Technicians may also be involved with maintaining the database for all of the incident reports. This may involve a report developed in-house, using a computer database such as Excel or Lotus, or a program specifically designed for the capture and analysis of medication incident data.

Total quality management

> *"Total quality management (TQM) is a relatively new approach to the art of management. It seeks to improve product and service quality and increase customer satisfaction by restructuring traditional management practices. The application of TQM is unique to each organization that adopts such an approach."*
>
> —Report of the U.S. General Accounting Office, May 1991[14]

W. Edwards Deming

When World War II ended, the U.S. government asked a statistician named Dr. W. Edwards Deming to go to Japan to assist in the recovery of the Japanese economy. Deming taught the Japanese a management theory and some techniques that resulted in their phenomenal economic rise. It wasn't until the 1980s that Americans appreciated Deming's work. American businesses started to incorporate the principles initiated by Deming, and his ideas continue to be used and expanded.

Deming Principles[15]

- Continuous improvement: the belief in "if it's not broke, don't fix it" had to end. Instead it is important to continuously improve. (This concept is referred to as continuous quality improvement or CQI.)

- Customer focus: the focus for improvement is the customer (both internal and external). By asking the customer what they need, an organization learns what to supply and in many cases what they no longer need to supply. (An internal customer is a concept that most people have trouble understanding. A hospital example would be to consider the nurse as a customer of the pharmacy. The nurse needs to receive the medications in a timely and accurate manner from the pharmacy in order to supply her customer—the patient—with the dose of medication.)
- Optimization: everyone in the organization needs to know the goals of the organization and how they fit into that goal. The idea is to optimize the system, not just the individual parts.
- Innovation: the organization is always looking for new ideas for meeting or exceeding the customer's expectations.
- Continuous learning: a culture must be developed in which staff members are constantly learning. Resources are made available to employees to foster this learning process.
- Knowledge: decisions are based on knowledge obtained through facts (data) collection. An understanding of variation and statistics is needed.

It is important to realize that the people who can best improve a process are the individuals responsible for that process. The organization must make it possible for people to be creative and enjoy their work.

Healthcare organizations have incorporated the quality improvement movement more slowly than the industrial portion of the U.S. economy. There are a number of reasons for this, which probably include the fact that healthcare organizations were already involved in a number of quality improvement programs and did not see the need to try new ones. Physicians are considered to be the leaders of the healthcare team; however, they are usually not employed by the hospital in which they practice. This makes it more difficult to start programs involving employees from the top on down. The legal system in the United States makes members of the healthcare team fear exposing any problem that might make them liable for a lawsuit.

Employing Deming Principles usually involves the use of Quality Action Teams (QATs). This concept involves training staff members to develop skills used to correct and prevent quality problems. QATs require the support of the entire management structure of the organization. A problem-solving mechanism is taught that involves learning to define a problem, gathering baseline data, developing an implementation plan to solve the problem, executing the plan, and monitoring the plan to determine its effectiveness. Teams should include those staff members who are involved with the problem area. In many healthcare organizations, this means that staff people from multiple departments are working together to solve issues that individual departments had not been able to affect in the past.

Pharmacy technician involvement in Quality Action Teams

A pharmacy technician's involvement in a QAT can vary. If QATs are active in their organization, technicians will be affected by it. Frequently, new employees are taught techniques involved in QAT participation so that, if invited to participate on a team, they are ready to do so. If a team is developed, participation is frequently voluntary. For a technician who is not a member of a team, involvement may include collecting data that the QAT needs to determine the next course of action. The team usually reports the results of their "data collection" in the form of charts and graphs, which are displayed in the work area. The results of a QAT will likely bring changes to the way the work is performed. A technician should be willing to accept change as needed and hopefully participate in future team activities.

Conclusion

Pharmacy technicians play valuable roles in improving the quality of the service their pharmacy delivers. By reporting problems and potential problems, collecting data for DUE and on ADRs, and participating in quality improvement activities, the pharmacy technician can positively impact the operations of a pharmacy and make it safer for patients to receive medications.

References

1. Joint Commission on Accreditation of Healthcare Organizations, www.jcaho.org. July 3, 2000.
2. Cohen, M., "Current Issues in Medication Safety," University of Michigan College of Pharmacy Annual Spring Seminar, Ypsilanti, MI, May 10, 1996.
3. "1999 accreditation standards address public concerns, says NCQA," *American Journal of Health-System Pharmacists,* Bethesda, MD, Vol. 55, pp. 2221-2225, Nov. 1, 1998.
4. *Quality Review,* The United States Pharmacopeial Convention, Inc., Rockville, MD, No. 57, January 1997.
5. Institute of Medicine's Recommendations for Medication Errors, *Pharmacists Letter,* www.pharmacistsletter.com/detailsearchend.asp, Feb. 16, 2000.
6. ASHP Guidelines on Medication-Use Evaluations, Best Practices for Health-system Pharmacy 1998-1999, American Society of Health-System Pharmacists, Bethesda, MD, pp. 70-72.
7. ASHP Guidelines on Adverse Drug Reaction Monitoring and Reporting, Best Practices for Health-system Pharmacy 1998-1999, American Society of Health-System Pharmacists, Bethesda, MD, pp. 77-79.
8. Bates, S. et al., "Incidence of Adverse Drug Events and Potential Adverse Drug Events," *Journal of the American Medical Association,* New York, NY, Vol. 274, No 1, pp. 29-34, July 5, 1995.
9. "Drug-related problems in spotlight again," *Pharmacy Today,* Washington, D.C. Vol. 4, No. 5, pp. 1-2, May 1998.
10. Clinical Therapeutics and the Recognition of Drug-Induced Disease, A MedWatch Continuing Education Article, Food and Drug Administration, U.S. Government, June 1995.
11. Hartwig, S.C., Denger, S.D., Schneider, P.J., "Severity-indexed, incident report-based medication error-based medication error-reporting program," *American Journal of Hospital Pharmacists,* Bethesda, MD, Vol . 55, pp. 2611-2616, December 1991.
12. Allan, E.L., Barker, K.N., "Fundamentals of medication error research." *American Journal of Hospital Pharmacists,* Bethesda, MD, Vol. 47, pp. 555-571, March 1990.
13. Ryan, K.D., "Driving fear out of the medication-use process so that improvement can occur," *American Journal of Health-System Pharmacists,* Bethesda, MD, Vol. 56, pp. 1765-1769, Sept. 1, 1999.
14. Chang, Y.S., Labovitz, G., Rosansky, V., Making Quality Work: A Leadership Guide for the Results-Driven Manager, Harper Business, New York, NY, 1993, p. 1.
15. Walton, M., Deming Management at Work, G.P. Putnam's Sons, New York, NY, 1990.

About the author

Judith Fedchenko received her bachelor's of science in pharmacy from the University of Michigan College of Pharmacy in Ann Arbor, Michigan, and a master's of science from Wayne State University College of Pharmacy & Allied Health Professions in Detroit, Michigan. She has been employed by St. Joseph Mercy Hospital in Ann Arbor, Michigan, for more than 30 years. Fedchenko currently holds the position of Coordinator for Quality Improvement in the Pharmacy Department. She is also an adjunct clinical assistant professor of pharmacy at the University of Michigan. Her auxiliary interests include the field of herbs and nutritional supplements. She has delivered numerous presentations to medical professionals and the community.

Self-assessment questions

1. JCAHO stands for:
   a. Japanese Care and Health Organization.
   b. Joint Commission on Accreditation of Healthcare Organizations.
   c. Judicial Committee for Analysis of Hospitals and Others.
   d. Joint Committee on Approval of Healthcare Organizations.
2. JCAHO accreditation is important to a healthcare organization because:
   a. the healthcare organization won't need a license to operate.
   b. the healthcare organization will be able to participate in Medicare without a yearly Medicare survey.
   c. it may cause the liability insurance premium to rise.
   d. JCAHO presents continuing education programs to the staff.
3. Which of the following questions might a JCAHO surveyor ask a pharmacy technician?
   a. What is the proper antibiotic to use to treat a patient with an anaerobic infection of the abdomen?
   b. Where is the closest fire extinguisher?
   c. What is your hospital policy on the use of restraints?
   d. What is the dose of warfarin for a patient with an INR of 1.5?
4. The criteria used to select medications for DUE reporting include:
   a. the least frequently used medications.
   b. medications which have never been known to cause an adverse reaction, interact with other medications, food, or diagnostic procedures.
   c. drugs that are potentially toxic at normal doses.
   d. drugs that have been removed from the formulary.
5. An example of adverse drug reaction is:
   a. when the administered medication allows the patient to go home in fewer days than the average length of stay.
   b. when it is necessary to change an oral tablet dosage form to a liquid form because the patient can't swallow a tablet.
   c. when an antibiotic is discontinued because the patient developed an allergic reaction.
   d. when the patient won't take the medication because it tastes bad.
6. Type A adverse drug reactions are:
   a. usually serious and life threatening.
   b. the possible cause of birth defects.
   c. infrequent and not predictable.
   d. frequent and often predictable.
7. Type B adverse drug reactions are:
   a. infrequent and not predictable.
   b. expected from the known properties of the drug.
   c. usually called a drug "side effect."
   d. frequent and often predictable.
8. Pharmacy employees may fear reporting a medication error because:
   a. they would have to get a job with a government healthcare organization.
   b. their employer would give them a raise.
   c. they would have to return to college and take a one-year remedial education course.
   d. they don't want their reputation damaged.
9. Total Quality Management or TQM involves:
   a. expensive training programs for employees.
   b. following a list of rigid specifications.
   c. improvement in product and service quality.
   d. a decrease in customer satisfaction.
10. Deming principles include the following *except*:
    a. continuous improvement.
    b. customer focus.
    c. continuous learning.
    d. continuous inspection of finished products to eliminate errors.

CHAPTER 27

ASEPTIC TECHNIQUE AND STERILE PRODUCT PREPARATION

Laura A. Thoma, Pharm.D.

Learning objectives:

Upon completion of this chapter, the technician should be able to do the following:

- List three reasons why a drug is given parenterally instead of orally.
- List four major routes of parenteral administration.
- List three advantages of parenteral administration.
- List three disadvantages of parenteral administration.
- Define *pyrogen*.
- Define *aseptic technique*.
- Define a *Class 100 area*.
- Explain how a laminar airflow hood works.
- Explain the difference between working in a horizontal flow hood versus a vertical flow hood.
- Describe the appropriate garb for the controlled area.
- Explain how to sanitize the laminar flow workbench (LFW).
- List four examples of critical sites.
- Explain the proper procedure for withdrawing a liquid from an ampule and a vial.
- Describe an intravenous (IV) piggyback.
- List the visual checks that must be made on a parenteral solution.
- List some major components of parenteral nutrition solutions.

Introduction to parenteral products

Parenteral products are products administered by injection and therefore bypass the gastrointestinal (GI) tract. Parenteral products must be sterile (free of all living microorganisms), free of pyrogens (fever-inducing substances), and free of particulate matter. Drugs that are destroyed when taken orally, inactivated in the GI tract, or poorly absorbed can be given by a parenteral route. Parenteral routes of administration may also be used when the patient being treated is uncooperative, unconscious, or unable to swallow. This route is also used when rapid drug absorption is essential, such as in emergency situations.

Parenteral routes of administration

There are a number of routes of administration for parenteral products. Some commonly used routes of administration include intravenous, intra-arterial, intradermal, subcutaneous, and intramuscular.

Intravenous route

An intravenous (IV) medication is administered directly into the vein. The IV route gives a rapid effect with a predictable response because the medication is rapidly diluted with blood. The IV route has less volume restriction than other parenteral routes. Drugs given by the intravenous route may be given as a bolus, an intermittent infusion, or a continuous infusion. A bolus is an injection of a drug into the vein over a short period of time. A bolus is used to administer a relatively small volume of solution and is often written as "IV push" (IVP). It is often used in emergency situations where rapid effect is desired. Many drugs can cause adverse effects to the patient if given too quickly. Intermittent infusions are used for drugs that require being given at defined time intervals to be most effective. Intermittent infusions are used to administer a relatively small volume of solution over a specified amount of time, at specific intervals. One type of intermittent infusion, the piggyback, is a second medication solution that is infused through an established primary IV administration set. Usually piggybacks are 500ml or less. Antibiotics, for example, are commonly piggybacked. A piggybacked medication eliminates the need for another needle stick and further dilutes the medication to help reduce irritation of the vein.

A continuous infusion refers to the introduction of larger volumes of solution, given over a longer period of time. A continuous infusion is used to administer a large volume of solution at a constant rate.

Intramuscular route

An intramuscular (IM) medication is injected deep into a large muscle mass, such as the upper arm, thigh or buttocks. The medication is absorbed from muscle tissue, acting more quickly than when given by the oral route, but not as quickly as a medication given by the IV route. Typically, no more than 2.5ml of medication may be administered intramuscularly as a solution or suspension. A sustained-release action can be achieved with certain drugs that have low solubility as they are released from muscle tissue at a prolonged rate. IM injections are often painful, and reversing adverse effects from medications given by this route is very difficult.

Subcutaneous route

Subcutaneous (SC or SQ) injections of solution or suspension are given beneath the surface of the skin. Medications administered by this route are not absorbed as well and have a slower onset of action than medications given by the IV or IM route. The volume of solution or suspension that can be injected subcutaneously is 2ml or less. Patients can be easily taught to give themselves SQ injections and many patients (e.g., diabetics) routinely administer medication in this manner.

Intradermal route

An intradermal (ID) injection is injected into the top layer of the skin. The injection is not as deep as a SQ injection. Medications used for diagnostic purposes such as a tuberculin (TB) test or allergy test are often administered by this route. The volume of solution which can be administered intradermally is limited to 0.1ml. The onset of action and the rate of absorption of medication from this route are slow.

Miscellaneous parenteral routes of administration

An *intra-arterial* medication is injected directly into the artery, delivering the medication directly to the desired location. One use for this route of administration is to introduce radio opaque materials (e.g., a dye that can be seen on an x-ray) for diagnostic purposes such as arteriograms (a tracing of the wave from an arterial pulse).

- An *intra-articular* medication is injected into a joint such as the elbow or knee.
- An *intracardiac* medication is injected directly into the heart muscle.
- An *intraperitoneal* medication is injected into the peritoneal or abdominal cavity.
- An *intrapleural* medication is injected into the sac surrounding the lungs.
- An *intraventricular* medication is injected directly into a ventricle of the brain.
- An *intravesicular* medication is instilled into the urinary bladder.

- An *intravitrial* medication is injected into the eye.
- An *intrathecal* medication is injected into the space around the spinal cord.

Advantages of parenteral administration

Medications given parenterally usually have a quicker onset of action and a more predictable absorption into the blood. Patient compliance is usually enhanced with the parenteral route. The parenteral route is used to correct fluid and electrolyte imbalances, and can be used to provide nutrition to the patient when food cannot be taken by mouth or tube feedings. Patients who are unable to swallow medications may receive their medication by the parenteral route. This route is required for medications that are not effective orally or that are destroyed by digestive secretions. Parenteral administration can also be used to provide a local effect for medications when desired, as in dentistry and anesthesiology.

Disadvantages of parenteral administration

Parenteral medications are not easily self-administered and, therefore, must be administered by trained personnel. This type of administration requires more time than other administration routes and is also more costly. Once a medication is injected parenterally, stopping all of its effects, including the undesirable ones, is difficult. IV injections are usually painful. Because there is always a risk of infection whenever the skin is punctured, strict adherence must be given to aseptic technique, which is discussed later in this chapter.

Intravenous bottles and bags

Intravenous solutions can be supplied in four types of containers. A glass container with an air tube is sometimes referred to as an *open system* because unfiltered air enters the container, requiring a non-vented administration set (Figures 1 and 2). The closure of an open system has two openings—one is the airway tube and the other receives the spike from the administration set. The closure is covered with a thin rubber diaphragm. Check to make sure there are small indentations in the seal over the holes, as this indicates that the vacuum is present in the bottle. If the bottle has lost its vacuum, it should be discarded immediately. Medications can be added to the bottle by injecting them through the additive injection port or through the seal covering the hole for the spike. Medication should never be added to the air tube. The seal on the closure is removed just before the bottle is spiked.

Figure 1 An open system

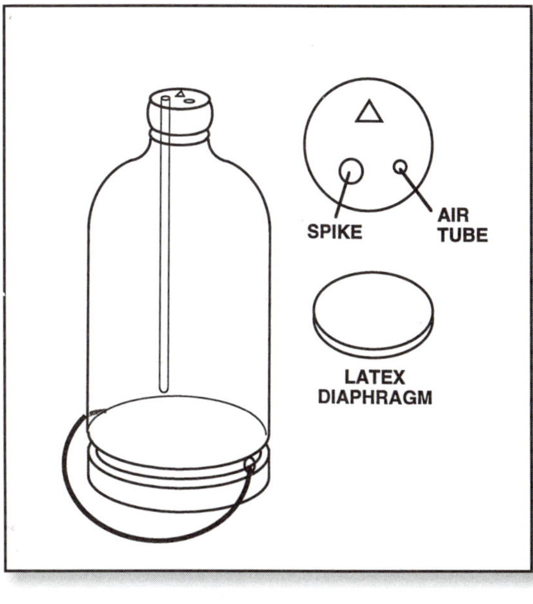

Figure 2 Non-vented administration set

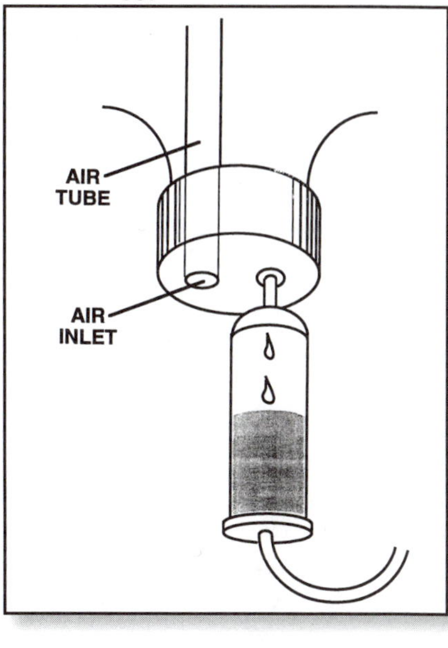

Figure 3 A semi-closed system

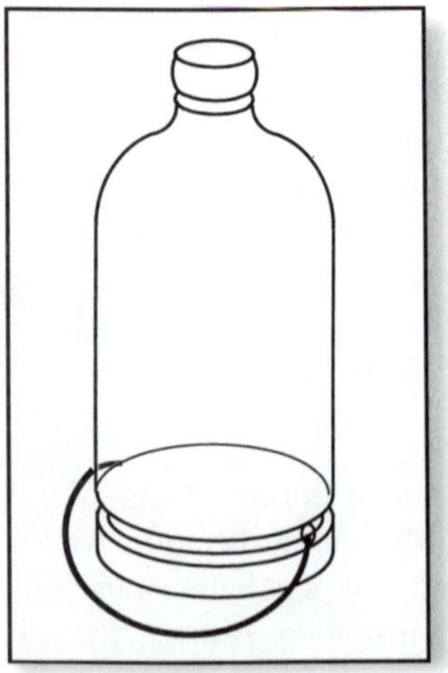

A glass container without an air tube contains a vacuum and is sometimes called a *semi-closed system* because the air that enters the container is filtered (Figure 3). This system requires a vented administration set. The air vent contains a 0.2-micron hydrophobic (water-hating) filter (Figure 4). This sterilizing filter allows air to pass into the bottle while preventing bacteria from entering. The closure is a solid rubber stopper. The target area in the center, where the closure is thinner, allows the injection of medication or spiking the administration set through this area.

Figure 4 Vented administration set

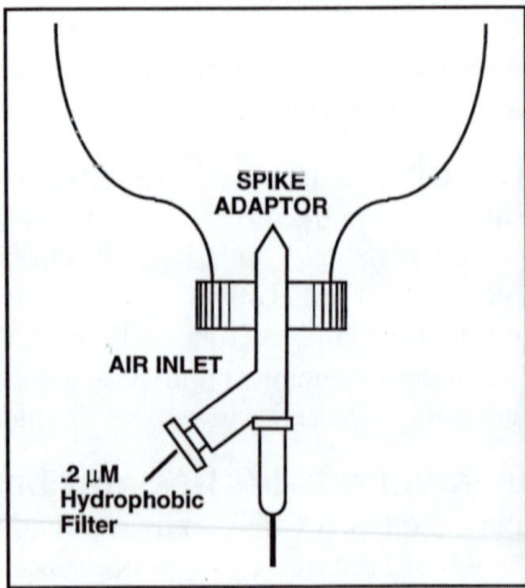

A flexible plastic bag is referred to as a *closed system* because the bag collapses to prevent air from entering the system (Figure 5). There are two ports on the bag. One port is covered with a plastic cover that is removed to accept the spike of the administration set. The other port is the injection port with a gum rubber covering used for the addition of medication to the bag. This system requires a non-vented set.

Figure 5 A closed system

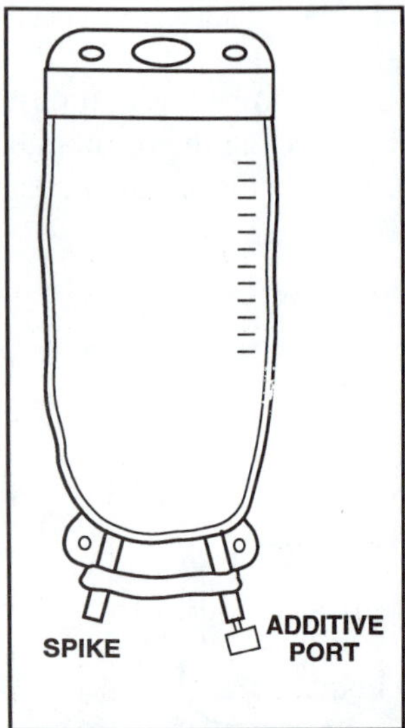

Sterilization by filtration

Filtration is the most common method of sterilization in a pharmacy. Filters come in various pore sizes and configurations; however, a sterilizing filter pore size must be 0.2 microns. A sterilizing filter is one that, when challenged with a solution of *Brevundimonas diminuta* at a concentration of 10^7 CFU (colony-forming units) per cm^2 of filter surface area, will give a sterile effluent discharge. A larger pore size filter (e.g., 0.45, 0.8, 1.2 and 5 microns) is used for clarification of the solutions. A 5-micron filter needle is not a sterilizing filter, but is acceptable for filtering a solution from an ampule. When selecting a filter, it is important to know if the solution is aqueous or non-aqueous and to know the volume of the solution being filtered. An aqueous solution requires a hydrophilic (water-loving) filter and a non-aqueous solution needs a hydrophobic filter. When selecting a filter, one must consider the pore size, the compatibility of the solution with the filter membrane and filter housing, the volume of solution to be filtered, and the amount of particulate of the solution. Filter suppliers are a great source of help in filter selection.

Methods of sterilization for products and devices include cold sterilization and heat sterilization. *Cold sterilization* uses chemicals (e.g., ethylene oxide gas), radiation, or ultrasonic process. *Heat sterilization* uses steam and pressure (as with an autoclave) or a hot air oven (in which high temperatures sterilize products or devices).

Pyrogens

Like bacterial contamination, pyrogen contamination is a concern when preparing products for parenteral administration. Pyrogens are substances that produce fever. One type of pyrogen, endotoxin, is a lipopolysaccharide (a large molecule of lipids and sugars joined by chemical bonds) shed from a gram-negative bacteria cell wall. An endotoxin can also be released when bacteria die. Pyrogens are not removed with a 0.2-micron filter and are not destroyed by autoclaving. Products contaminated with pyrogens must be thrown away. The *bacterial endotoxin test* determines the amount of endotoxin in a parenteral product. When commercially prepared sterile products are used and aseptic technique is observed, pyrogens will not be of concern, as long as good aseptic technique is used. However, if a sterile product is being compounded from a non-sterile product, one must check for pyrogens before releasing the product.

Aseptic technique glossary

Aseptic technique is a means of manipulating sterile products without contaminating them. Bacteria are everywhere, and contamination can come from the environment, equipment and supplies, or personnel. The following definitions and terminology are used to describe aseptic compounding of pharmaceutical products:

Admixture: a parenteral dosage form made from combining several drug products for administration as a single entity.

Class 100 area: an area in which there are no more than 100 particles, 0.5 microns and larger, per cubic foot of air.

Class 10,000 area: an area in which there are no more than 10,000 particles, 0.5 microns and larger, per cubic foot of air.

Class 100,000 area: an area in which there are no more than 100,000 particles, 0.5 microns and larger, per cubic foot of air.

Controlled area: also called a *buffer area*, the area in which the laminar flow workbench is located. It is the area in the pharmacy that is second in cleanliness to the laminar flow workbench.

Critical site: any opening or surface that can provide a pathway between the sterile product and the environment. Examples of critical sites are the hub of the needle, the tip of the syringe, the open neck of the ampule, the top of the vial closure, and the ribs of the plunger on a syringe.

Figure 6 Horizontal laminar flow workstation

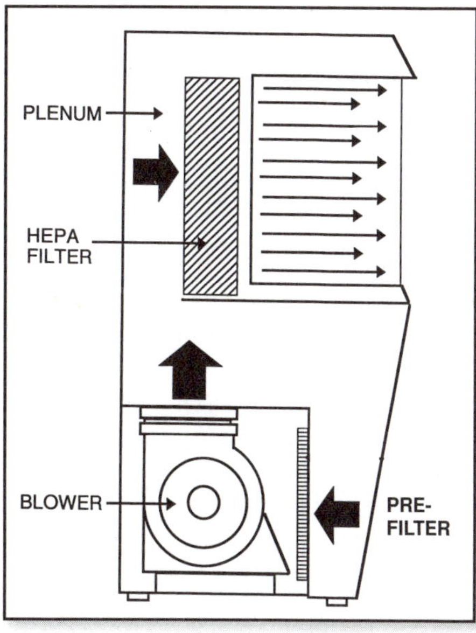

Laminar flow: air in a confined area moving with uniform speed along parallel lines. Air flow in a laminar flow workbench (LFW) must have a velocity of 90 feet/minute plus or minus 20 percent. A LFW can be a horizontal flow where the air flows towards the operator, or a vertical flow where the air flows down towards the bench.

The *horizontal laminar flow workstation* (HLFW) draws air in through a pre-filter (Figure 6). The pre-filtered air is pressurized in the plenum for even distribution of air to the high efficiency particulate air (HEPA) filter. The plenum of the hood is the space between the pre-filter and HEPA filter. The air is blown across the work surface toward the operator. The pre-filter in the laminar flow workstation protects the HEPA filter from premature clogging. Pre-filters are similar to furnace filters and must be checked regularly. The HEPA filter consists of banks of filter medium separated by corrugated aluminum pleats. The separators act as baffles to direct air in a laminar flow. The HEPA filter is 99.97 percent efficient at removing particles 0.3 microns and larger. To put this in perspective, the smallest particles visible to the human eye are about 40 to 50 microns in size.

The *vertical laminar flow workstation* (VLFW) is similar to a HLFW in that air is drawn in through the pre-filter, pressurized in the plenum, and pushed through the HEPA filter (Figure 7). However, the air is blown down from the top of the workstation onto the work surface, not across it. Working in vertical laminar flow (VLF) requires different techniques than working in HLF. In VLF, the hands of the operator or any object must *not be above* an object in the hood. In HLF, the hands of the operator or any object must not be *in back* of another object. The hands of the operator must never come between the HEPA filter and the object. Remember, always protect the critical site.

Figure 7 Vertical laminar flow workstation

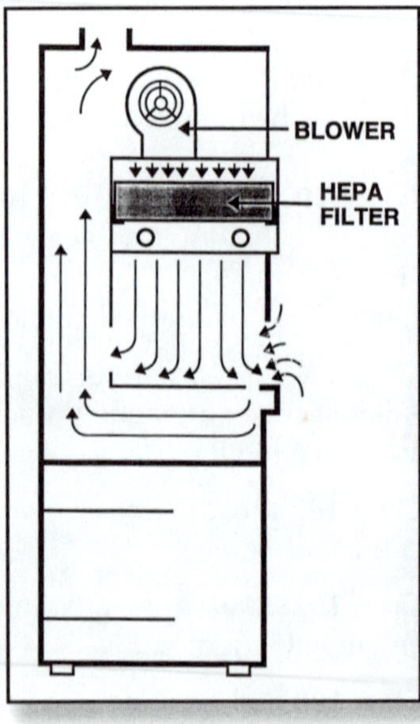

Sterility: the state of being "free of all living microorganisms." It does not mean that the solution is free from pyrogens or viruses. Compounding sterile products takes place in a Class 100 area. Usually the Class 100 area is only in the LFW; however, some institutions have a Class 100 room.

Validation: establishing documented evidence that provides a high degree of assurance that a specific process will consistently produce a product that meets predetermined specifications. In other words, validation is documentation or evidence that you are producing what you say you are producing.

Buffer area

Because overcoming a velocity of 90 feet/minute is very easy, the LFW must be placed in a controlled environment called a buffer area. The buffer area, which is second in cleanliness to the LFW, is enclosed from other pharmacy operations, preferably with walls. In some situations, curtains are acceptable. The LFW must be located away from excess traffic, doors, air vents, or anything that could produce air currents that may introduce contamination into the hood. Any air currents or movements greater than the velocity of the airflow from the HEPA filter may introduce contaminants into the hood. Some examples are coughing or sneezing into the hood and quick movements in and out of the hood.

Surfaces in the buffer area should be smooth, non-porous, non-shedding, and easily cleaned or disinfected. Cracks, crevices, and seams must be avoided. Cracks and crevices are hard to keep clean and are a perfect place for microorganisms to flourish. Ledges or other places where dust may collect should also be avoided. The buffer room should meet the requirement of at least a Class 100,000 clean room; in some cases a Class 10,000 clean room is recommended. This room must have positive (greater) pressure in relationship to the rest of the pharmacy to prevent dirty air from entering the clean room. Access to the buffer area must be restricted to only qualified personnel who must be properly scrubbed and gowned. Housekeeping of the buffer area must be kept at high standards. The cleaning tools and supplies must be kept separate and only used in the buffer area. The cleaning personnel must be trained in the appropriate procedures.

Anteroom

The anteroom is an area of high cleanliness separated from the buffer area by a barrier. Preferably this barrier is a wall, but in some cases a curtain is acceptable. The anteroom is used to decontaminate supplies, equipment, and personnel. Hand washing, gowning, and unpacking supplies from cardboard boxes is done in the anteroom to reduce the number of particles in the buffer area. Clean and sanitized supplies can also be stored in this area. Like the buffer area, the anteroom is constructed from non-shedding, easily cleaned material. Ideally, this room is less positive in pressure than the buffer area, but still positive to the rest of the pharmacy.

The dirty side of the anteroom is clearly separated from the clean side by a line on the floor, or a bench across the room. This line easily identifies the stock room and anteroom. Equipment and supplies do not cross this line without being sanitized.

Preparation of supplies

Large-volume parenteral products (volume greater than 100 milliliters), small volume parenteral products (volume of 100 milliliters or less), devices, and other supplies must not be in the buffer area in shipping cartons. Cardboard sheds many particles. Supplies must be unpacked in the anteroom on the dirty side, wiped with a non-lint-producing wipe soaked with a sanitizing agent, and placed on a cart for transfer into the buffer area.

Preparation of pharmacy technicians and pharmacists

The operators (pharmacy technicians and pharmacists) must minimize the introduction of contaminants into the buffer area. The operator must be properly scrubbed and gowned before entering the buffer area. Proper preparation of the operator is a critical key to maintaining a controlled environment. The greatest source of contamination in a clean room is the people in the area. A person sitting down releases 100,000 particles per minute. A person moving at two miles per hour releases five million particles into the air each minute.

Operators scrub from the elbow to hands for an appropriate amount of time with antimicrobial skin cleanser. Hands are dried using a forced air dryer or disposable, non-shedding towels. After scrubbing, frequent use of a foamed sanitizing agent or sterile 70% isopropyl alcohol during the shift and before entering the hood is essential.

Optimally, the operator does not wear jewelry or makeup when working in the buffer area. Before entering the buffer room, the operator dons a hair cover, shoe covers, clean knee length non-shedding gown or coverall, and sterile gloves. The sterile gloves are put on aseptically, with the cuffs of the gown inside the gloves. Once the gloves are out of the package they are no longer sterile. The purpose of the gloves is to contain the particles shed from the operators' hands, not to replace good aseptic technique. To maintain glove surfaces as free from contamination as possible, frequently rinse the glove with a sanitizing agent. Before working in the hood, the operator dons a face mask.

Only pharmacy technicians and pharmacists highly skilled in aseptic technique may enter the buffer area. Before compounding sterile products, an operator must be validated by successfully completing three consecutive "media fills." After completing the initial validation, personnel must be revalidated according to the written policy and procedure in their practice site. It is recommended that all personnel revalidate at least once a year; some facilities revalidate quarterly. Media is used to compound the sterile product instead of the drug and diluent. The process is as complicated as the most complex item compounded now or in the future. The media is incubated for 14 days and then inspected for growth. One container with growth constitutes a media fill failure. If a media fill fails at any time, the operator must successfully revalidate with three consecutive media fills.

Preparation of LFW

The blower to the LFW always remains in operation. If the hood is shut off, it must be turned on for at least 30 minutes (or according to the manufacturer recommendations) before use. The hood is wiped with a sanitizing agent such as sterile 70% isopropyl alcohol. Begin by wiping the HLFW bar first, using a non-shedding wipe soaked with the sanitizing agent, followed by wiping the sides of the hood. Start at the end closest to the filter, working outward, and wipe from the top edge of the side to the bottom. The bench top is cleaned last. Starting closest to the filter, wipe from side to side, from the filter to the outside. Work from the cleanest part outward. The LFW is wiped at the beginning of the shift and after any spill (at least). Spraying the sanitizing agent increases the chances of wetting the HEPA filter. Do not spray sanitizing agent into the hood; it is better to pour the agent from a bottle onto the wiping material. A wet HEPA filter could easily develop a pinhole.

To ensure its proper working condition, a LFW should be certified every six months, every time the HEPA filter is wetted, or every time the LFW is moved. A reputable testing company may be used to test the velocity of the laminar flow and the integrity of the HEPA filter. The velocity of the air from the HEPA filter is checked by using a velometer. The average air velocity is 90 linear feet per minute (ft/min), plus or minus 20 percent. No one measurement may be less than 72 ft/min. The integrity of the HEPA filter is checked by introducing aerosolized Emery 3004 or a similar agent into the plenum of the LFW while monitoring for penetration of the Emery 3004 on the downstream side of the HEPA filter. The aerosol has an average particle size of 0.3 microns. No more than 0.01 percent of the upstream concentration may be detected downstream of the HEPA filter.

Working in the LFW

An operator must always use good aseptic technique to compound sterile products. Working in a LFW may give an operator a false sense of security concerning the sterility of the products prepared. Products and supplies not in an overwrap are first wiped with isopropyl alcohol before being placed in the hood. An LFW *does not* remove microbial contaminants from the surface of containers or other items placed in the workstation. LFW is not a sterilization process. An LFW must be properly maintained and used correctly to provide a Class 100 area.

Any items not in a protective overwrap (e.g., ampules, vials, IV bags and bottles) must be wiped with a non-lint-producing wipe soaked with sterile 70% isopropyl alcohol before being placed in the hood. Check all containers for cracks, tears, and particles before using them to compound IV admixtures. If an item is in a protective overwrap, it may be taken from the overwrap at the edge of the hood and placed in the hood. One exception to this practice is the needle, which is not removed from its overwrap until immediately before its use. Needles are placed in the first six inches of the hood until they are ready to be removed from their wrap and used. Items in a horizontal laminar flow station are placed left or right of the critical work area. The critical sites must be in laminar air flow at all times. The operator must work without placing a hand or object behind a critical site.

All work done in the HLFW must be done at least six inches inside the hood. Room air can be carried into the front of the hood from the turbulence created as the laminar flow air passes around the person working at the hood. It must be remembered that a HLFW is not a means of sterilization. It only maintains an area free of microorganisms, contaminants, and particulate matter when it is properly maintained, prepared, and used by operators with good aseptic technique. An HLFW will not compensate for bad aseptic technique.

When an item is in the HLFW, it disturbs the laminar flow of air. The air flow is disturbed downstream of the object, for approximately three times the diameter of the object. If the item is flush with the side wall, it will disturb the laminar flow for approximately six times the diameter of the object (Figure 8). Any non-sterile object has the potential to contaminate articles downstream with particles. It is very important that a direct path exists between the HEPA filter and the critical site.

Figure 8 Downward view of a laminar-air-flow hood

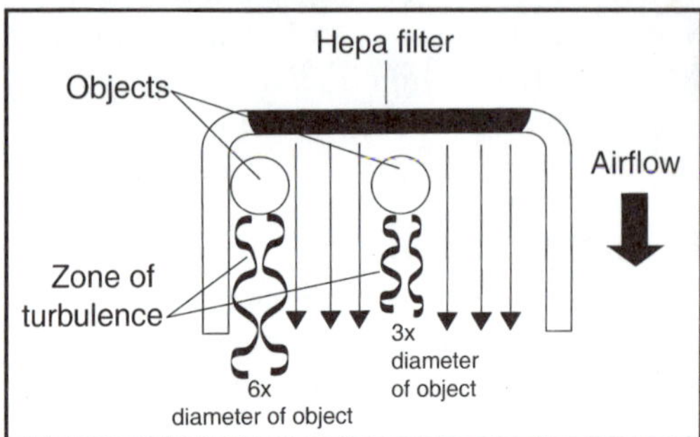

In a VLFW, supplies are placed so that the operator may work without placing a hand or object *above* the critical site. Movements in and out of the hood must be minimized. All items needed for the aseptic manipulation are introduced into the work area at one time. Articles to be thrown away may be dropped over the edge of the hood into the trash or they may be left in the first six inches of the hood until the manipulations are complete, then thrown away in the trash or a container for sharp contaminated objects.

Needles

Sterile needles are wrapped in rigid or semi-rigid plastic covers. This wrap must be inspected before using the needle; tears or pinholes in the wrap will compromise the sterility of the needle. Needles come in a variety of sizes. The gauge of the needle refers to the outer diameter of the needle—the larger the number, the smaller the bore of the needle. The smallest is 27 gauge, and the largest is 13 gauge. Most facilities use an 18-gauge to 21-gauge needle. The needle length is measured in inches. Commonly used are 1-inch and 1.5-inch lengths.

Figure 9 Basic parts of a needle

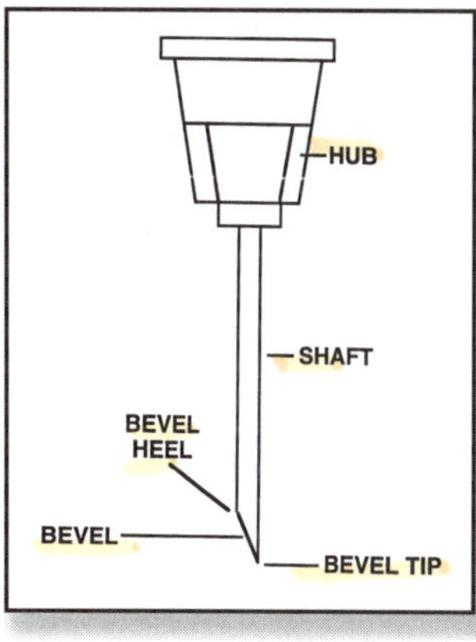

The basic parts of a needle include the hub, needle shaft, bevel, bevel heel, and tip (Figure 9). The needle shaft is encased in a rigid plastic sheath by which the needle is handled. This sheath is left on until the needle and syringe are used. The needle shaft is *never* swabbed with alcohol, as it is usually coated with silicone to allow for easy penetration of the rubber. The critical sites on a needle are the needle hub and the tip.

Syringes

Syringes can be made of plastic or glass. Disposable plastic syringes are now used most often in the preparation of sterile products. They are sterile, pyrogen-free, and packaged in either paper or a rigid plastic container. Inspect the syringe wrap carefully to assure that the syringe is intact and sterile. The basic parts of a syringe are the barrel, plunger, the rubber tip of the plunger (piston), and the tip (Figure 10). The critical sites on the syringe are the plunger and the tip of the syringe.

Figure 10 Basic parts of a syringe

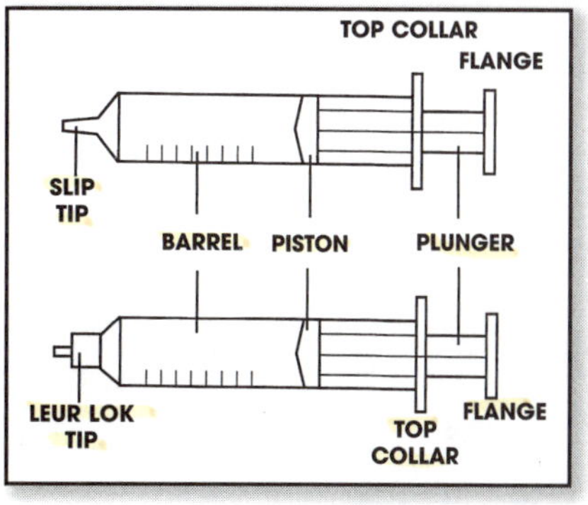

Syringes have either a Luer Lok tip or a slip tip (friction fit tip) (Figure 10). The Luer Lok tip is threaded, and the needle is tightened on the threaded tip. The friction tip needle simply slides onto the tip of the syringe. It is held in place by friction.

A protective cover is usually on the tip of the syringe. This cap remains on until the needle is attached.

Figure 11 Syringe markings on the barrel with 2ml withdrawn

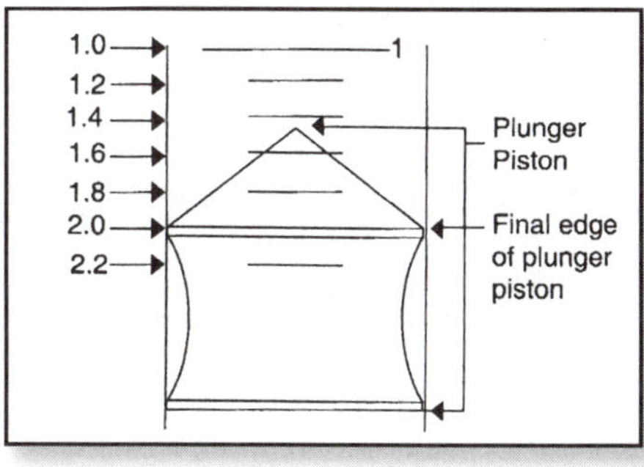

Calibration marks are on the barrel of the syringe. The larger the syringe, the larger the increments on the barrel of the syringe. These marks are accurate to one-half of the interval marked on the syringe. For the sake of accuracy, the operator should use the smallest syringe available to hold the amount of solution needed. To deliver a given volume in a syringe, the final edge of the rubber tip of the plunger that comes in contact with the syringe is lined up with the calibration mark that corresponds with the volume of fluid desired (Figure 11).

Gowning

To begin gowning, select a clean hair cover and put it on with little or no touching of the hair (Picture 1). Scrub the hands and forearms to the elbow for at least 30 seconds with a sanitizing soap and a brush (Picture 2). Rinse arms and start the hand dryer with an elbow (Picture 3). Select two clean shoe covers. Sit on the bench with feet on the "dirty side." Open the shoe cover using three fingers of each hand to protect the clean fingers as the cover is placed on the shoe (Pictures 4 and 5). Once the shoe cover is on, swing the foot over the bench to the clean side. Repeat for the other foot. Select a clean non-linting coat and put it on, zipping it all the way up (Picture 6). Open the appropriate size gloves, remove them from the package, and unfold the inner package. Pick up the first glove by the folded down cuff of the glove (Picture 7). The hand is now touching the inside of the glove. The ungloved hand should never touch the outside of the glove (Picture 8). Do not fully pull off the cuff of the glove at this time. Insert two fingers of the gloved hand into the cuff of the other glove. The gloved hand is now touching the outside of the glove (Picture 9). Pull the glove on and pull the cuff up over the sleeve of the gown. Pull the cuff of the second glove over the coat (Picture 10). Before working in the hood, the face mask must be on. Place the top inside of the mask (wire band) over the bridge of the nose. Fit the mask to the head (Picture 11). Tie the top strings tightly in a bow at the crown of the skull (Picture 12). Pull down gently on the lower edge of the mask, and tie the bottom strings loosely (Picture 13).

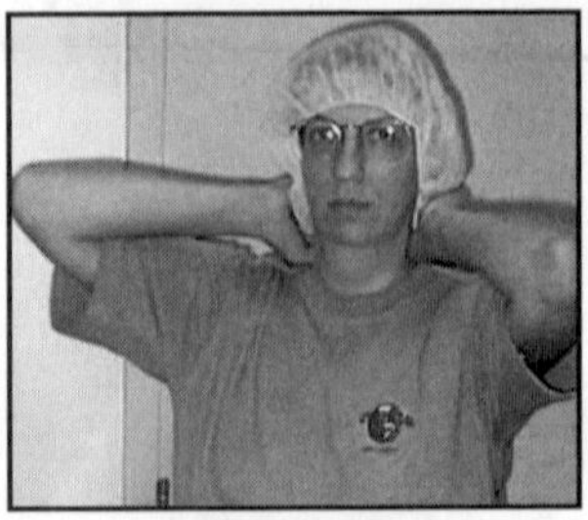

Picture 1

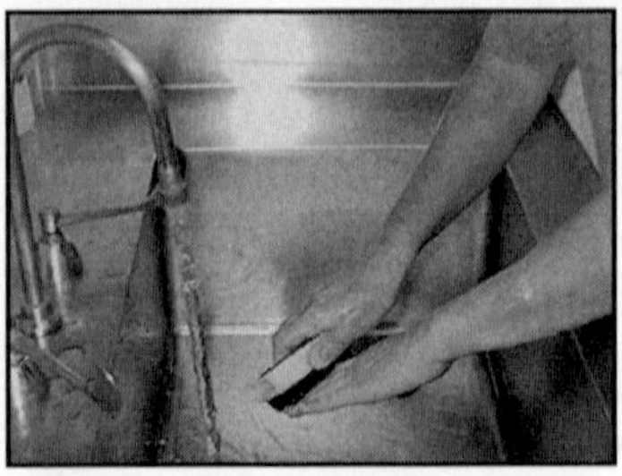

Picture 2

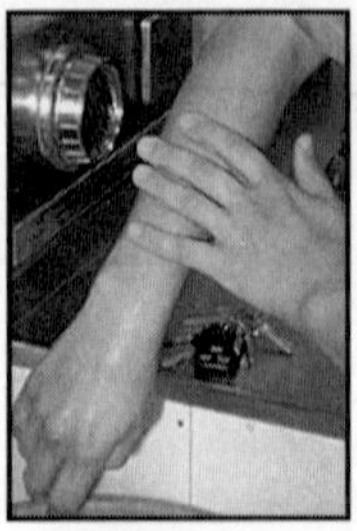

Picture 3

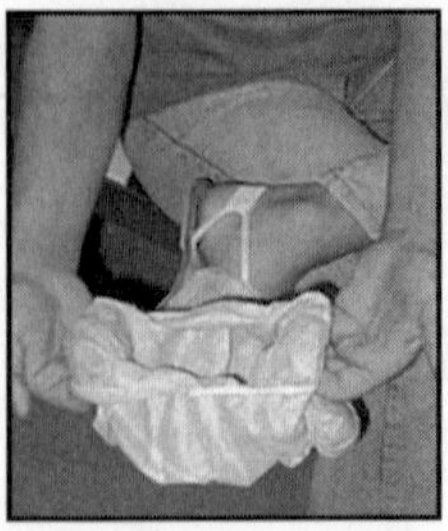

Picture 4

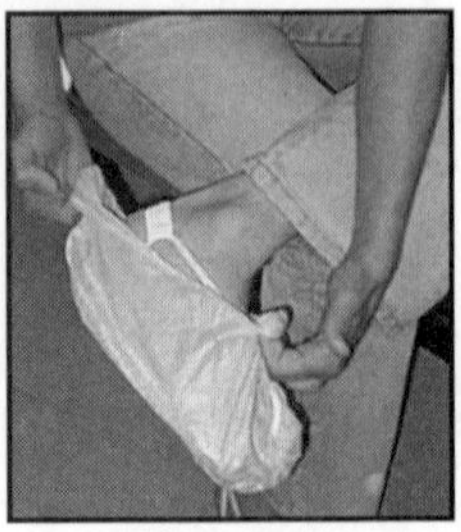

Picture 5

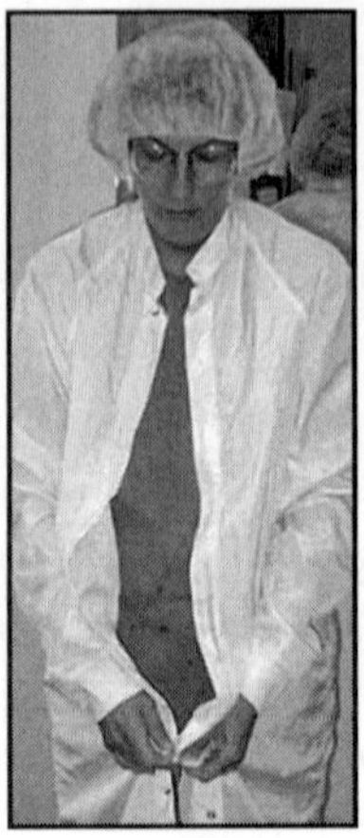

Picture 6

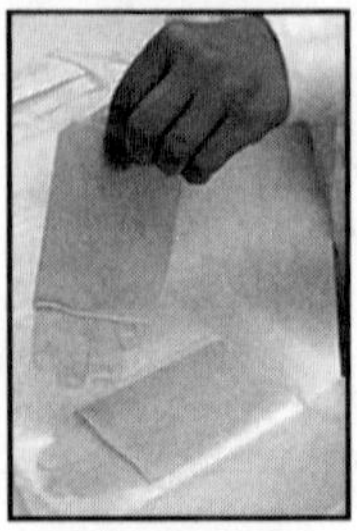

Picture 7

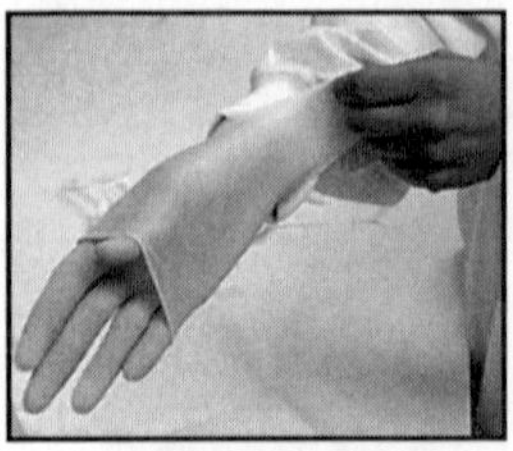

Picture 8

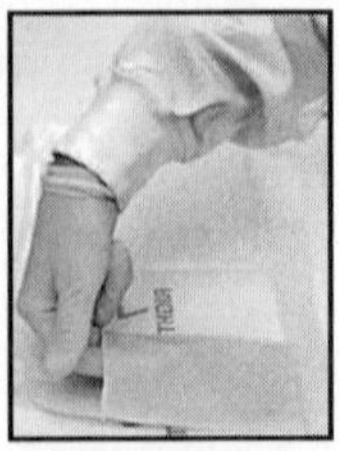

Picture 9

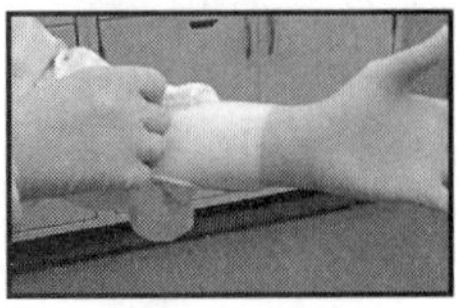

Picture 10

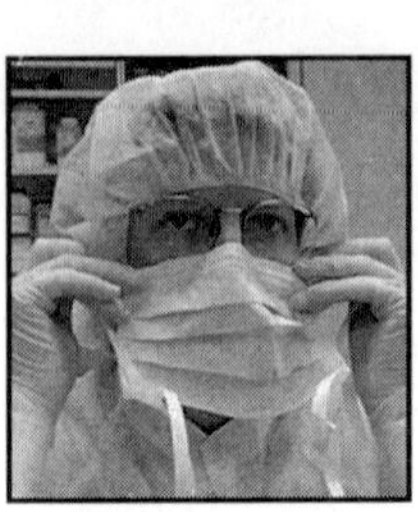

Picture 11

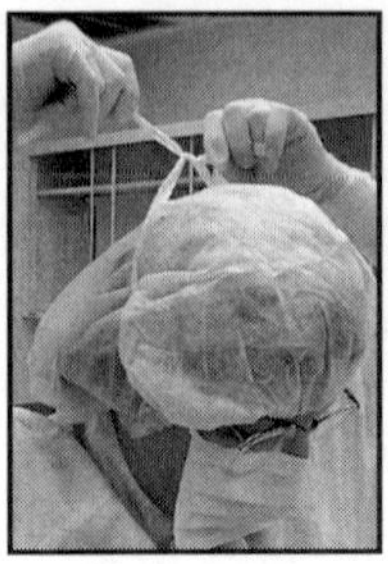

Picture 12

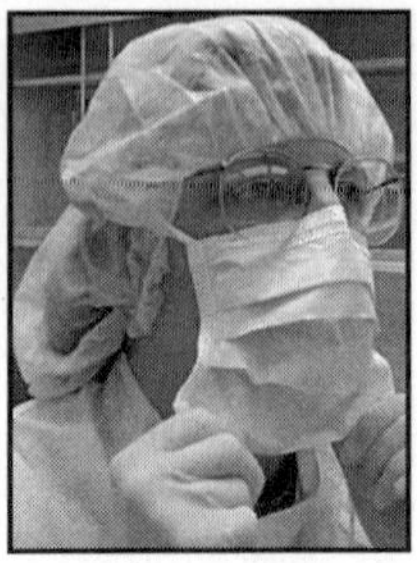

Picture 13

Preparing the horizontal laminar flow workbench

When preparing the HLFW, the hood is sanitized with sterile 70% isopropyl alcohol. Pour isopropyl alcohol on the stainless steel counter in the hood (Picture 14). Wet the sterile non-linting wipe with the isopropyl alcohol. Wipe the bar of the hood first (Picture 15). Next wipe the side walls. Wipe up and down, from front (closest to the HEPA filter) to back, not going back, over wiped surfaces (Pictures 16 and 17). The last thing to be wiped is the counter. Start in the back corner by the HEPA filter and wipe all the way across the bench (Picture 18). Go from side to side, working from the HEPA filter to the edge of the counter (Picture 19).

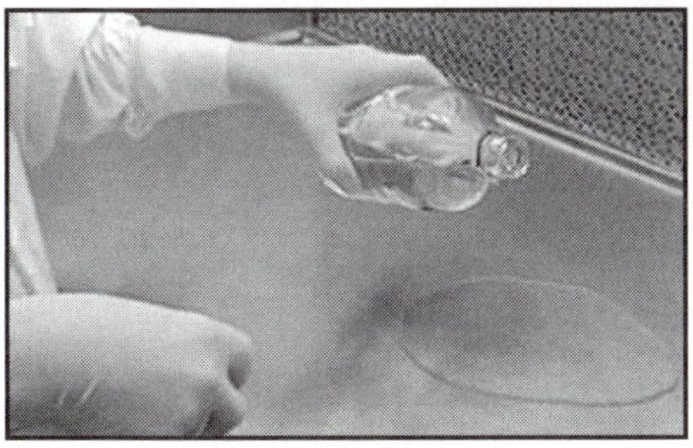

Picture 14

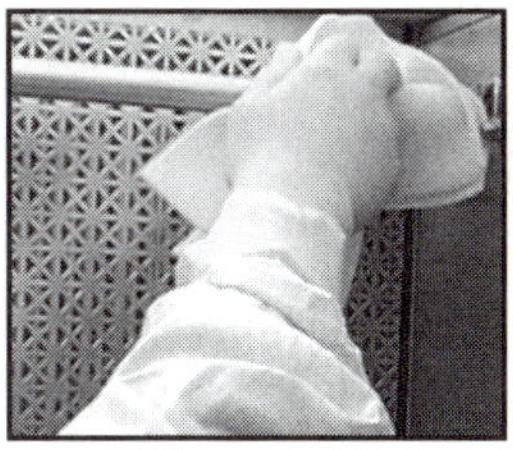

Picture 15

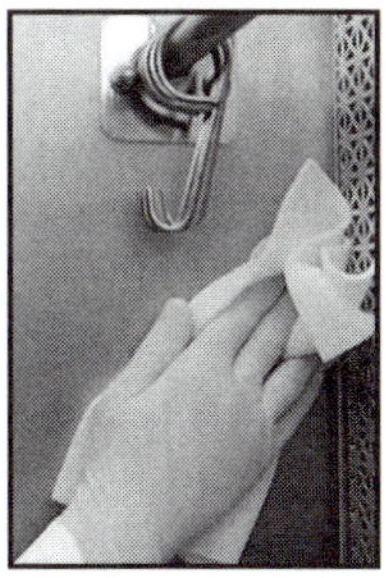

Picture 16

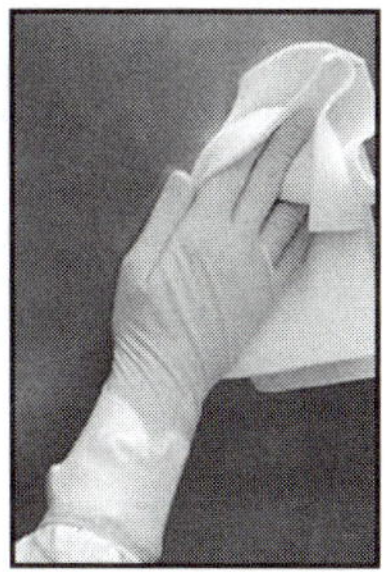

Picture 17

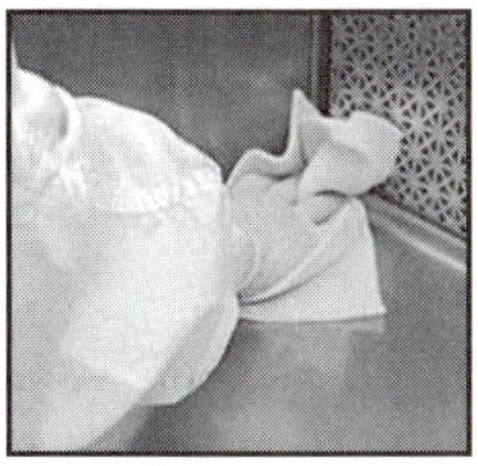

Picture 18

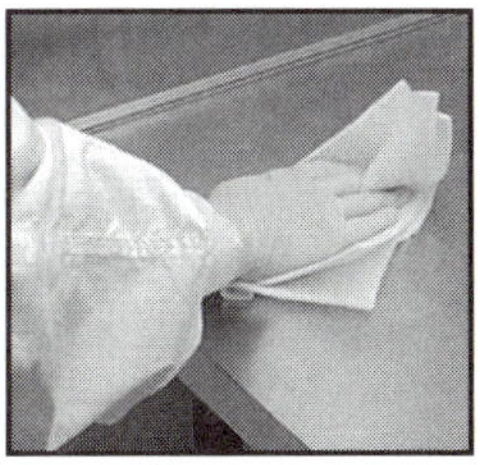

Picture 19

Putting the needle on a syringe

To put a needle on a syringe, select the appropriate size syringe large enough to accommodate the volume required. Inspect the integrity of the outer wrap for defects such as holes or tears in the package. At the edge of the hood, peel the paper on the syringe and place the syringe in the hood (Picture 20). Do not push the syringe through the paper wrap, because tearing the paper generates many particles. Select the needle and examine the package for defects. While pointing the hub of the needle toward the HEPA filter, peel back the wrap (Picture 21).

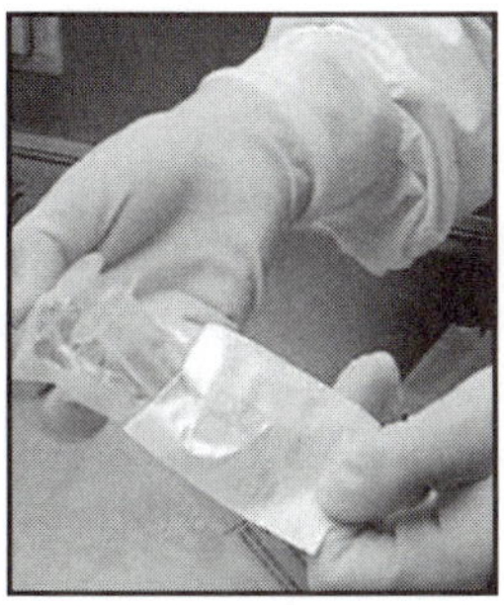

Picture 20

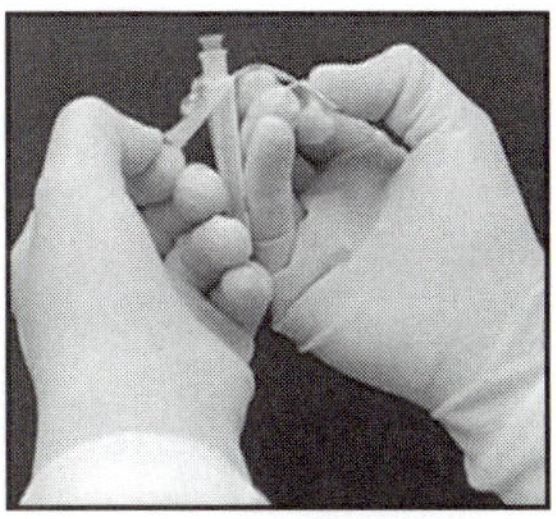

Picture 21

(The following instructions are given for a right-handed person. If the technician or pharmacist is left-handed, simply reverse the directions.)

Hold the needle between the thumb and first finger on the left hand (Picture 22). Take the syringe in the right hand, and take hold of the protective tip of the syringe with the thumb and first finger of the left hand (Picture 23). Twist the syringe to remove the protective tip. Rotate the left hand and attach the hub of the needle to the tip of the syringe (Picture 24). Push the plunger down to the tip of the barrel while keeping the needle cover on to unlock the syringe (Picture 25).

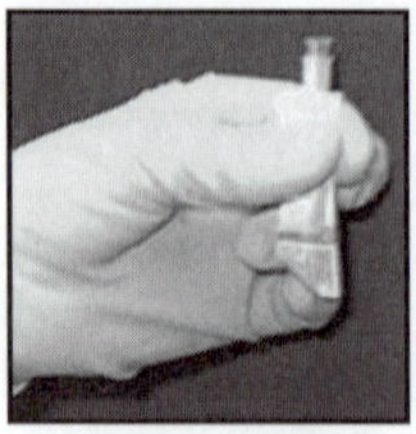

Picture 22

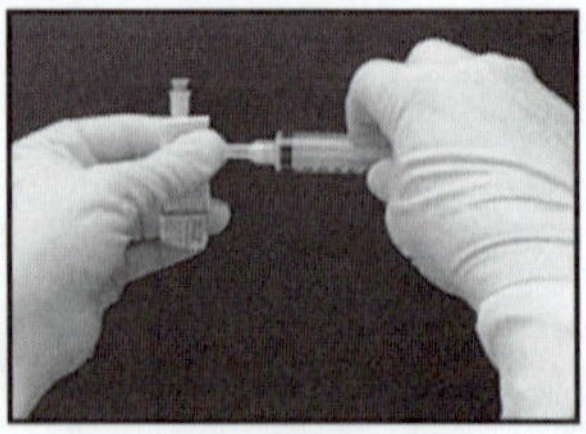

Picture 23

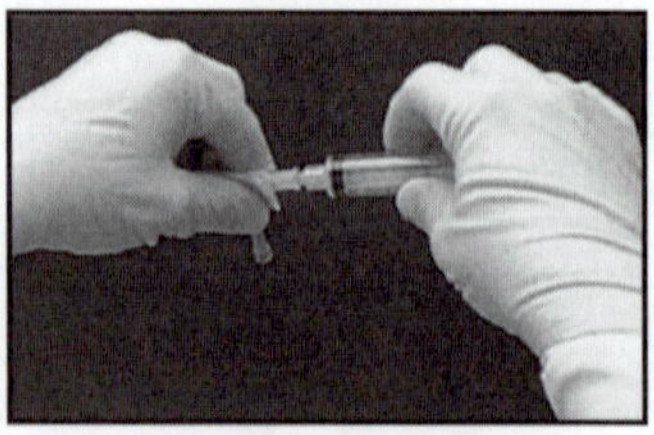

Picture 24

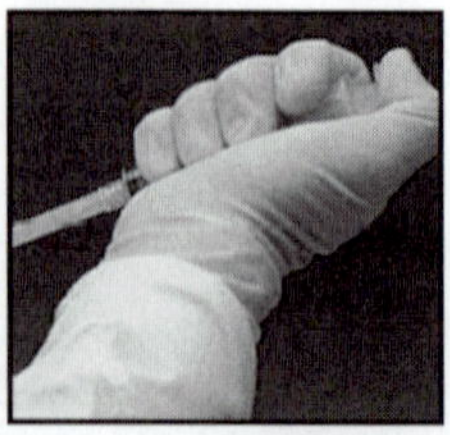

Picture 25

Withdrawing from an ampule

Ampules are single-dose containers. Once the tip is broken open, the ampule is an open system with air passing freely in and out of the container. Wipe the ampule with a wipe soaked in sterile 70% isopropyl alcohol before placing in the HLFW (Picture 26). With the ampule in an upright position, tap the neck to release solution trapped in the end of the ampule. Wipe the neck of the ampule with a sterile alcohol pad to further clean the neck of the ampule, as glass particles will fall into the solution when the ampule is broken (Picture 27). Make sure the ampule is dry so your hands do not slip while attempting to break it open.

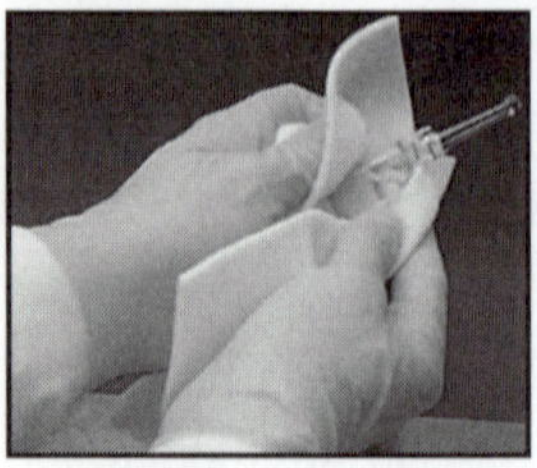

Picture 26

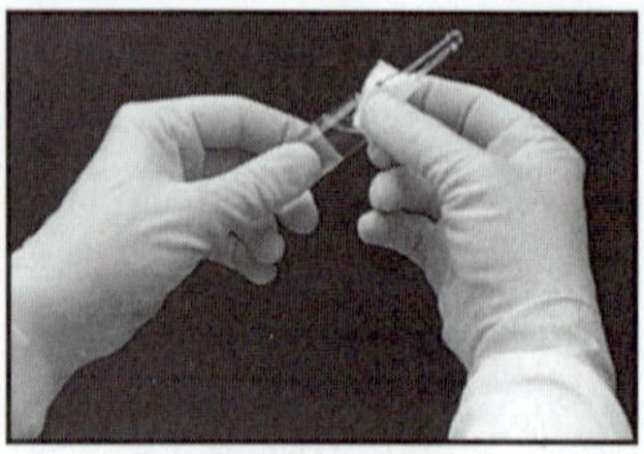

Picture 27

Position your thumbs about one-half inch apart on either side of the constricted neck of the ampule to apply pressure with the fingers, as if breaking a pencil in half (Picture 28). Break the ampule toward the side of the hood, not toward the HEPA filter. Glass particles and drops of fluid are dispersed when the ampule is broken. If the ampule does not break easily, rotate it one-half turn and try again. Lay the top to the side in the bench and place the ampule in laminar air flow (Picture 29). Remove the needle cover from the needle and syringe. Place it either between the ring finger and little finger (Picture 30), or lay it on a sterile alcohol prep pad pointing toward the HEPA filter.

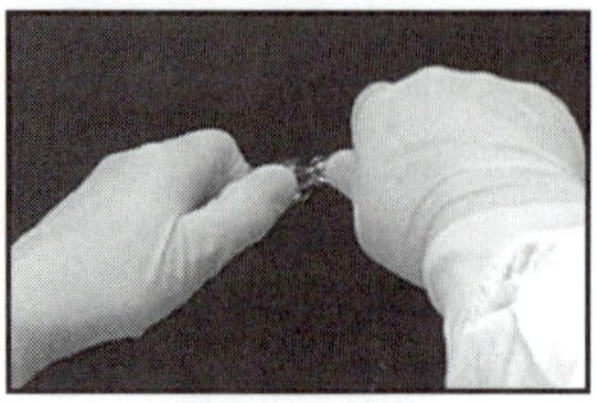

Picture 28

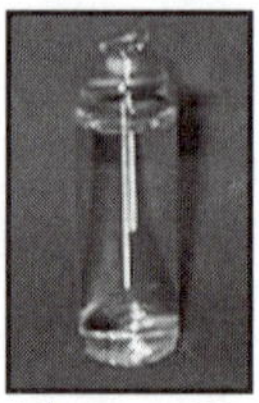

Picture 29

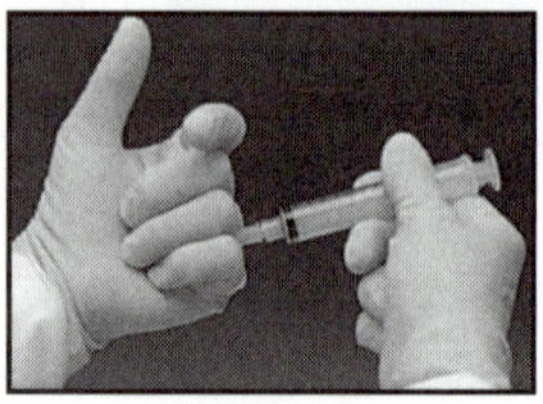

Picture 30

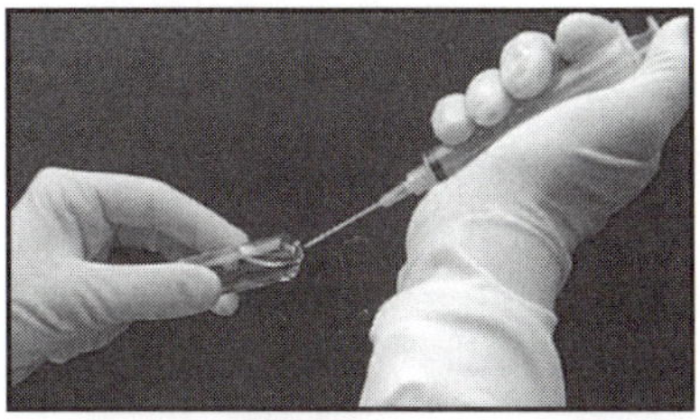

Picture 31

Pick up the ampule and insert the needle bevel down into the shoulder of the ampule (Picture 31). Tilt the ampule at an angle to keep the tip of the needle in the solution. When inserting the needle into the ampule, do not let the needle touch the outside edge of the ampule. If this does happen, replace the contaminated needle with a new needle on the syringe. The opening of the ampule and the tip of the needle are *critical sites*; therefore, take care to keep them in uninterrupted laminar air flow.

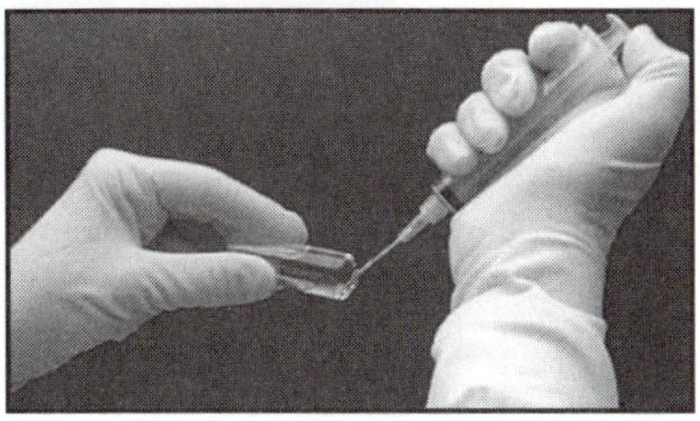

Picture 32

Hold the syringe by wrapping the fingers around the barrel and pulling back the plunger with the thumb (Picture 32). Do not contaminate (by touch) the ribs of the plunger. Another safe method is to use the index finger to push the plunger out and withdraw the fluid from the ampule. Discard any unused solution in the ampule.

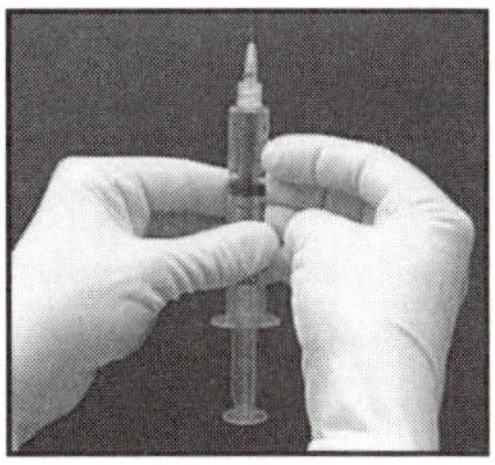

Picture 33

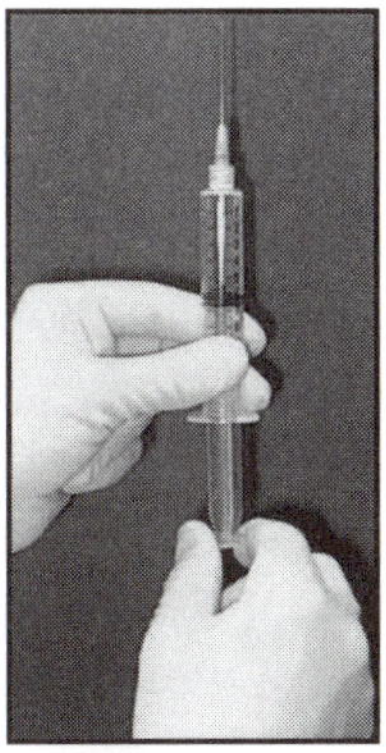

Picture 34

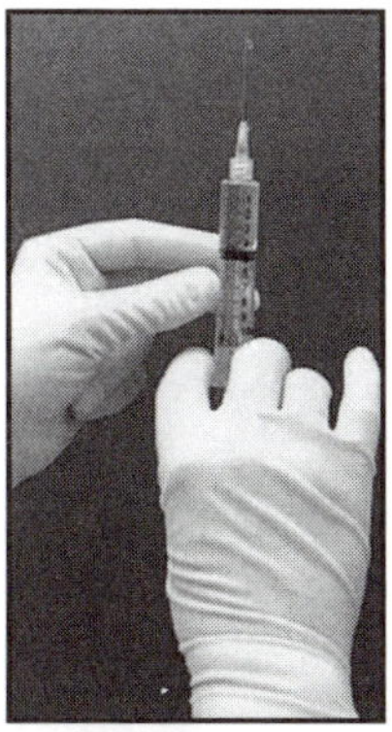

Picture 35

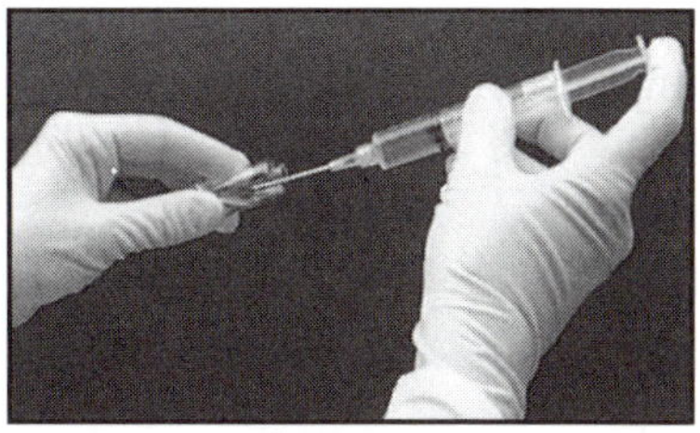

Picture 36

If air is in the syringe, hold the syringe with the needle up and tap the syringe firmly to allow the air bubbles to rise (Picture 33). Draw back on the plunger to get the drop of fluid out of the hub of the needle, then gently push up on the plunger to expel all the air in the syringe (Pictures 34 and 35). To adjust the volume in the syringe to the correct amount, move the edge of the rubber plunger closest to the tip to the correct calibration mark. Any excess solution is put back into the ampule (Picture 36).

Any solution taken from an ampule must always be filtered because glass particles can fall into the ampule when it breaks open. The solution is filtered when withdrawing from an ampule by using a filter needle, a filter disk, or a filter straw. The filter is discarded and replaced by a clean needle before injecting.

Withdrawing solution from a vial

Vials are molded glass or plastic containers with rubber closures secured in place with an aluminum seal. Vials can be filled with dry powders, sterile solutions, or lyophilized (freeze-dried) medications; a vial could also be an empty, evacuated container. Vials may be single-dose or multiple-dose containers. A multiple-dose container has preservatives and can be entered more than once. Usually each practice site has a written policy about the use of multi-dose vials after the initial entry. Because single-dose vials contain no preservatives, pharmaceutical manufacturers recommend entering each vial only once. Generally, the standard of practice is that a single-dose vial may be used for 24 hours after the initial entry, as long as the vial remains in the laminar flow workstation. It is imperative that the first person opening and using a single-dose vial labels the vial with the date and time of initial entry and his or her initials.

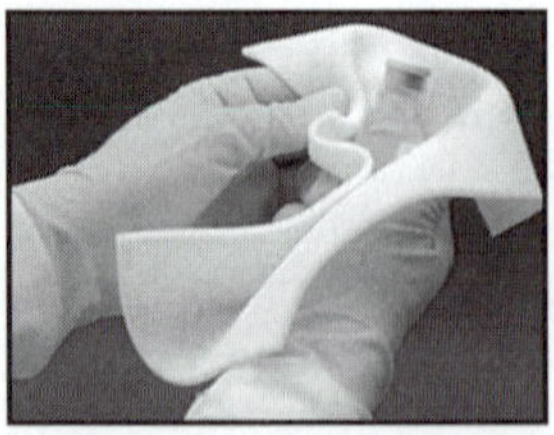
Picture 37

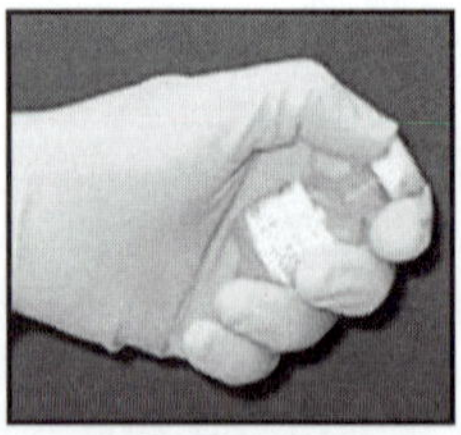
Picture 38

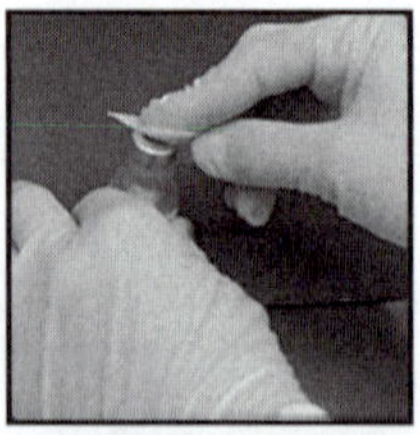
Picture 39

Using a non-lint-producing wipe soaked in isopropyl alcohol, wipe the vial before placing it in the hood (Picture 37). Remove the flip-top seal from the vial and swab the closure with a sterile alcohol pad, wiping in one direction with several strokes (Pictures 38 and 39). Wiping the closure with the sterile 70% isopropyl alcohol helps clean and sanitize the surface of the closure. While the alcohol on the surface of the closure is drying, assemble the needle and syringe.

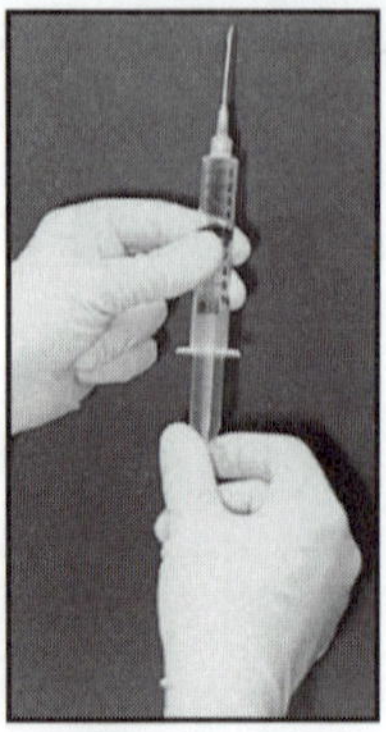
Picture 40

Remove the needle cover and place it between the ring finger and little finger or lay it on a sterile alcohol pad with the opening pointing toward the HEPA filter. Air must be injected into the vial so fluid may be withdrawn because the vial is a closed system. Draw in an amount of air equal to the volume of solution needed (Picture 40).

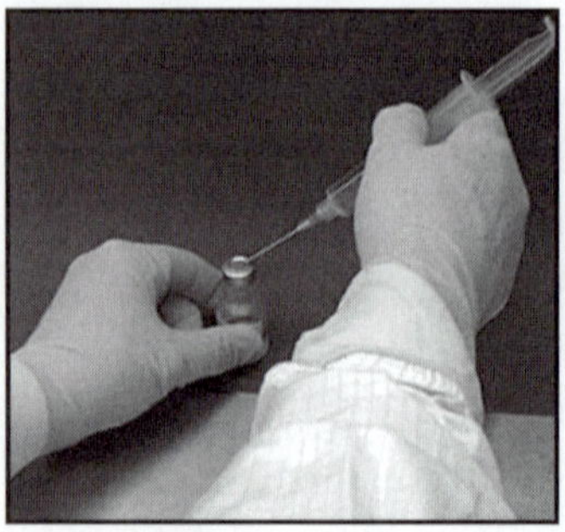
Picture 41

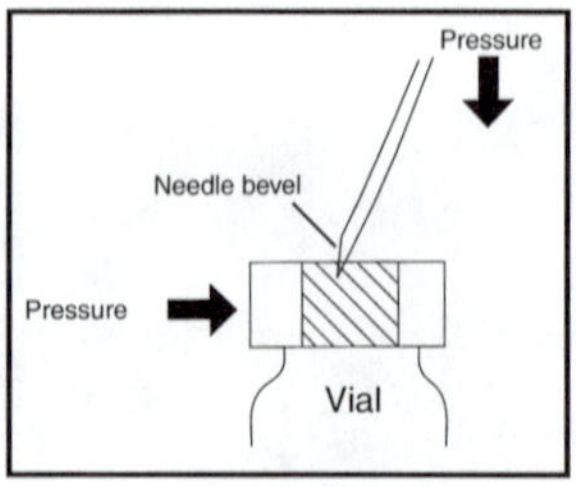

Figure 12

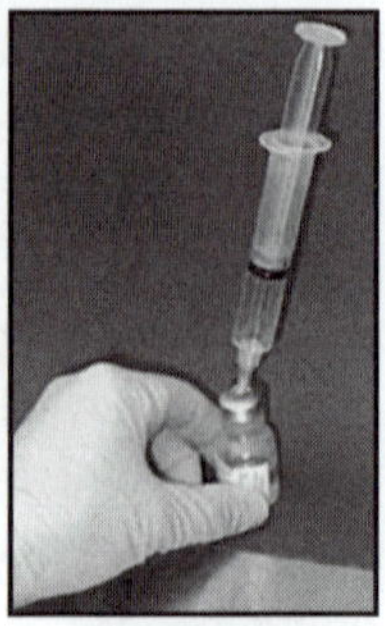
Picture 42

Grasp the base of the vial in one hand. Hold the syringe at an angle of approximately 60 degrees with the bevel of the needle up (Picture 41 and Figure 12). As the closure is penetrated, elevate the needle to a vertical position while exerting lateral (sideways) pressure on the needle. Be sure the critical sites are in direct laminar air flow (Picture 42).

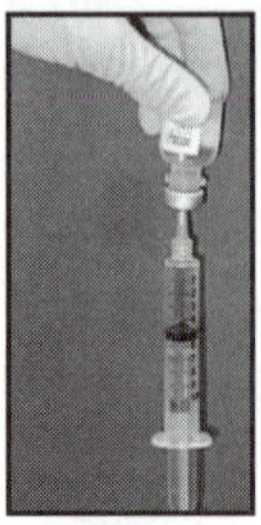
Picture 43

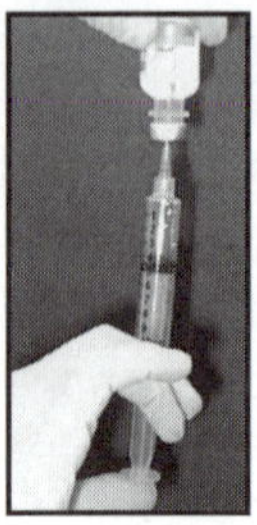
Picture 44

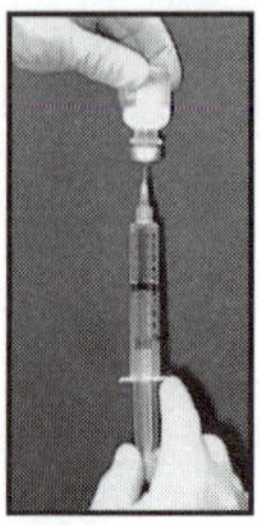
Picture 45

Invert the vial and syringe and inject air into the vial by depressing the plunger (Pictures 43 and 44). Let the solution run back into the syringe as air is injected into the vial. Hold the flat top of the plunger with the middle finger and thumb, and push against the collar of the syringe with the index finger to pull back on the plunger. Pull back to an amount slightly larger than desired (Picture 45).

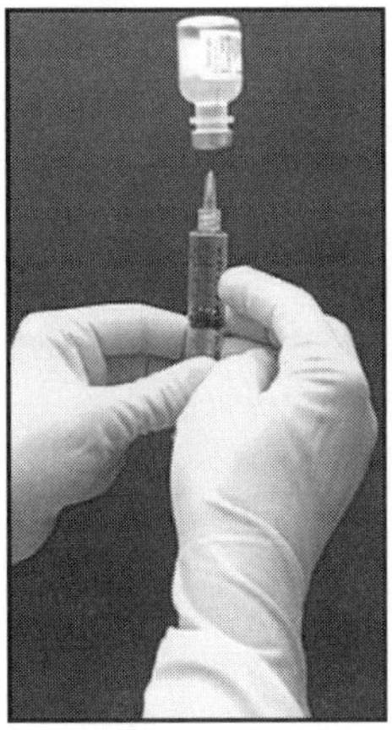

Picture 46

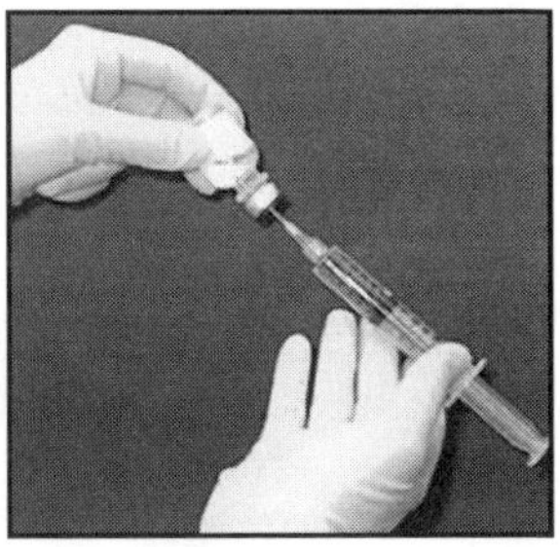

Picture 47

Firmly tap on the syringe to dislodge any air bubbles (Picture 46). Push the plunger to dispel the air, and adjust the plunger until the appropriate amount of solution is in the syringe. While holding the inverted vial with one hand, hold the syringe barrel with the other and turn the vial and syringe over (Picture 47). When turning the syringe, use care to keep hands away from the HEPA filter and the critical site. Withdraw the needle and syringe from the vial.

Reconstitution of a sterile powder

Reconstitution is the process of adding a liquid, the diluent, to the powdered solid to yield a solution. The medication is in powder form because it usually has limited stability in solution. The *diluent* is a fluid solvent that is added to a solid to render it a solution. Always read the label to determine the proper diluent and the volume needed before reconstituting.

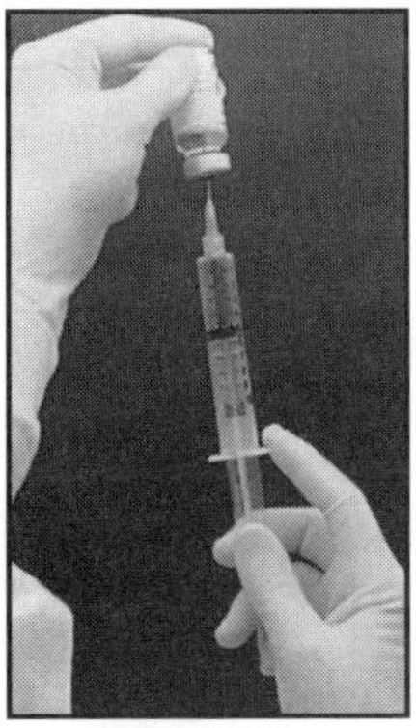

Picture 48

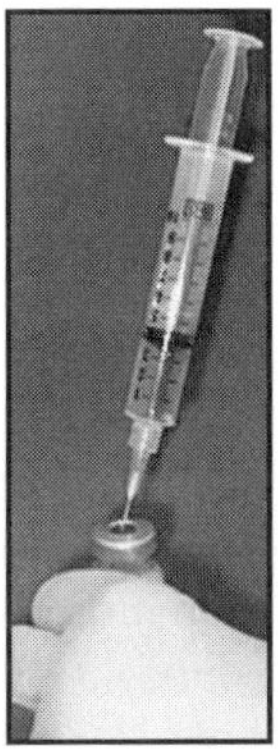

Picture 49

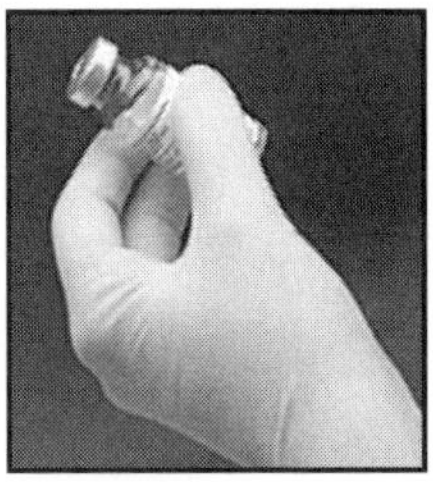

Picture 50

Using aseptic technique, withdraw the correct amount of diluent from the ampule or vial (Picture 48). Inject the diluent into the vial of powder. Allow the air to go back into the syringe so the vial will not contain positive pressure (Picture 49). If this is not done, some of the vial contents may be forced out from the vial due to the positive pressure in the vial when the needle is removed. Shake the vial to make sure that the medication is completely dissolved before withdrawing the necessary amount of drug solution (Picture 50). The reconstituted solution does not need filtering unless, upon inspection of the vial, a particle or a rubber core is floating in the solution.

Visual inspection of parenteral solutions

Each completed parenteral admixture solution must be inspected and verified by a pharmacist before it is delivered to the nursing unit for administration to the patient. The operator also checks the completed admixture immediately after it is prepared. The following checks for accuracy must be made on every completed admixture:

- The label is complete and free from errors.
- The correct intravenous solutions, including strength and quantity, have been used.
- The correct drug additives, including strength and quantity, have been used.
- The admixture is clear and free from particulate matter, crystals, and precipitation.

When checking for particulate matter, invert the solution and swirl it gently. Vigorous shaking may produce some air bubbles. Hold the solution in front of well-illuminated light and dark backgrounds to detect particles of different colors. It is sometimes hard to distinguish between air bubbles and particles; however, air bubbles will rise and particles will sink.

Parenteral nutrition

Parenteral nutrition is an intravenous feeding, containing high concentrations of dextrose, amino acids, electrolytes, vitamins, trace elements, and sometimes insulin. A lipid (fat) emulsion may be mixed in the same bag with the amino acids and dextrose, or it can be administered separately. Lipids provide calories and help to treat or prevent essential fatty acid deficiency. The parenteral nutrition solution is designed to provide adequate caloric intake while keeping the volume of solution administered to a minimum. The nutrition solution is administered through a large vein, such as the subclavian (by the base of the neck), over eight to 24 hours. Parenteral nutrition is used when a patient cannot tolerate an oral feeding or when it is necessary to bypass the gastrointestinal tract. A full discussion of compounding of parenteral nutrition solutions is beyond the scope of this chapter.

Chemotherapeutic agents

Concern exists that handling, preparation, and administration of chemotherapeutic agents may constitute an occupational hazard. When handling chemotherapeutic agents, personnel need to be concerned about using good aseptic technique to keep the product sterile and must take measures to minimize unnecessary exposure to these agents.

Pharmacy technicians and pharmacists working with antineoplastic agents should receive special training and be informed of the potential risks involved. All mixing of antineoplastic drugs should be performed in a certified Class II biological safety cabinet. No other IV admixtures should be prepared in the biological safety cabinet designated for the mixing of cytotoxic drugs. The viewing window is lowered when compounding cytotoxic drugs. Disposable gloves and protective barrier garments with a closed front, long sleeves, and closed cuffs are worn for all procedures. Syringes and IV sets with Luer Lok fittings are used whenever possible. A sterile, plastic-backed absorbent drape is placed on the work surface of the safety cabinet during mixing procedures. It is exchanged after significant spillage or at the end of each production sequence.

Vials must be vented with hydrophobic filters. Many compounding devices now prevent the buildup of positive pressure inside the vial. Final medication measurement must be performed before removing the needle from the stopper of the vial. Because the medication is contained, it decreases the operator's exposure to the medications. Written special procedures must be followed in case of a major spill or acute exposure. All disposable items that have potential contact with antineoplastic drugs during compounding or administration must be disposed of in specifically designated containers with a biohazard symbol on them. All of these hazardous waste containers must be disposed of by proper methods.

Conclusion

The parenteral administration of medications involves a variety of routes, but must always utilize products that are as sterile and free of undesired substances as possible. Following aseptic technique to ensure parenteral products do not become contaminated is of the utmost importance. Technicians must know the proper procedures for preparing parenteral products and maintaining the equipment used to prepare them. When handling chemotherapy medications, special care must be taken to minimize exposure to such products.

Bibliography

American Society of Health-System Pharmacists, "ASHP Guidelines on Quality Assurance for Pharmacy-Prepared Sterile Products," *American Journal of Health-System Pharmacists,* Vol. 57, pp. 1150-69, 2000.

Bryan D., Marback R., "Laminar airflow equipment certification: What the pharmacist needs to know," *American Journal of Hospital Pharmacists*, Vol. 42, pp. 1343 and 1348, 1984.

Clean Room and Work Station Requirements, Controlled Environment, Federal Standard 209E, Government Printing Office, Washington, D.C., September 1992.

Pharmacopeial Forum, "Sterile Preparations – Pharmacy Practices," The Pharmacopeial Forum, Vol. 26, pp. 812-832.

United States Pharmacopeia, Quality Assurance for Sterile Drug Compounding An Education Source, 1998.

Additional reading

Akers M., Sterile Preparation for the Hospital Pharmacist, Ann Arbor Science Publishers Inc., Ann Arbor, MI, 1981.

Hunt M.L., Training Manual for Intravenous Admixture Personnel, 4th edition, Baxter Health Care Corporation, 1984.

Turco S., Sterile Dosage Forms: Their Preparation and Clinical Application, 4th edition, Lea & Febiger, Malvern, PA, 1994.

About the author

Laura A. Thoma received her bachelor's degree in pharmacy from Briar Cliff College in Sioux City, Iowa, and her Doctor of Pharmacy degree from the University of Tennessee in Memphis. Dr. Thoma is the assistant professor of pharmaceutical sciences and the director of the Parenteral Medications Laboratories at the University of Tennessee Health Science Center. Her research interests include parenteral processing and process development, container and closure compatibility studies and the compatibility and stability of combinations of parenteral medication in IV admixtures. She has extensive experience in providing training of pharmaceutical and biotech industry personnel in all procedures and methods used in the preparation and quality control of sterile products. Dr. Thoma is also responsible for training hospital and home healthcare pharmacists in the application of aseptic procedures in preparing sterile products.

Self-assessment questions

1. A properly functioning laminar flow workstation will filter out all particles that have a diameter of ___or larger.
   a. 1 micron
   b. 0.5 microns
   c. 0.3 microns
   d. 0.8 microns

2. The pore size of a sterilizing filter is:
   a. 0.2 microns.
   b. 0.45 microns.
   c. 0.12 microns.
   d. 5 microns

3. An intradermal injection is injected into which of the following?
   a. Loose tissue below the skin
   b. Deltoid muscle
   c. Subclavian vein
   d. Top layer of the skin

4. Working in a laminar flow workstation often gives the operator a false sense of security concerning the sterility of the product being prepared. Please choose the incorrect statement.
   a. LFW removes microbial contaminants from the surface of containers or other items placed in the workstation.
   b. A LFW is not a sterilization process – what you put in there is not sterilized.
   c. A LFW must be properly maintained and used correctly in order for it to provide a Class 100 area.
   d. Items in an overwrap must be taken out of the overwrap as they are placed in the hood.

5. A *sterile product* is one that is:
   a. free from all pyrogens.
   b. free from all viruses.
   c. free from all microorganisms.
   d. all of the above.

6. In the definition of a Class 100, Class 10,000, and Class 100,000 area, the size of the particles per cubic foot of air are:
   a. 0.2 microns and larger.
   b. 0.5 microns and larger.
   c. 1.0 microns and larger.
   d. 1.5 microns and larger.

7. The major source of contamination in a clean room is:
   a. the ventilation system.
   b. the IV supplies.
   c. the IV supply boxes.
   d. the people in the room.

8. Proper technique when working in a Horizontal Laminar Flow Workstation includes:
   a. spraying a sanitizing agent into the hood.
   b. working within the hood at least six inches from the front edge.
   c. arranging objects behind each other within the hood.
   d. arranging objects along the walls of the hood.

9. Which of the following is ***not*** an example of a critical site?
   a. The hub of the needle
   b. The open neck of the ampule
   c. The laminar flow workbench
   d. The ribs of the plunger on a syringe

10. Chemotherapy drugs should be prepared in a:
    a. vertical flow hood.
    b. horizontal flow hood.
    c. Class II biological safety cabinet.
    d. parenteral work station.

CHAPTER 28

OPERATIONS AND MEDICATION CONTROL

Paul W. Bush, Pharm.D., MBA

Learning objectives

Upon completion of this chapter, the technician should be able to do the following:

- Explain the concept of a *pharmacy formulary.*
- Identify sources of medication.
- Explain the medication purchasing process.
- List concepts of inventory management.
- Explain special handling requirements needed for select pharmaceuticals.
- Identify medication storage requirements for pharmaceuticals.
- Identify the functions of a medication package.
- Explain the difference between pharmacy *compounding* and *manufacturing.*
- List the concepts of good manufacturing practices.
- Explain important aspects of weighing pharmaceuticals.
- Explain important aspects of measuring liquid pharmaceuticals.
- Explain the concept of *reconstitution.*

Introduction

The high cost of medications is a contributing factor for the need to utilize specific methods of operation within a pharmacy. Formularies help dictate which medications the pharmacy will use, while inventory regulations and procedures allow the pharmacy to properly account for its stock and handle medications that require special attention. When prescriptions are not commercially available, pharmacies must create them via compounding by following a set of established practices and documentation requirements.

Formulary system

The formulary system is a method for evaluating and selecting suitable drug products for the formulary of an organized health setting (e.g., hospital, managed care plan). The formulary is a list of drugs that are considered by the professional staff of that setting to be the most useful in patient care. Pharmacies located in hospitals, clinics, or Health Maintenance Organizations (HMOs) utilize this list of approved medications for stocking medications and dispensing them to their patients.

Automatic therapeutic interchange for certain types of medications may be a standard practice in some inpatient settings. An automatic interchange substitutes one medication for another that is not generically equal but has the same therapeutic effect. One example might be substituting ranitidine if famotidine is prescribed. Both of these medications are classified as histamine-2 receptor antagonists, but are not generically equivalent. Therapeutic interchanges are only allowed within the specific institution at which the interchanges are established.

Most ambulatory (community) pharmacies are not required to adhere to a formulary, so they stock and dispense those medications that are commonly prescribed by physicians located in their area. In the ambulatory setting, reimbursement from prescription plans may be limited to a specific formulary of medications, or as an alternative, non-formulary medications may be reimbursed if the patient pays a higher co-pay.

Medication purchasing and inventory control process

A pharmacy obtains medications from a variety of sources. Technicians play an important role in maintaining and obtaining the medication inventory, including recording items in short supply, contacting suppliers, preparing purchase documents, receiving medication orders, and placing the medications in proper storage for later distribution.

The pharmacy technician has an active and important role in inventory management. The technician can monitor usage, help establish minimum stock levels, reduce the number of "look-alike" medications that are stored in close proximity, and ensure that adequate stock is available to meet patient needs. The technician, through his or her daily duties, most often identifies fluctuation in medication use. A technician who can identify usage trends, and thus avoid potential out-of-stock situations, is a highly valued member of the pharmacy team. One of the most frustrating situations in a pharmacy is when a medication is out-of-stock because someone forgot to reorder it. Every pharmacy employee is responsible to identify when an item needs reordering. Pharmacies often use a "want book," kept in a convenient location, to list medications that are used and low in stock. This manual system, which is only as good as the person using it, is frequently used in conjunction with another inventory management system to be the basis for placing an order.

Some pharmacy computers track medication use to assist with ordering. A minimum level of stock is established for each medication so that the computer will trigger an automatic reorder of the product when stock levels go below that minimum. For more information on how to calculate an inventory turnover ratio and use other inventory management systems, please refer to the bibliography at the end of this chapter. Several other approaches to inventory management exist, including the following:

- *Just in time:* This system keeps little inventory on hand, but arranges for delivery of stock as the name implies.
- *Pareto's Law or 80/20 analysis:* This system examines the frequency of ordering and tries to maximize inventory "turn over" of high usage items. The numbers "80" and "20" refer to the goal of having 80 percent of the pharmacy's sales come from 20 percent of the pharmacy's inventory.

A pharmacy technician may place a direct order of medications with the pharmaceutical manufacturer if the pharmacy's account is established. Advantages of direct orders include being able to purchase medications at the lowest price and purchase larger quantities if desired. Disadvantages of direct ordering include minimum order requirements set by the manufacturer (especially if the pharmacy only needs a small quantity) and increased paperwork (if frequent orders must be placed).

A pharmacy may also purchase medications from a drug wholesaler. Wholesalers will resell, at an increased price, pharmaceuticals they have purchased directly from the manufacturer. Wholesalers do not manufacture pharmaceuticals; they are an intermediary in the distribution process. Advantages to purchasing from a wholesaler include quick delivery of medications and no minimum order, which gives a pharmacy the ability to purchase small quantities. A disadvantage of using a wholesaler may be the increased price over a direct purchase. Drug wholesalers may enter into a prime vendor agreement with a pharmacy. Under a prime vendor agreement, the wholesaler agrees to provide pharmaceuticals to a pharmacy at the direct order purchase price, plus a very small markup, in exchange for the pharmacy's commitment to buy most of its drugs through that wholesaler. Advantages to this arrangement include quick deliveries, no minimum orders, less paperwork and a price very close to the direct order price.

Pharmacies may form a group purchasing organization (GPO) or be part of an organization that combines the purchasing power of the individual members (a cooperative buying group). These purchasing groups request bids for reduced prices on multi-source medications (such as ampicillin) from the manufacturers in return for the purchasing group's commitment to buy the manufacturer's product. A pharmacy's prime vendor will also honor these negotiated contract prices.

Technicians are actively involved with the drug procurement or purchasing process in every pharmacy. The purchasing process is followed whenever stock runs low and needs replacement. Ordering is the first step of purchasing. Orders may be placed directly to the manufacturer or to the drug wholesaler. Orders can be communicated in a variety of ways—telephoned to the company, transmitted by facsimile machine (FAX), transmitted via modem/computer, mailed, or given directly to the sales representative. Purchase orders are business forms utilized to record the details of the order, including the purchase order number, the name of company, the date of order, the product ordered, quantity ordered, and price. The purchase order also provides information such as payment terms and shipping addresses. The purchase order number is used as a reference number when the invoice requesting payment is sent to the pharmacy.

Once the order is shipped to the pharmacy, the technician is involved in receiving the product. The technician responsible for receiving stock will be asked to sign a manifest (receipt) indicating the shipment was received at the pharmacy. When signing a manifest, the technician must verify the number of boxes received, look for damages or leaks, and identify any shortages. As the order is unpacked, the technician compares each item received against the purchase order for correctness of item and quantity shipped. Each item is inspected for damage and expiration date. The technician documents on the purchase order and packing slip any inaccuracies from the shipment. The technician then brings the inaccuracies to the attention of the pharmacist so that no incorrect medications enter the dispensing area that could bring about a possible medication error.

Technicians perform important duties while placing medications into the pharmacy's drug stock. New stock should be put away in its correct place, whether in the active dispensing area or in a storage area. Rotating the stock by placing the newest medications behind existing stock reduces unnecessary outdating of medications. The technician should also inspect existing stock for outdated medications to help prevent expired medications from being dispensed. If the new stock is from a different manufacturer, the technician can prevent medication errors by identifying "look-alike" products that may be located on the shelf near its location.

Record completion is the last part of the purchasing process. After all shortages, breakages, and mis-shipments are noted on the purchase order, the packing slip and the invoice are attached to the purchase order and processed by the accounts payable clerk so payment may be made to the manufacturer or wholesaler.

Borrowing pharmaceuticals

Occasionally, a pharmacy is out of a specific medication and needs to obtain a small quantity in an emergency to begin treatment for a patient. The pharmacy may arrange to borrow it from another pharmacy if wholesalers are closed or the manufacturers cannot supply it. Borrowing from one pharmacy to another is discouraged and used only in urgent situations. A detailed record of borrowed or loaned medication is essential. Regulations limit the quantities that may be borrowed. Recalled medications are harder to track if borrowed. Since contracts often restrict the resale of medications to other pharmacies, borrowed medications are not purchased by a pharmacy but replaced (to the original pharmacy) once regular stock is obtained.

Managing expired medication, credits and returns

Each drug has an expiration date established by its manufacturer. Pharmacy technicians involved with dispensing functions are actively involved with monitoring medication stock for being "in-date." Once a pharmaceutical product has reached its expiration date, it must be removed from active stock and placed in a designated area in the pharmacy for disposal processing.

Occasionally, pharmacies may have to return a product to the manufacturer. The item may have been ordered in error or in too large a quantity, or may be outdated. Credit and return policies vary greatly with each company and should be checked before a product return is attempted. Returns of expired medications are sometimes handled by return goods specialty companies that charge a fee for handling a pharmacy's expired drugs. Handling of expired medications is an important part of inventory management and proper medication control. Expired medications must be disposed of properly to ensure safety.

Recalled medications

The Food and Drug Administration (FDA) is one of the government agencies that regulates and monitors the pharmaceutical industry. If a product in use is deemed unsafe or has reported problems, the FDA may issue a recall of the reported drug or a specific manufactured batch of the product. Recalled medication should be isolated and prepared for return to the manufacturer. All paperwork involving recalled medications is kept in pharmacy records. The technician may be involved with checking stock for recalled medications and processing the returns.

Medication storage

Pharmacy technicians contribute significantly to the quality of the pharmacy service by helping to ensure that medications are stored properly. Items that require refrigeration are labeled as such and should be refrigerated promptly to maintain full potency. Pharmaceutical products that are light sensitive are also labeled in their original protective packages. Controlled substances need secure storage locations and should not be left unattended. Oncology materials need appropriate handling. Chemicals and flammable items should be stored in safe places to avoid accidents. If a technician is uncertain about product storage requirements, he or she should review the policy and procedure with the pharmacist.

Controlled substances

All controlled substances have special requirements for ordering, inventory maintenance, record keeping, storage, and disposal. Descriptions of the laws regulating controlled substances are reviewed in the *Controlled Substance Manual for Pharmacists*, published by the U.S. Justice Department. One should note that narcotics (Class II Controlled Substances) require a special Drug Enforcement Administration (DEA) order form that must be signed by an authorized individual given power of attorney for that pharmacy. Since this form must be processed manually, delays in obtaining new stock may be several days. Every technician handling controlled substances should have knowledge of the pharmacy's rules on correct procedures for dispensing, record keeping, and related duties.

Investigational medications

Investigational medications may only be used for those patients enrolled in a controlled study and may not be used on other patients. Procedures for handling investigational drugs resemble those of dispensing controlled substances. Dispensing records and dose accountability is required for investigational medications. A specially trained pharmacy technician may be involved in the inventory control, protocol management, and distribution of these medications. Borrowing or loaning investigational medications is not permitted. Investigational drugs are supplied directly from the manufacturer. Restocking of investigational drugs may take longer, since the investigating physician or a medical center's Investigational Drug Service usually orders these medications.

Medication samples

Medication samples are supplied by pharmaceutical manufacturers to introduce a new product, promote an existing product, or provide a supply for an indigent patient on an interim basis. Medication samples, which are ordered by a physician for personal dispensing in his or her professional practice, become the property of the physician. Institutions often have clinics or other ambulatory centers where a physician practices to keep these samples for use. Control of these samples is important, and each institution has established procedures for their use. Pharmacy technicians may come in contact with these samples during routine inspection of these units for outdated medications. Samples are not part of pharmacy stock and must not be used in pharmacy dispensing; they cannot be sold to a patient.

Packaging

Packaging pharmaceuticals for patient use is an important aspect of any pharmacy service. Drug packages must provide several functions. The package identifies the drug completely and precisely; prevents deterioration of the drug from the surrounding environment; protects the drug from breakage, contamination, or other damage; and allows safe and ready access to the drug packaged. The packaging process must have good controls throughout all phases. Breakdown in packaging controls can lead to serious medication errors or product deterioration.

Bulk package: a large container of medication (e.g., bottle of 1,000 tablets) purchased from the manufacturer by the pharmacy to obtain the lowest price. Bulk packages are not intended for direct dispensing to the patient.

Dispensing package: a smaller container of a medication that is packaged to contain enough medication to complete a typical therapy (e.g., a methylprednisolone dosepak, or 100ml of cephalexin suspension). Also known as a unit-of-use package.

Prepackaging: medications individually (single tablet or dose) packaged by the manufacturer and sold to a pharmacy in prepackaged, unit-dose packages.

Repackaging: through a controlled process, a bulk medication (e.g., tablet, liquid) is sealed in a single dose package for use in unit-dose dispensing systems. Technicians can manually repackage a medication or use a unit-dose packaging machine.

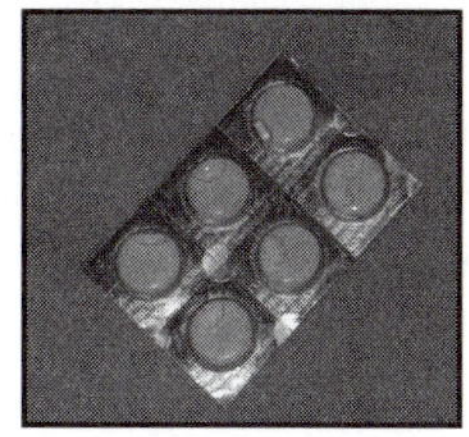

Unit-dose package: the common term for individually packaged drugs. Conceptually, a unit-dose package provides one dose of a medication. The package could actually contain two tablets (e.g., acetaminophen 650mg dose, two acetaminophen 325mg tablets are packaged together). A more proper term is a single unit-of-use package.

Batch repackaging: the task of repackaging a large number of doses into unit-dose (single-unit) packages (e.g., 500 tablets in one session). Extemporaneous repackaging refers to the task of doing a smaller quantity (e.g., 20 tablets) to provide only a few days' supply. Repackaging is not limited to tablets and capsules. Liquids, ointments, powders, respiratory products, etc., may be repackaged into unit dose containers. Proper procedures of repackaging (regardless of the dosage form) must be followed to ensure that the final package has the same product in a properly labeled, appropriate package. Proper record keeping, which is often the responsibility of a well-trained pharmacy technician, is essential for inventory control, recall tracking and patient safety.

Compounding

Pharmacy compounding refers to the task of preparing and packaging a prescription order for a specific patient. In this process, a product is compounded (e.g., two ointments are mixed together) in the pharmacy and labeled with the specific patient's name . Pharmacy compounding is also referred to as "extemporaneous compounding."

Bulk compounding (or bulk manufacturing) refers to preparing and packaging a pharmaceutical product for use by more than one patient. This process involves compounding pharmaceuticals in advance of their need (the patient is not yet known). The amount to be compounded can be determined by assessing the prior history of amount dispensed. The product is compounded in the pharmacy from a detailed formula that contains directions on how to prepare, store, and label the final product (e.g., 3% acetic acid solution). Because pharmacy-manufactured items are not commercially available, their preparation records must be retained in the pharmacy, they must have lot numbers assigned to them, and they must have expiration dates put on the labels of the new containers. These bulk compounded items are only used within the institution where they are prepared. This type of compounding is generally not considered commercial manufacturing when, in accordance with state laws, the pharmacy practice license requires extemporaneous compounding. Specially trained pharmacy technicians may be used in manufacturing or compounding under certain policies and procedures.

Compounding for sale to other pharmacies

To produce commercially manufactured pharmaceuticals designed for sale to other pharmacies, an institution must be registered with the FDA as a manufacturer. Pharmaceutical manufacturers operate under the FDA-mandated Good Manufacturing Practices (GMP). The *U.S. Pharmacopeia-National Formulary* lists GMP categories and their related requirements. Those key categories are as follows:

- Organization and personnel
- Facilities
- Equipment
- Control of components and drug product containers and closures
- Production and process controls
- Packaging and labeling controls
- Holding and distribution
- Laboratory controls
- Records and reports

Details within each GMP category can be obtained from the USP. While these regulations are directed primarily at pharmaceutical manufacturers, the principles of GMP are expected to be followed at each pharmacy practice site.

Pharmaceutical compounding techniques

Good compounding practices should include use of clean and appropriate equipment. Only one item should be compounded at a time in a clean work area. Formulas should be established and followed carefully. All ingredients of the pharmaceutical product must be checked carefully. Expiration dates of individual ingredients must be carefully checked prior to compounding, as the final expiration date cannot be later than the expiration date of any individual ingredient. Labels should contain complete information and be checked prior to compounding. Appropriate repackaging materials should be used. Repackaging materials for oral solids are classified by their moisture permeability (Class A is the least permeable and Class D is the most permeable). Repackaging materials for liquids are classified by their inertness. A newly compounded item should be held until all quality control checks have been completed. Any report of problems with a compounded pharmaceutical is evaluated while the suspected batch is held from active distribution.

Weighing powders, crystals, ointments, or other solid substances is done on a prescription balance. A *Class A* prescription balance can accurately weigh from 120 milligrams (mg) to 15 grams (gm), while a *Class B* prescription balance can accurately weigh from 650mg to 120gm. A *Class A* balance

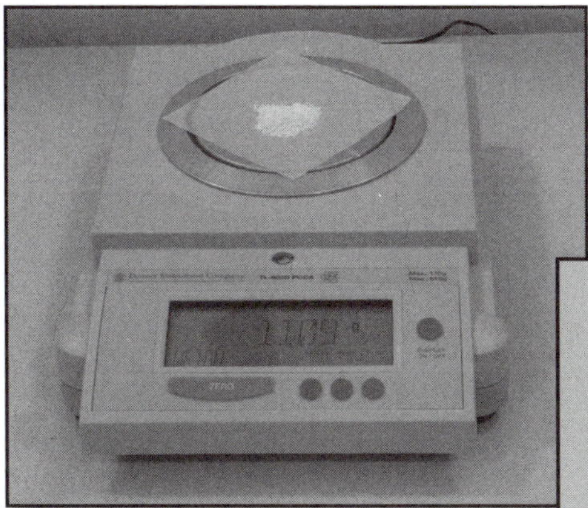

Electronic balance

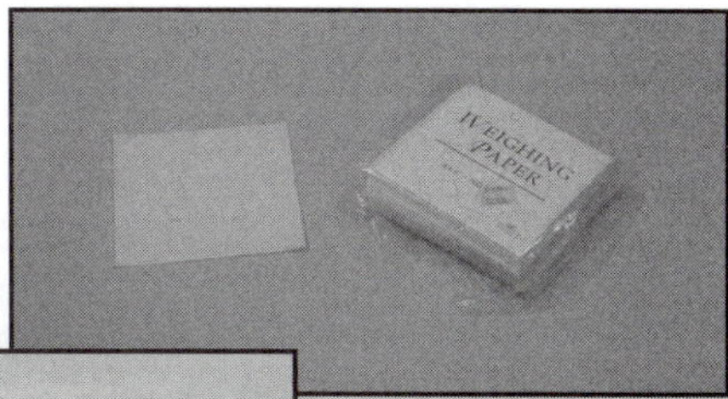

Glassine papers

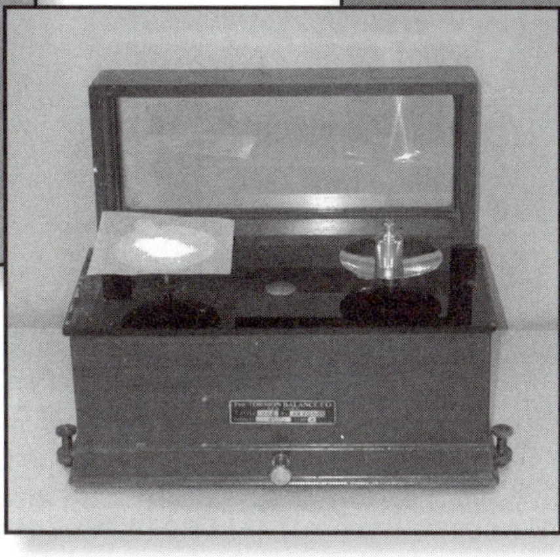

Manual balance

is more sensitive and has greater accuracy than a Class B balance. When using a prescription balance, one should make sure that the balance is sitting on a level, stable surface away from pedestrian traffic or air current such as from a fan or air vent. Equal size glassine papers are placed on each of the pans of the balance to protect the pans from the product being weighed. The balance must then be "zeroed out" or leveled until the indicator on the balance shows both pans are of even weight. Once this is done, weighing the solid product may begin, balancing the amount needed in one pan against a certified metal weight in the other pan. A prescription balance is handled delicately to maintain its accuracy.

Pharmaceutical liquids are measured in glass or plastic graduates of various sizes and shapes. Conical graduates are easier to handle and clean. Cylinder graduates are more accurate because of their consistent and usually smaller diameters. All graduates are labeled *TD* (to deliver) or *TC* (to contain). A *TC graduate* indicates that the volume measured on the scale is equal to the volume of liquid inside the graduate. A *TD graduate* allows one to measure the amount of liquid needed by considering the residual amount of liquid that is left inside the graduate once the liquid is poured out. An aqueous or alcohol liquid poured in a cylindrical shaped graduate forms a meniscus, a concave surface that looks like a double line. To accurately read a graduate scale, one must read the level at the bottom of the meniscus while holding the graduate at eye level.

Calibration of equipment is essential during compounding or repackaging operations. Automated equipment is frequently used to assist these operations and must be assessed for accuracy at each use. Peristaltic pump tubing (for repackaging liquids) may stretch and cause the volume delivered to vary. Other electrical equipment is subject to power surges that could cause inaccuracies.

Reconstitution of certain pharmaceutical products may be necessary. Many pediatric antibiotic liquids are sold to a pharmacy in a powder form for better product stability. These products must have a specific volume of water added to the bottle to reconstitute the medication (to liquid form) before the medication is dispensed to the patient. The time and date of reconstitution must be noted on the bottle while a new, shorter expiration date is calculated and posted on the label. Reconstituted liquids usually need to be refrigerated to prolong stability. Such refrigeration requirements should be indicated on the label.

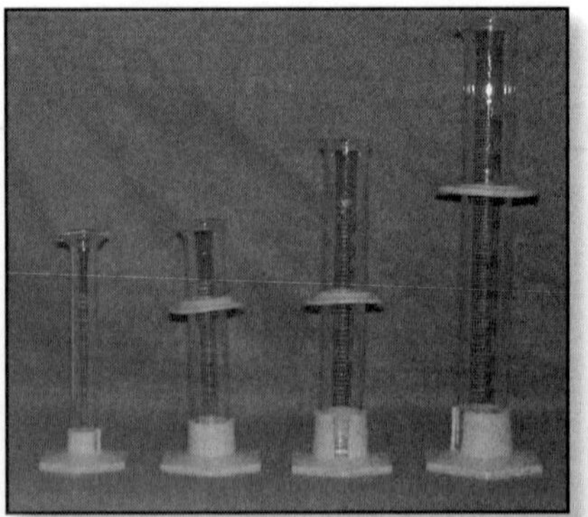

Graduates

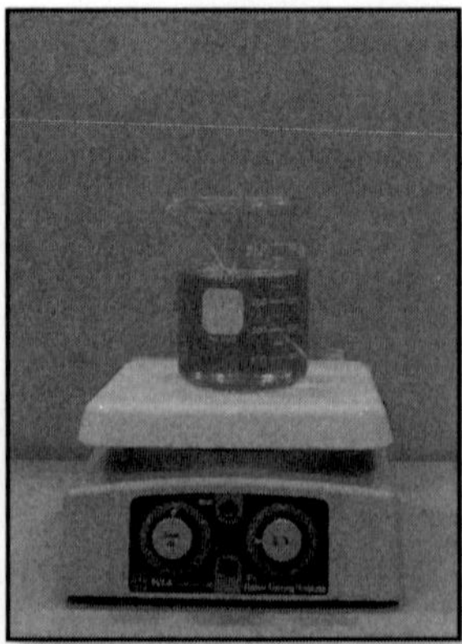

Beaker on a hot plate with a magnetic stirrer

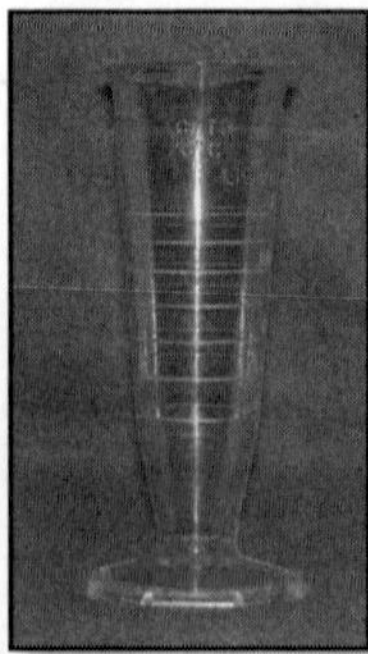

Graduate

Documentation and record keeping is important for each step of the compounding process in detail sufficient so that preparations can be replicated and the history of each ingredient can be traced. Records should be kept of (1) compounding formulas and procedures, (2) all compounded items including batch records and sample batch labels, (3) equipment maintenance, and (4) ingredients purchased, including certificates of purity for chemicals and material safety data sheets.

Documentation should include a record of who prepared the product, lot numbers, quantities of ingredients used, the assigned beyond-use date, and any special storage requirements.

Conclusion

As more pharmacists spend their time counseling patients on their medication usage, pharmacy technicians are being relied upon to handle the roles of managing the pharmacy's inventory and compounding medications. Technicians need to practice their profession according to the laws, rules, policies, and procedures as they relate to such areas of practice as borrowing pharmaceuticals, storing medications, handing expired and recalled products, documenting compounded medications, and other areas of pharmacy operations and medication control. By being thorough when dealing with medications in all steps of the procurement and preparation processes, pharmacy technicians help to enable pharmacists to provide patients with the highest level of care.

Acknowledgment

The author and publisher wish to acknowledge Gordon Naruta, R.Ph., M.A., for his extensive contributions to this chapter in the previous edition of this manual.

Bibliography

American Society of Health-System Pharmacists, ASHP guidelines on formulary system management, *American Journal of Health-System Pharmacy*, Vol. 49, pp. 648-52, 1992.

American Society of Health-System Pharmacists, ASHP technical assistance bulletin on compounding nonsterile products in pharmacies, *American Journal of Health-System Pharmacy*, Vol. 51, pp. 1441-8, 1994.

Bicker W.J., Gagnon J.P., "Purchasing and inventory control for hospital pharmacies," *Topics in Hospital Pharmacy Management,* Vol. 7, No. 2, pp. 59-74, 1987.

Effective Pharmacy Management, Fourth Edition, Marion Laboratories, Kansas City, MO, 1987.

Henry B., Auberman J., "Unit-dose prepackaging: A guide for development of policies and procedures," *Hospital Pharmacist,* Vol. 15, pp. 357-363, 1980.

Pharmacy Certified Technician Training Manual, 7th edition, Michigan Pharmacists Association, Lansing, MI, 1997.

Soares D.P., "Quality assurance standards for purchasing and inventory control," *American Journal of Hospital Pharmacy,* Vol. 42, pp. 610-620, 1985.

U.S. Department of Justice Drug Enforcement Administration, Pharmacist's Manual: An informational outline of the Controlled Substances Act of 1970, 5th edition, Washington, D.C., April 1986.

U.S. Pharmacopeia Convention: US Pharmacopeia-National Formulary, USP XXII-NF, XVII, U.S. Pharmacopeia Convention, Rockville, MD, 1990.

About the author

Paul W. Bush received his bachelor's degree in pharmacy from the University of Michigan College of Pharmacy in Ann Arbor, Michigan, and Doctor of Pharmacy and MBA from Wayne State University (WSU) College of Pharmacy & Allied Health Professions in Detroit, Michigan. Bush is currently Director of Pharmacy Services and Clinical Assistant Dean of Pharmacy for the Medical University of South Carolina (MUSC) in Charleston, South Carolina. At MUSC, Bush directs pharmacy services for the 701-bed academic medical center and teaches pharmacy administration for the College of Pharmacy. Previously, he was Director of Pharmacy Services for St. John's Hospital and Medical Center in Detroit, Michigan, Chairman of the Pharmacy Management Council for the St. John's Health System, and an adjunct professor of pharmacy practice at WSU. While at WSU, he was coordinator for the financial management course in the Master's in Health System Pharmacy Management Program. Bush has also held positions with Horizon Health System as Corporate Director of Clinical Pharmacy Services and Director of Pharmacy Services.

Self-assessment questions

1. A drug formulary is ***not***:
   a. a list of drugs that are considered by the professional staff of an institution to be the most useful in patient care.
   b. a list of medications that has been approved for prescribing to patients within a given institution.
   c. utilized in hospitals, clinics, or Health Maintenance Organizations.
   d. a list of the newest therapies for every disease state or condition.

2. All of the following are advantages to having a prime vendor agreement with a wholesaler *except*:
   a. quick deliveries.
   b. minimum orders.
   c. less paperwork.
   d. prices very close to the direct order price.

3. When a technician receives a shipment made to the pharmacy, which of the following is ***not*** part of the technician's responsibilities?
   a. Accept incorrect medications
   b. Check for damages or leaks
   c. Identify any shortages
   d. Sign a manifest

4. Which of the following requires a special Drug Enforcement Administration (DEA) order form when ordering?
   a. Class II controlled substances
   b. Class III controlled substances
   c. Class IV controlled substances
   d. Class V controlled substances

5. What is the correct procedure upon discovering the expiration date has been exceeded on a medication?
   a. Relabel with a new expiration date.
   b. Sell at a reduced price.
   c. Rotate the medication to the front of the stock so that it will be used first.
   d. Remove from active stock for proper disposal.

6. Which of the following is a function of medication packaging?
   a. Incompletely identifies the drug
   b. Allows deterioration of the drug
   c. Protects the drug from breakage
   d. Disallows access to the packaged drug

7. A unit-dose package contains:
   a. enough medication for one course of therapy.
   b. one dose of the drug.
   c. one-week supply of medication.
   d. one-day supply of medication.

8. Which of the following would be an appropriate balance on which to weigh a 50-gram substance?
   a. Class A prescription balance
   b. Class B prescription balance
   c. Class C prescription balance
   d. Zeroed prescription balance

9. The most accurate way to read a graduate scale is to:
   a. read the bottom of the meniscus holding the graduate at eye level.
   b. read the top of the meniscus holding the graduate at eye level.
   c. read the top of the meniscus viewing from the top of the graduate.
   d. read the bottom of the meniscus looking upward from the bottom of the graduate.

10. A reference that could be used to list key areas of good manufacturing practices is the:
    a. U.S. Pharmacopeia-National Formulary.
    b. American Hospital Formulary Service.
    c. Facts and Comparisons.
    d. Physicians Desk Reference.

CHAPTER 29

POLICIES AND PROCEDURES

Scott R. McCreadie, Pharm.D., MBA

Learning objectives

Upon completion of this chapter, the technician should be able to do the following:

- Define the term *policy*.
- Define the term *procedure*
- Explain why policies and procedures are needed and important.
- Describe the benefits of policies and procedures.
- Explain how a policies and procedures manual is organized.
- Describe the benefits of online policies and procedures.

Introduction

Policies and procedures in a pharmacy setting are a collection of documents designed to ensure safe and effective operations in the preparation and use of drug therapy and to ensure consistency in how situations are handled. They are a collection of decisions made in the past about the way the pharmacy will operate. Specifically, a *policy* is "a definite course or method of action selected from among alternatives and in the light of given conditions to guide and determine present and future decisions."[1] In a pharmacy setting, a policy broadly defines what needs to be done and sets limits or boundaries around decisions that are to be made. For example, policies will tell one the expected rules of attendance or criteria for using certain drug products. A *procedure* is defined as "a particular way of accomplishing something."[1] A procedure is a "how-to" guide to look at a process in a step-by-step approach. Examples include mixing a certain intravenous (IV) medication or handling chemotherapy wastes. A procedure will describe the steps to be taken to accomplish what is stated in the policy. Policies and procedures are found in all types of pharmacy settings from inpatient pharmacies to ambulatory care pharmacies to community-based pharmacies. Each workplace should have policies and procedures geared toward that work environment.

Policies and procedures are required by pharmacy professional organizations and regulatory agencies. Since 1950, the American Society of Health-System Pharmacists (ASHP), the American Pharmaceutical Association (APhA), the American Hospital Association (AHA), and the Catholic Hospital Association have required policies and procedures as minimum standards in hospitals.[2] The Joint Commission on Accreditation of Healthcare Organizations (JCAHO) also requires certain policies and procedures for the hospital to be accredited. This accreditation is needed for hospitals to receive reimbursement from some of the federal healthcare programs. A few examples of these required policies include the handling of food-drug interactions, drug recalls, medication errors, and adverse drug reactions. Most of these agencies recommend an annual review of the department's policies and procedures.

Many policies and procedures are needed to cover all of the different situations faced in pharmacy operations. Due to the large number of documents, they are usually bound together in manuals or placed online. Each policy and procedure is coded or numbered, and each manual typically has an index to assist in locating the specific document.

Benefits of policies and procedures

Policies and procedures provide many benefits to daily pharmacy practice by providing standards for the way the pharmacy operates. These documents will list the functions of the pharmacists and technicians on a daily basis, as well as list other special operations that might be seen on the job. This becomes valuable when an unusual or infrequent situation occurs so one can refer to the policy to see what should be done. These documents also help communication within the department because employees have a standard to use and don't have to rely on their memory or that of someone else. Policies and procedures can help to coordinate resources such as personnel, supplies, and equipment to operate efficiently by reducing waste and unnecessary work.

The policy and procedure manual will help a pharmacist or technician during orientation. This allows for a standardized reference when learning a new job. A new position is often complicated and confusing at first. Pharmacists and technicians frequently use the policies and procedures when starting a new position because things aren't very familiar. Many jobs require the review of the policy and procedure manual to occur during the first few weeks of a new job. Supervisors may also go through a checklist of the policies to ensure that new employees understand them and are able to perform the duties and activities set by the policy.

Policies and procedures can help promote safety in the workplace. Documentation of safety measures to protect the workers and the patients are found in the policies and procedures. The steps to be taken to ensure safety in the workplace and welfare for the patients will be listed. An employee should always rely on a policy or a procedure to guide work patterns when safety is an issue and not rely on someone else's short-cut method.

Contents of a policy and procedure manual

Policies and procedures should be current and reliable. Day-to-day operations change in pharmacy practice with new drugs, technology, and regulations; therefore, the policy and procedure manual should be updated frequently. A three-ring binder is commonly utilized to allow policies to be added, deleted, or revised when needed. Many organizations are now making policies and procedures available online through the Internet or an intranet for better access by employees. Online policies and procedures are especially easy to search because you only need to supply a few key words. Online versions can also be updated more easily by management and don't require someone to manually change sheets in a binder for new or changed policies. This saves paper and allows updates to be inserted quickly. Usually, the director of pharmacy or a corporate authority approves changes to the manual. Technicians know the specifics of their job very well and may be valuable in suggesting updates and changes. Policies and procedures are arranged by general subject matter. Some examples of subjects are listed below.

Table 1 Subjects for policy and procedure manuals

1. Departmental organization
2. Information system use
3. Drug distribution and control
4. Parenteral/enteral solution compounding
5. Pharmacy and Therapeutics Committee

Policies and procedures should address ***all*** areas of pharmacy practice. Included in this are the clinical or direct patient care activities of the pharmacist and the functions related to dispensing. Technicians usually work in areas supporting the dispensing role of pharmacy. Policies and procedures of interest to technicians will focus on drug distribution. Some of the policies and procedures useful for drug distribution are listed in the Table 2.

Table 2 Policies and procedures useful for drug distribution

- Procedure for handling medication orders
- Computer entry of orders
- IV admixtures
- Labeling, including accessory, cautionary, and expiration labels
- Removal of expired or improperly labeled drugs
- Recall of drugs
- Reporting of drug product defects
- Handling of drug samples
- Use of investigational agents
- Restricted drugs
- Safety information

A sample policy and procedure is found in Figure 1 at the end of this section. At the top is the code or number used to identify the document, followed by the subject of the policy. This number comes from the numbering of the subject and a sequential numbering of the various policies under that subject. The subject is usually a short description or title of the policy. The stated policy *(course of action)* is next and the procedure *(how-to)* is listed below it. The procedure will typically have many steps to ensure that the policy statement is fulfilled. At the bottom of the policy will be the original date of the document and any date(s) of revision. The person approving the policy signs at the very bottom. All policies and procedures within a manual should follow the same format. This enables the users to quickly locate the specific information needed.

Using the policy and procedure manual

A current policy and procedure manual or access to the online version should be available in all pharmacy areas where employees work. A table of contents or index helps to find the specific policy or procedure needed. For example, the proper and safe way to dispose of intravenous chemotherapy waste might be found in the section that covers intravenous solutions. If the pharmacy works with chemotherapy, there may be an entire section of the policy and procedure manual devoted to the handling of these drugs. Finding topics in the manual will get easier once the employee becomes more familiar with its layout.

The policy and procedure manual is a useful tool for looking at the functions that make up a job. Both pharmacists and technicians should be familiar with the layout and content of policies and procedures. Many employers require that pharmacists and technicians demonstrate competency in the areas covered by the policies and procedures (see Figure 2). The information contained within the policies and procedures, along with the employee's knowledge and experience, will help create a safe and effective work environment for the employees and the patients of pharmacy.

Figure 1 Sample policy and procedure

GENERAL MEDICAL CENTER
DEPARTMENT OF PHARMACY SERVICES

CODE: 6:1234

SUBJECT: Solutions — Deliveries and Return

POLICY: The technician sets the delivery cart, delivers solutions to patient care units, and returns the reusable solutions to the pharmacy.

PROCEDURE:

A. Preparing Delivery Cart
   1.0 All solutions that are checked and scheduled for the next delivery are placed on a delivery cart by technicians in groups according to units.

B. Solution delivery
   1.0 The technician proceeds to all units even if there are no solutions for delivery.
   2.0 Solutions are delivered to the correct patient care unit and double checked at that unit to ensure that no solution is left on the wrong unit.
   3.0 The small volume intravenous piggyback solutions (IVPB), total parenteral nutrition (TPN) solutions, and irrigation solutions are stored in the refrigerator. Solutions not needing refrigeration are placed in the appropriate bin next to the refrigerator.
   4.0 Solutions remaining in the refrigerator, or in the bin from a prior delivery, are retrieved by the technician and returned to the pharmacy for credit and/or reuse.
   5.0 Expired solutions are not returned to the pharmacy. These solutions are appropriately disposed by nursing personnel.

C. Upon return to the pharmacy with solutions, the technician:
   1.0 Discards any expired or unusable solutions.
   2.0 Places large volume parenterals (LVP) in the appropriate section of the recycling cart for reuse.
   3.0 Places IVPBs in the designated refrigerator box for recycling.

ORIGINATION DATE: January 14, 1990

REVISION DATES: 6/90; 2/92; 10/95; 2/98; 1/00

APPROVAL:______________________________

Director of Pharmacy Services: ____________________ Date: __________

Figure 2 Sample competency checklist

Competency Checklist
Solutions — Deliveries and Return

✔ Check if tasks are completed satisfactorily

Delivery Cart

___ Ensured that the IV labels were clear and firmly attached to the IV.

___ Correctly placed IV solutions on cart according to nursing unit of delivery.

___ Pulled discontinued orders from cart before the run.

Delivery

___ Went to all units to deliver IV solutions

___ Retrieved any discontinued IV solutions from units to be credited in the pharmacy

___ Assured that the IV solutions were delivered to the correct units.

___ Delivered solutions to the appropriate location on the nursing unit.

___ Placed solutions requiring refrigeration in the appropriate refrigerator.

___ Did not refrigerate solutions that do not require refrigeration.

___ Ensured that expired solutions were destroyed and not returned to pharmacy.

Return

___ Stored any recyclable solutions appropriately.

___ Credited any reusable solutions to the patient's account correctly.

Employee Signature ______________________________ Date__________

Supervisor Signature______________________________ Date__________

Conclusion

Following established policies and procedures helps to ensure that all pharmacy staff members adhere to the same guidelines when performing their duties. This leads to improved patient and employee safety, as well as reduced legal liability. Understanding how to use a policy and procedure manual allows pharmacy technicians to easily find guidelines to follow when unusual situations arise.

References

1. Webster's Ninth New Collegiate Dictionary, Merriam-Webster, Springfield, MA, 1988.

2. "American Society of Health-System Pharmacists guidelines: Minimum standard for pharmacies in institutions," *American Journal of Hospital Pharmacy*, Vol. 42, pp. 372-375, 1985.

Bibliography

"American Society of Health-System Pharmacists guidelines: Minimum standard for pharmacies in institutions," *American Journal of Hospital Pharmacy*, Vol. 42, pp. 372-375, 1985.

Hethcox, J.M., "The policy and procedure manual," Handbook of Institutional Pharmacy Practice, 3rd edition, American Society of Health-System Pharmacists, Bethesda, MD, 1992.

Neubrecht, F., Pharmacy Technician Policy and Procedure Manual, 1st edition, Pharmacy Services Inc., Lansing, MI.

Webster's Ninth New Collegiate Dictionary, Merriam-Webster, Springfield, MA, 1988.

About the author

Scott R. McCreadie received his Doctor of Pharmacy degree from the University of Michigan and then completed a pharmacy administrative residency at Detroit Receiving Hospital in Detroit, Mich. Dr. McCreadie has also earned an MBA from Oakland University in Rochester, Mich. He currently is a Strategic Project Coordinator at the University of Michigan Health System in Ann Arbor, Mich. Dr. McCreadie has worked at the Detroit Medical Center as a clinical specialist in the areas of trauma and surgery and then in management and coordinator positions involving information systems standardization and the development of an intranet knowledge system. These efforts led the Southeastern Michigan Society of Health-System Pharmacists to award Dr. McCreadie with their 1999 Innovative Practice Award.

Self-assessment questions

1. Where is a policy and procedure manual best placed?
   a. In your supervisor's office
   b. In the library
   c. In the workplace
   d. With whoever writes it

2. What section of the policy and procedure manual contains information on IV admixtures?
   a. Interdepartmental Policies and Procedures
   b. Parenteral/Enteral Solution Compounding
   c. Department Organization
   d. Drug Distribution and Control

3. If a policy and procedure does not reflect common practice in a work environment, you should:
   a. notify your supervisor.
   b. cross off the parts that are wrong.
   c. rewrite the policy and procedure yourself.
   d. ignore all policies and procedures because they're probably all wrong.

4. How does a supervisor usually measure whether an employee understands and follows policies and procedures?
   a. Performs a competency evaluation
   b. Takes the employee's word that they read the manual
   c. Assumes that the employee will learn it by working in the pharmacy
   d. Asks the employee's coworkers

5. What is ***not*** a benefit of putting policies and procedure online?
   a. Easier to search using keywords
   b. Can be updated easier by management
   c. Policy can be just a summary of the whole policy
   d. Reduces the amount of paper use in the department

Part V:
Professional Conduct

Chapter 30

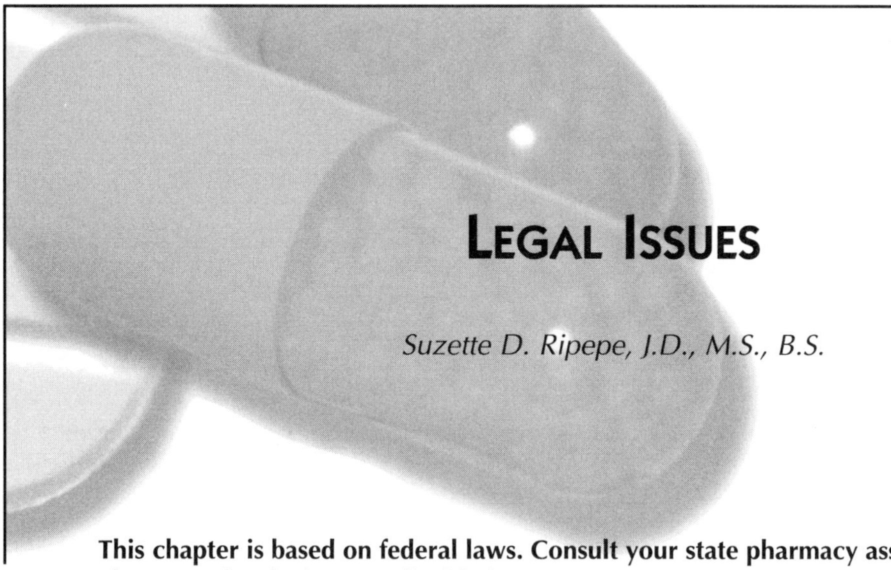

Legal Issues

Suzette D. Ripepe, J.D., M.S., B.S.

This chapter is based on federal laws. Consult your state pharmacy association or board of pharmacy for the laws applicable in your state.

Learning objectives

Upon completion of this chapter, the technician should be able to do the following:

- Name two federal agencies that develop and enforce drug product regulations.
- Explain the difference between a prescription-only (legend) and nonprescription (over-the-counter) drug.
- Describe the role of the Food and Drug Administration with regard to ensuring drug efficacy and safety.
- Describe the classes of drug recalls.
- List the required documentation for investigational drug therapy.
- Define each class of controlled substances and give examples.
- List the record keeping requirements for controlled substances.
- Identify and confirm a Drug Enforcement Agency prescriber registration number.
- Define a *hazardous substance.*
- Define *tamper-resistant packaging.*
- Define *child-resistant packaging* and give examples of exempted drugs.
- Describe the provisions of the Nonprofit Institutions Act.
- Describe the main provisions of the Prescription Drug Marketing Act.
- Define the drug use review requirements under the Omnibus Reconciliation Act of 1990 (OBRA '90).
- Describe the areas of prospective drug review by the pharmacist under OBRA '90.
- Discuss the state agencies and laws that affect the practice of pharmacy.
- List the four elements of a malpractice lawsuit.
- Describe different acts of negligence by a pharmacist or pharmacy technician that can lead to a malpractice lawsuit.
- Discuss the role of the pharmacy technician in maintaining patient confidentiality.

Introduction

Laws are enacted by elected officials (legislators) to provide rules and protect society. Crimes are divided into felonies and misdemeanors that are punishable by fines and/or imprisonment. Examples of criminal acts that may apply to pharmacy technicians include making false claims to Medicare/Medicaid and stealing narcotics from the workplace. Civil law covers various disputes between people in society. The remedy in a civil lawsuit is monetary damages. Examples of civil liability that may apply to pharmacy technicians include negligence and intentional torts, such as false imprisonment and assault and battery. Some actions can lead to both civil and criminal liability (such as assault and battery). The legislature delegates authority to administrative agencies that issue and enforce regulations. Pharmacy is highly regulated by numerous state and federal laws to protect the public from harm when taking medications.

Federal laws and regulations

The major federal laws affecting pharmacy practice are the Food, Drug, and Cosmetic Act (FDCA), the Controlled Substances Act (CSA), the Poison Prevention Packaging Act (PPPA), and the Omnibus Reconciliation Act of 1990 (OBRA '90). State laws affecting pharmacy are found in the state Public Health Code and state laws relating to pharmacy.

While federal and state laws regarding pharmacy overlap in many areas, a simplistic way of describing the two systems of law is that the federal government regulates the manufacturing and marketing of drugs, while the states regulate the practice of pharmacy and dispensing functions. For example, the federal government decides what drugs can be used as prescription drugs in the United States, in contrast to state government, which determines who can dispense prescription drugs in that state.

To determine if a federal or state law prevails in a given situation, the general rule requires following the more strict law, or the law with the greatest (highest) requirements. If a state law or regulation conflicts with a valid federal law or regulation and does not require at least what the federal law requires, the state law must yield to the federal law.

Pharmacies in healthcare institutions are subject to regulations from federal and state laws, national and state organizations, such as the Joint Commission on Accreditation of Healthcare Organizations (JCAHO), state public health departments, and other local agencies that have a direct influence on healthcare institutions.

Food, Drug and Cosmetic Act (FDCA)

The FDCA of 1938, with amendments, is the law that regulates drug quality. "Food," defined by the FDCA, is any substance used for food or drink by man and animals, and includes chewing gum. A "drug" is described as a substance, recognized in an official reference, used in diagnosis, cure, mitigation treatment or prevention of disease in man or animals. A drug affects the structure or function of the body of man or other animals. A "cosmetic" is defined under the FDCA as any substance applied externally to the human body for cleansing, beautifying or affecting appearance.

"Dietary Supplement" has replaced the word "vitamin" in the FDCA. The term "dietary supplement" includes vitamins, minerals, herbs, and nutritional supplements.

Dietary supplements are now regulated under the Dietary Supplement Health and Education Act of 1994 as a special class of foods. The Food and Drug Administration (FDA) must prove a dietary supplement unsafe before it can be removed from the market. Dietary supplements cannot make health claims of treating a specific disease (for example, "may alleviate depression") on its label without prior review by the FDA, but it can indicate how it may affect the normal structure or function of the human body (for example, "helps stabilize mood") that is affected by the herb.

New drugs can be marketed under the FDCA only after proven safe for use under conditions described on the label and approved by the FDA. The FDCA applies to pharmacies and pharmacists, as they sell drugs to patients.

Prescription Drug Amendment

The Prescription Drug Amendment, enacted in 1951, creates two classes of drugs: prescription and nonprescription. Nonprescription drugs (also known as over-the-counter drugs) are those believed by experts in the field to be safe and effective when used as labeled *without* medical supervision. Prescription drugs are also safe and effective when used as intended, but because of potential harmful effects, require medical supervision. A patient can obtain a prescription-only drug after receiving a written order from a licensed prescriber. All prescription drugs are labeled with specific labeling (called a *legend* or *caution statement*): "*Caution: Federal law prohibits dispensing without a prescription.*" This labeling requirement will be phased out (by February 19, 2003) to simplify the label and is being replaced by the following, much shorter statement: "Rx only."

Drug Efficacy Amendment

The Drug Efficacy Amendment (do not confuse this with the Drug Enforcement Agency) was enacted by Congress in response to the thalidomide disaster, where thousands of infants were born with seal-like limbs (phocomelia). Even though the FDA prevented the marketing of thalidomide in the United States, the fear of a similar disaster occurring in the United States led to the enactment of this amendment to make the new drug approval process much stricter. A pharmaceutical manufacturer must prove a new drug to be not only safe, but also effective. The efficacy requirement was made retroactive to all drugs marketed between 1938 and 1961. Nonprescription drug efficacy, safety, and labeling are also regulated through the FDA.

Food and Drug Administration

The Food and Drug Administration (FDA) is the administrative agency that enforces the FDCA. The FDA can force a violator of the FDCA to cease its illegal activity and can begin criminal proceedings (fines and/or imprisonment) against a violator. The FDA may also, with court approval, seize any adulterated (contaminated or not manufactured appropriately) or misbranded (mislabeled) food, drug, or cosmetic.

The FDA approves new drug entities after reviewing a manufacturer's New Drug Application (NDA). The NDA is filed after studies are done under an Investigational New Drug (IND) application on file with the FDA. The drug approval process must prove a drug to be safe and effective. INDs are drugs being used for experimental or investigational use. Physicians must generally seek approval to do research using an IND at a healthcare facility through the facility's Institutional Review Board (IRB).

Drugs classified as "investigational" are subject to required documentation: 1) an IND application filed by the investigator, 2) a consent form signed by the patient that is being treated with the IND (where written consent is required), and 3) perpetual inventory, lot numbers, and other investigative data usually maintained by the dispensing pharmacy.

Investigational drugs are studied under the following four phases:

Phase I: Clinical investigation in a small number of patients to determine the preferred route of administration and safe dosage.

Phase II: Clinical investigation on a limited number of patients for a specific disease treatment or prevention of disease to further determine the drug's safety.

Phase III: Clinical trials are expanded to further test for safety and efficacy of the drug.

Phase IV: Post-marketing surveillance continues after a drug is marketed. The manufacturer must report to the FDA all serious adverse drug reactions, along with other information including additional drug safety and efficacy data. The FDA may withdraw its approval of a new drug upon review of post-marketing information.

The FDA also approves the drug package insert labeling that accompanies a prescription drug product.

Generic drug entities are assigned a two-letter coding system in the FDA publication *Approved Drug Products with Therapeutic Equivalence Evaluations,* also known as the "Orange Book." Looking only at the first letter of the two-letter symbol, an "A" rating indicates drug products considered therapeutically equivalent. A "B" rating indicates that the FDA considers the drug products not to be therapeutically equivalent. Many states require a drug product to be "A" rated before it can be substituted as a generic equivalent for a brand name drug.

Drug advertising

The FDA requires manufacturers to include a summary of information such as side effects, contraindications, and effectiveness in all advertising of a prescription drug. Advertising can occur in journals, magazines, newspapers, radio, television and on the Internet. When advertising prescription drugs to the consumer or general public, information must be given on how to obtain additional information regarding the drug, such as dialing telephone and fax numbers, referring to print advertisements in commonly read publications, or referring to an Internet website. The Federal Trade Commission (FTC) and the FDA also monitor the advertising of over-the-counter drugs; information should not be misleading to a consumer.

Federal recall of drug products or devices

The FDA cannot order a product recall, but it can ask a manufacturer to voluntarily recall a product rather than be forced to cease making the product or have the FDA confiscate the product. The manufacturer must notify sellers of the recall; the sellers, in turn, must notify consumers. For example, if a pharmacist in a community pharmacy is notified of a recall, the pharmacist must then notify all patients who have current prescriptions filled at the pharmacy for the recalled product. Sellers are notified of a recall through letters, telegrams, e-mail, sales representatives, and listings in pharmacy publications. The three classes of recalls are listed from most serious to least serious:

Class I: Reasonable probability that the product will cause serious adverse health consequences or death.

Class II: Product may cause temporary or medically reversible adverse health consequences; probability of serious adverse consequences is remote.

Class III: Product not likely to cause adverse health consequences.

Healthcare institutions, such as hospitals, must document and maintain records on action taken with drug recalls. Be careful not to confuse recall classes and controlled substances schedules. It is easy to confuse these rating systems because they use a similar numbering scheme.

Controlled substance requirements

The federal government has classified certain drugs by abuse potential and has made regulations based on this classification under the Controlled Substances Act (CSA). The regulations cover buying, inventorying, prescribing, dispensing, storing, using, and destroying these drugs. The Drug Enforcement Agency (DEA), an agency of the U.S. Department of Justice, administers the CSA; coordination with the FDA is frequently required. Controlled substances are classified into five schedules that are:

Schedule I (C-I): *Drugs having no accepted medical use in the United States and having a high abuse potential.*

Examples: heroin, lysergic acid diethylamide (LSD), mescaline, peyote, tetrahydrocannibol (THC, marijuana)

Schedule II (C-II): *Drugs having an accepted medical use and a high abuse potential with severe psychic or dependence liability.*

Examples: amobarbital, amphetamines, cocaine, codeine (not in combination with other drugs), hydromorphone, meperidine, methadone, morphine, oxycodone, pentobarbital, secobarbital

Schedule III (C-III): *Drugs having an accepted medical use and an abuse potential less than those in Schedules I and II.*

Examples: barbiturates not in Schedules I or II, paregoric, combination narcotics (e.g., acetaminophen with codeine #2, #3, #4, etc.), anabolic steroids

Schedule IV (C-IV): *Drugs having an accepted medical use and an abuse potential less than those listed in Schedule III.*

Examples: alprazolam, chloral hydrate, diazepam, dextropropoxyphene, flurazepam, lorazepam, meprobamate, phenobarbital, phentermine

Schedule V (C-V): *Drugs having an accepted medical use and an abuse potential less than those listed in Schedule IV.*

Examples: cough preparations containing narcotics (e.g., guaifenesin with codeine), diphenoxylate and atropine sulfate

Every state also has additional controlled substances laws. Technicians need to know both state and federal laws. This chapter only addresses the federal law.

Bulk containers of controlled substances must be labeled with symbols for each class (e.g., C-II, C-III, etc.). All controlled substance prescriptions must contain the full name and address of the patient and the name, address, and DEA registration number of the prescribing practitioner. When controlled substance prescriptions are filled, they must indicate the number of units or volume dispensed, the date of dispensing, and a hand-written or typewritten name of the dispensing professional. Pharmacists may enter missing information on the prescription, if state law does not prohibit this activity.

Many Schedule V (C-V) controlled substances are available without a prescription. Some states may require a prescription for a C-V although the drug may not be classified as a prescription drug by the FDA. Dispensing a C-V as a nonprescription drug can only be done by a pharmacist, and in some states, pharmacy interns. Non-pharmacist employees, such as pharmacy technicians, are not allowed to dispense a C-V, even under a pharmacist's supervision. They may complete the sale transaction once the pharmacist requirements are completed. Some requirements may include: obtaining patient information, completing a C-V dispensing logbook with patient signature, and labeling the C-V with the date dispensed and the dispensing pharmacist's initials.

Documentation of use and inventory

Record keeping requirements are very important under the CSA. Records must be kept for inventory, drugs received, and drugs dispensed. An initial inventory of controlled substances must be taken when a pharmacy opens and then every two years. In some states, a controlled substance inventory is required every year. Since this is a "higher" requirement than the federal law, pharmacists in those states must comply by performing an annual inventory. Schedule II (C-II) controlled substances must be ordered by a pharmacy on a special DEA form (DEA Form 222-C) and C-II records must be kept separate from C-III, C-IV, and C-V records. Violation of record-keeping requirements can lead to imprisonment and/or fines.

The pharmacy site where a pharmacist practices must be registered with the DEA. With the exception of sole proprietorships, individual pharmacists do not need to be registered with the DEA. Individual practitioners such as physicians, dentists, veterinarians, and others allowed by the state (e.g., nurse practitioners, physician's assistants) must be registered with the DEA and obtain a DEA number to prescribe controlled substances. Exceptions to this include practitioners who are employed by a hospital or other healthcare facility, and prescribe controlled substances only for inpatients at that institution; these practitioners use the institution's DEA number. In some states, nurse practitioners and physician's assistants prescribe controlled substances under authority of a physician with a DEA number, so they do not have to obtain their own DEA number. All prescribers have two letters as a prefix to their DEA prescriber registration number. The first letter designates the classification of the practitioner and the second letter designates the first letter of the prescriber's last name. The accuracy of a DEA prescriber registration number can be confirmed using the following formula:

1. Add the first, third, and fifth digits of the DEA number;
2. Add the second, fourth, and sixth digits and multiply the sum by two;
3. Add the two numbers.
4. The last digit of this sum is the same as the last digit of the DEA prescriber registration number.

Example: DEA Prescriber Registration Number: 1234563

$1 + 3 + 5 = 9$

$(2 + 4 + 6) \times 2 = 24$

$9 + 24 = 33$

3 is also the last digit of 1234563, so the assumption can be made that this DEA number is valid.

Pharmacists dispense controlled substances under an individual controlled substance state license. Pharmacy technicians, pharmacy interns, and other ancillary personnel may dispense controlled substances under the supervision of a pharmacist **only** if allowed by state law. According to 21CFR§1306.04(a), pharmacists are required to assure that a controlled substance is prescribed for a "legitimate medical purpose" for a patient in the usual course of professional practice.

Prescription Drug Marketing Act

The Prescription Drug Marketing Act of 1987 (PDMA) was passed by Congress to prevent misbranding and adulteration of prescription drug products. The PDMA's intent is to assure the U.S. public that prescription drugs are safe and effective. To prevent the resale, relabeling, or adulteration of any prescription drug product sold outside normal channels, the PDMA requires several measures. The two most important measures involve manufacturer drug samples and purchases and resale by hospitals and healthcare facilities.

Drug samples cannot be sold, traded, or purchased. Samples can only be distributed to practitioners licensed to prescribe or to pharmacies of hospitals or healthcare entities at the written request of the prescriber. The PDMA requires certain information in the request and several record-keeping requirements after receipt of the samples. A community pharmacy (ambulatory, chain, corporate, or retail) **cannot** receive any sample drugs.

Hospitals and some healthcare entities can purchase drugs at large discounts. This may lead to the illegal resale of drugs from hospitals to other entities. Drugs sold in this manner are often improperly stored or labeled where the integrity of the drug product may be uncertain. The purchase of drugs outside normal purchasing channels leads to unfair competition by the pharmacies purchasing the drugs at discounted prices. The PDMA prohibits the sale, purchase, or trade (or offer to do so) of prescription drugs purchased by a hospital, healthcare entity or charitable organization. Some exceptions are:

1. Purchases by a hospital from a group purchasing organization for its own use;
2. Sales or purchases to nonprofit affiliates;
3. Sales or purchases for emergency medical reasons (e.g., a transfer between hospitals and from a hospital to a community pharmacy if there is a temporary drug shortage).

Federal Hazardous Substance Act (FHSA)

Under the Federal Hazardous Substance Act (FHSA), a *hazardous substance* is one that can cause injury or illness and potential danger, especially to children, if mishandled. Federal legislation covering hazardous substances does not include drugs, but regulates household items such as bleach, cleaning fluids, antifreeze, and drainpipe cleaners. Pharmacies must sell all hazardous substances covered by the FHSA only in the original containers labeled by the manufacturer or supplier, or label the product as outlined in the FHSA.

Tamper-resistant packaging

Effective February 1983, the FDA established requirements for tamper-resistant packaging. *A tamper-resistant package* provides a barrier to entry that clearly indicates to a consumer if some kind of tampering has occurred with the package. A tamper-resistant package may involve an immediate container-and-closure system, a secondary container or carton system, or any combination of systems intended to provide a visual indication of package integrity. These regulations were established after the tampering of nonprescription products led to at least seven deaths. However, some products are exempt from these packaging requirements.

Child resistant (safety) packaging

In April 1974 the FDA issued regulations regarding child-resistant containers to comply with the Poison Prevention Packaging Act (PPPA). The regulation requires that all prescription medications dispensed from a pharmacy or a hospital must be dispensed in child-resistant containers. This includes drugs dispensed from outpatient clinics and emergency rooms, or medications given to patients upon discharge. Child-resistant packaging requirements do not apply to medications administered within an institution. Unit-dose packaging does **not** qualify as safety packaging.

Several nonprescription drugs are covered under the PPPA. Both acetaminophen and aspirin-containing products intended for oral administration must be sold in child-resistant packaging (with some exemptions). Other examples of substances covered by the PPPA include furniture polish, methyl salicylate (oil of wintergreen), turpentine, methyl alcohol (methanol), ethylene, and ethylene glycol. Also, some iron-containing drugs and dietary supplements are listed in the PPPA.

Exemptions from safety packaging

Certain drugs are exempt from safety packaging. Patients may request that their prescription be filled in a non-child-resistant package. In these cases, the pharmacist should require the patient's signature for permission to dispense in a non-child-resistant package. Preferably, the signature should be obtained each time the prescription is filled. Examples of exempted prescription drugs that **do not** have to comply with the requirements of child-resistant packaging are listed below:

1. Sublingual dosage forms of nitroglycerin and isosorbide dinitrate
2. A potassium supplement in unit-dose forms, including individually wrapped effervescent tablets, unit-dose containers of liquid potassium and powdered potassium in unit-dose packets

3. Medically administered oral contraceptives in manufacturers' calendar-reminder dispensing packages.
4. Conjugated estrogen and norethindrone tablets when dispensed in mnemonic (memory-aid) dispenser packages
5. Medroxyprogesterone acetate tablets

Nonprofit Institutions Act

The Nonprofit Institutions Act exempts purchases by nonprofit institutions of supplies for their own use from the price discrimination provisions of the Robinson-Patman Act. This act allows institutions to purchase drugs and supplies at prices sometimes not available to the general retail industry. However, these products are subject to the limitation of use as described above. "Own use" (for pharmaceuticals) is defined by the United States Supreme Court as follows:

1. Drug products provided to the **inpatient, outpatient, or emergency room patient** when for personal use on the premises of the institution
2. Drug products provided to the above for personal use off the premises of the institution in **limited and reasonable quantities** (refills of these products **are not** considered **own use** by the institution)
3. Drug products provided by the institution for employees, students, volunteers, physician-staff members, and dependents when for personal use
4. Occasional patients in emergencies when no other pharmacy is available

Omnibus Reconciliation Act of 1990

Pharmacy practice has been influenced by major provisions under the Omnibus Reconciliation Act of 1990 (OBRA '90). Congress recognized the pharmacist as a healthcare professional who can improve the quality of drug therapy and, therefore, save healthcare costs.

The most important area of OBRA '90 for pharmacy is drug utilization review (DUR) for all Medicaid patients. States must require DUR under OBRA '90 for all Medicaid patients receiving prescription drugs in their state. Almost all states have expanded OBRA '90 requirements under their pharmacy practice statutes to all patients, not just Medicaid patients. Some states may require DUR for all Medicaid patients and varying levels of DUR to other patients. Other insurance companies may also require DUR as part of the provider contract. The DUR process has three parts: retrospective review, educational programs, and prospective review.

Retrospective review is done in each state by a DUR Board. Large amounts of data on drug use by Medicaid patients are reviewed to identify areas of improvement; topics for educational programs may be established.

Educational programs for pharmacists and physicians are the second area necessary for compliance under OBRA '90. The programs are focused on improvement of medication use and can be face-to-face visits by an expert with the pharmacist or physician, large educational meetings, or written materials sent to the pharmacist or physician.

Prospective Drug Utilization Review is the area required by each pharmacist when dispensing a prescription to a Medicaid patient. Prospective review includes: (1) a review of a patient's prescription drug therapy before dispensing, (2) patient counseling by the pharmacist, and (3) pharmacist documentation of patient information. Any changes made for the patient are best documented in the patient's medication use profile. Pharmacists review a patient's drug therapy before dispensing by screening for the following potential drug therapy problems:

1. therapeutic duplication (two drugs being used for the same purpose)
2. drug-disease contraindications (certain drugs not appropriate because of a patient's disease state)
3. drug-drug interactions (including interactions with nonprescription and dietary supplement drugs)
4. wrong drug dosage or length of drug therapy
5. clinical abuse/misuse (underuse or overuse of a drug)

To enhance patient compliance with medication use, the pharmacist must offer to counsel each Medicaid patient on the use of a dispensed prescription. Some states allow a non-pharmacist, such as a pharmacy technician, to offer counseling; however, a pharmacist must do the actual counseling. Although not mandatory, a patient signature can be obtained when the patient refuses counseling. Information discussed during patient counseling is left to the professional discretion of the pharmacist under OBRA '90. Suggested information for discussion during counseling includes:

1. the name and description of the medication
2. the dosage form, dosage, the route of administration, and duration of drug therapy
3. special directions and precautions for preparation, administration, and use by the patient
4. common severe side effects, adverse effects, or interactions and therapeutic contraindications that may be encountered, including ways to prevent them and the action required if they do occur
5. techniques for self-monitoring drug therapy
6. proper storage
7. prescription refill information
8. action taken in case of a missed dose
9. how to contact the pharmacist for questions or concerns

Giving the patient written information about their prescription **without** an oral consultation does **not** meet the counseling requirement under OBRA '90.

The last requirement pharmacists must comply with under OBRA '90 is to attempt to obtain patient specific information. States may allow non-pharmacist personnel, such as pharmacy technicians, to help the pharmacist in obtaining information from the patient. The minimum information obtained and recorded is: (1) name, address, telephone number, date of birth (or age), and gender; (2) individual histories where significant, including disease state or states, known allergies and drug reactions, and a complete list of current medications and relevant devices; and (3) pharmacist comments about the individual's drug therapy.

State laws and regulations

State law, not federal law, regulates professionals practicing in each state. Regulation is accomplished through professional licensure. Beyond the responsibility as an employee in any given situation, licensed professionals are also accountable to the state board that regulates their license to practice as professionals. Pharmacy practice statutes contain the state laws that regulate the practice of pharmacy. In most states, a board of pharmacy is the administrative agency designated to protect the public through enforcement of the pharmacy practice statutes, especially in granting licenses to pharmacists and pharmacies.

Utilization of pharmacy technicians

States regulate many details of the practice of pharmacy and regulations vary from state to state. Some examples of differing state regulations include the dispensing label of the prescription product, required controlled substance prescription forms, the pharmacist-to-technician ratio, and the functions a pharmacy technician is allowed to perform. Pharmacy technicians are utilized for as many functions as legally possible under state and federal law to allow pharmacists time to do screening, counseling, and monitoring functions. To comply with OBRA '90 counseling requirements, some states allow a pharmacy technician, or other designated person, to offer to counsel the patient, if the pharmacist does the actual counseling.

Several states are recognizing certified pharmacy technicians in various ways. Kentucky allows certified technicians to have a higher level of responsibilities than non-certified technicians. Tennessee allows a higher pharmacist-to-tech ratio if technicians are certified; the state allows more certified technicians to be assigned to each pharmacist. Some states such as Texas and Utah are requiring technicians to be certified in order to work as a pharmacy technician in their states.

Since state laws are very different, as discussed above, the reader is urged to consult the state pharmacy association or state board of pharmacy for the laws applicable in his or her state.

Malpractice

Malpractice falls under tort law, a type of civil liability. A tort involves causing injury or damage to another through negligence or intentional action. Anyone can be considered negligent if they do or do not perform an act that a reasonable person would have done in a similar situation, and that action or inaction causes some type of harm.

Malpractice, or professional negligence, involves the following elements: (1) a duty owed by the defendant (healthcare professional); (2) the defendant (healthcare professional) has to breach (or not adhere to) their duty, (3) the plaintiff (patient) has to be injured, and (4) the injury has to be caused by the breach of the duty. A duty by the defendant (healthcare professional) is determined by state and federal law, professional group standards, and expert witness testimony. Courts of law have traditionally made the pharmacist responsible only when committing a dispensing error that causes patient harm. Examples of dispensing errors include giving the patient the wrong drug, the wrong strength of the drug, or incorrect directions on how to take the drug. New requirements under OBRA '90 and state law have courts expanding the responsibility of pharmacists to include a duty to recognize potential drug therapy problems and warning the patient and/or physician of the potential problem. An example of this type of error includes not warning the patient and/or physician of a possible severe drug interaction between two drugs that are dispensed together.

Pharmacists can be responsible for malpractice, and the state board can take disciplinary actions against their license for the same act.

Since pharmacy technicians are not generally licensed by the state, their primary accountability is to their employer as supervised by licensed pharmacists. Employers are responsible for their employees (and their negligent acts) as long as the employee is acting within the scope of their employment. It is important for the pharmacy technician to follow policies and procedures (see Chapter 29), and never to act in place of a pharmacist. Pharmacy technicians are frequently asked to testify in medication error and other types of pharmacy lawsuits. Several insurance companies now provide malpractice insurance policies for pharmacy technicians. The issue of having malpractice insurance is a personal one, and the pharmacy technician should seek out legal advice if they are unsure in this area.

Patient confidentiality

A patient's medical record is a confidential, legal document. Most states have laws that make it a crime to falsify a patient's medical record. Health professionals can also be held liable under civil law for falsifying a patient's medical record. The institution (hospital, doctor's office, etc.) owns the patient's medical record, but a patient has the right to request a copy and/or view their medical record. Care must be taken when providing family prescription reports in an ambulatory setting. Both spouses and older children should sign the request for a family report.

Most states consider the pharmacy prescription record a medical record, and laws protecting medical records also apply to pharmacy prescription records. Even if a state does not recognize a pharmacist-patient relationship to include confidentiality of patient information, pharmacists and pharmacy technicians have an ethical duty to maintain patient confidentiality (see Chapter 31). Some exceptions to patient confidentiality in different states include mandatory reporting of suspected child abuse and certain communicable diseases (such as tuberculosis). Patients with healthcare insurance plans agree that healthcare providers can give medical information to their insurer.

Computerized medical records must also be kept confidential. There is a lot of concern in this area and federal guidelines are expected to be developed and enforced. Employees of pharmacies are usually required to sign a confidentiality agreement upon hire. Employees must access computerized records only when necessary to perform their job. Also, computer screens and written medical records need to be kept out of the public's view.

The most common breach of patient confidentiality includes verbal slips. These can occur in the elevator, cafeteria, or lobby of a hospital. Also, when interviewing or counseling a patient regarding their medication, care should be taken that other patients cannot hear the discussion. Speakerphones should also be discouraged from use to prevent others from overhearing a conversation. Another type of confidentiality breach includes discussing patients with family and friends. A recent Michigan case illustrates this problem. A man with AIDS sued a chain pharmacy because he claims a pharmacy technician employee told her son that the man had AIDS. The patient had not told his children yet about his illness, but claims the technician's son taunted his children at school, calling one of them an "AIDS baby." The case settled for an undisclosed amount of money.

Conclusion

It is important that all pharmacy technicians know and understand the laws and regulations governing pharmacies, pharmacy personnel, and pharmaceuticals in order to ensure that patient safety and confidentiality are not compromised. Technicians play important roles when dealing with the ordering of and filling prescriptions for controlled substances. Because this text only discusses federal laws, technicians should consult their respective boards of pharmacy to obtain a copy of laws that will apply to pharmacy and pharmacy personnel in their state. Additionally, pharmacy technicians have the responsibility of acting within the scope of their practice as outlined by state laws and their pharmacy's policies, as well as preserve the confidentiality of their patients' records.

Bibliography

Abood, R.R., Brushwood, D.B., Pharmacy Practice and the Law 2nd Edition, Aspen Publications, Gaithersburg, MD, 1996.

Fink, J.L., Vivian, J.C., Reid, K.K., Pharmacy Law Digest, Facts and Comparisons, St. Louis, MO, 1999.

Younger, P., Conner, C., Cartwright, K.K., and Kole, S.M., Pharmacy Law Answer Book, Aspen Publishing, Gaithersburg, MD, 1996.

About the author

Suzette D. Ripepe received her bachelor's of science in pharmacy from Ferris State University College of Pharmacy in Big Rapids, Michigan. She also received a master's of science in hospital pharmacy administration and a juris doctor from Wayne State University in Detroit, Michigan. She has worked primarily at hospital pharmacy locations in the southeastern Michigan area. Her areas of expertise include hospital pharmacy management, medication error and adverse drug reaction monitoring, drug use evaluation, and pharmacy technician education. She is an advocate for and has lectured to pharmacy technicians for several years. Ripepe also teaches medical law to allied health program students and works as a pharmacy law consultant.

Self-assessment questions

1. Which of the following statements is true regarding federal and state laws affecting pharmacy practice?
   a. When there is a conflict, federal law always prevails over state law.
   b. A state law cannot be more strict than a federal law.
   c. Licensure of professionals is regulated by federal law.
   d. Pharmacy technicians are licensed under federal law.

2. The Food and Drug Administration:
   a. may seize any adulterated or misbranded food, drug, or cosmetic without a court order.
   b. does not review drug product advertising.
   c. approves new drug entities through review of a manufacturer's New Drug Application.
   d. enforces the Controlled Substance Act.

3. All of the following are true about the publication *Approved Drug Products with Therapeutic Equivalence Evaluations except:*
   a. it is published by the FDA.
   b. it is also known as the "Orange Book."
   c. it is also known as the "Red Book."
   d. it is gives therapeutically equivalent drug products an "A" rating.

4. The FDA enforces drug advertising laws by:
   a. allowing advertisements only in magazines.
   b. requiring manufacturers to include summary information of side effects and contraindications.
   c. monitoring prescription-only drug advertising and not monitoring over-the-counter drug advertising.
   d. charging a fee for each advertisement that is televised.

5. The most serious type of drug recall that may cause serious harm to the patient is:
   a. Class I.
   b. Class II.
   c. Class III.
   d. Class IV.

6. Record keeping requirements under the Controlled Substance Act include all of the following *except:*
   a. records of inventory.
   b. records of all state prescriber DEA numbers.
   c. records of drugs received.
   d. records of drugs dispensed.

7. Drugs having no accepted medical use in the United States and having a high abuse potential are classified as:
   a. Schedule I.
   b. Schedule II.
   c. Schedule III.
   d. Schedule IV.

8. Which of the following is a legitimate DEA prescriber registration number?
   A. 2453161
   B. 2453162
   C. 2453163
   D. 2453164

9. Child (safety) resistant packaging is:
   a. not necessary for a prescription drug when a patient requests a non-child-resistant container.
   b. required of all nonprescription drugs.
   c. required for drugs administered within a healthcare institution such as a hospital.
   d. not applicable when a prescription is dispensed from a hospital outpatient clinic pharmacy.

10. The regulation which prohibits the sale, purchase, or trading of drug samples is the:
    a. Nonprofit Institutions Act.
    b. Prescription Drug Marketing Act.
    c. Controlled Substances Act.
    d. OBRA '90.

11. The regulation which requires pharmacists to perform drug use reviews for all Medicaid patients is the:
    a. Nonprofit Institutions Act.
    b. Prescription Drug Marketing Act.
    c. Federal Hazardous Substances Act.
    d. OBRA '90.

12. Under the requirements of OBRA '90, a pharmacy technician may:
    a. counsel a patient regarding drug therapy.
    b. screen patient profiles for drug-disease contraindications.
    c. call a prescriber and recommend a different drug dosage.
    d. make the offer to have the pharmacist counsel a patient, if permitted by state law.

13. A pharmacy employer is responsible for the negligent acts of a pharmacy technician when:
    a. the pharmacy technician pays the pharmacy employer for protection.
    b. the pharmacy technician ignores policies and procedures.
    c. the pharmacy technician acts as a pharmacist when the pharmacist is at lunch.
    d. the pharmacy technician is acting within the scope of his or her employment.

14. A pharmacy technician may do which of the following with a patient's computerized prescription record?
    a. Look at a patient's prescription record to enter a new prescription dropped off by the patient.
    b. Look at every patient's record who lives on your street even though you are not processing prescriptions for them.
    c. Look at a record upon patient request and yell across the counter, "Nope, you don't have any refills left on your birth control pills."
    d. Tell their spouse that you saw the patient profile of a local judge and he had a prescription filled for an anticancer drug.

15. A breach of a patient's confidentiality occurs when:
    a. pharmacists are discussing a patient's drug therapy inside the hospital pharmacy department.
    b. pharmacy technicians are complaining on the hospital elevator about how many times they had to run emergency drugs to Mrs. Wilson's room on 4 West today.
    c. a pharmacist is entering a new prescription for a patient into the computer.
    d. a pharmacist is counseling a patient in a private counseling room.

Chapter 31

Ethics

Jesse C. Vivian, R.Ph., J.D.

Learning objectives

Upon completion of this chapter, the technician should be able to do the following:

- Explain how professional ethics establish normative behavior and provide guidelines for resolving ethical dilemmas.
- Cite relevant codes of ethics for pharmacists and technicians.
- Understand how legal and ethical principles interact to regulate and guide behavior in pharmacy practice.
- Name and discuss the most common ethical principles used in analyzing ethical issues in pharmacy practice.
- Describe and utilize a problem-solving technique for resolving ethical conflicts.

Introduction

The practice of pharmacy and our nation's system of drug distribution are the subjects of intense legal regulation. Of all the health professions, pharmacy is without doubt the most highly regulated. Even so, the law does not dictate all behaviors for pharmacists and technicians. Likewise, the law does not provide answers to many questions encountered in daily practice. Occasionally, an application of the law will cause an undesirable outcome for a patient. The use of common sense and adherence to ethical values might even suggest that unlawful conduct will provide a better result for the patient's well-being. For example, consider the situation when a patient's prescription refill expires for a medication that she takes regularly to prevent angina (heart pain), and the doctor is not available to extend or renew the prescription. In the vast majority of states, the law prohibits pharmacy from dispensing the medication under these circumstances. Failure to provide the medication, however, will result in significant discomfort or even harm for the patient. The compassionate, albeit technically unlawful, response would be to deliver at least some of the medication to her until the physician can be contacted. The argument in favor of "breaking the law" in order to protect the patient's well-being might not be as compelling if the expired refills were for something like birth-control pills or Viagra®.

More commonly, practitioners are faced with multiple alternative behaviors and find almost no guidance in vague laws that are subject to differing interpretations. As an example, consider what should be done when a husband asks for a copy of his wife's prescription records. This seemingly innocent request has multiple implications and consequences. This request may facilitate an income tax deduction or to make a claim for reimbursement on an insurance policy. There could, however, be a more sinister motivation for the request. The couple might be divorcing or engaged in a child custody battle that might be affected by the wife's use of psychotropic drugs. Or it could be that the husband is concerned that the wife is being treated for a sexually transmitted disease. In any event, does the wife have an expectation that her prescription records are confidential, even against her own husband's request? Does a husband have the legal or *moral* right to know the medications his spouse is using? Does your state law clearly address these kinds of questions or are there several ways to interpret the law? Does the pharmacy profession have any guidelines for helping make decisions with this type of request? (These situations are discussed further under applicable sections of the **Code of Ethics**.) While laws may have some application to these situations, there are often no clear answers.

Many pharmacy practitioners might dismiss these dilemmas as not the kind of moral questions that should be addressed by pharmacy technicians. After all, if the technician is only there to assist the pharmacist, are not the decisions on how to go about answering the issues fully the responsibility of that pharmacist? While this position might ultimately be correct, it is too simplistic in this day and age of intensely busy and highly technical pharmacy practices. Technicians are interacting with patients more frequently and in much greater depth than even a few years ago. The scope of assistance that technicians provide to pharmacists is also increasing rapidly. This means that technicians are more likely to encounter ethical questions and moral dilemmas on a first-hand basis. Technicians may be of great assistance in gathering facts and clarifying issues so that those individuals who do have ultimate decision-making authority will be able to optimize the care of our patients. Knowing the framework of ethical analysis and the kinds of issues that might be faced will help pharmacists, technicians, patients, prescribers, caregivers, and anyone else involved make the best decisions possible. Furthermore, a pharmacist might not always be present to decide how to act or what to say in a situation that requires an immediate decision by the technician. In these rare but very realistic situations, the technician might have to decide what to do without the availability of any authority figure. Hopefully, exposure to some of the ethical considerations addressed in this chapter will ease the technician's burden and provide some guidance in how to behave appropriately and professionally.

At the outset, it is important to realize that many practice-based decisions are left up to *professional discretion* where there is no single *right* or *wrong* solution. These are sometimes called the *gray* areas because there is no clear rule of behavior. In these situations, rather than relying solely on personal values to make judgment calls, pharmacists and technicians may wonder what other pharmacy practitioners would do under the circumstances. These are the types of dilemmas that are the subject matter of professional ethics.

Background

Ethics is a branch of philosophy that studies and describes right and wrong conduct. It also suggests explanations or justifications for the moral choices that people make.[1] The values and principles that individuals follow in making moral decisions are founded in their upbringing, usually from parents, their education, religious training, and the environment around them as they mature. All social groups, whether a large national concern, an ethnic division, a small fraternity, or just a group of friends, exhibit *norm*ative behavior that suggests what kinds of conduct within the group are both acceptable and unacceptable. Unlike legal standards, which are enforced by a governmental entity, ethical *norms* within a group are followed voluntarily. With some exceptions, these ethical behavioral patterns are not formally enforced. Individuals who do not conduct themselves within the behavioral expectations of the group are ostracized or shunned.

The language of ethics is sometimes confusing because we often use the same words to mean different things. Or different words are used interchangeably when they might have different meanings to different people. As used in this chapter, *ethics* and *morals* are words used to mean the same thing.[2] Morality might refer to very different concepts depending on the context in which the term is used. *Personal morality* refers to the values and duties that the individual finds important. *Social morality* deals with the values of a much larger group of individuals and uses a common denominator to measure acceptable group behavior. The society could be that of a community, a state, a nation, a particular religious denomination, or a culture or an ethnic group. *Group morality* sets forth the ethical norms for a societal subgroup that an individual joins or is eligible to join by virtue of some qualification. The healthcare professions and the subgroups, such as pharmacy, satisfy this category. It is often easy to confuse personal values with group and societal values. One of the most pressing questions of ethics is, "What happens when a member of a group has different values or ranks certain behavior as more important than those of the group?" If this question is ever to be answered, the ethics of both the group and the individual must be fully understood. Most of the rest of this chapter is about the ethics of the pharmacy profession.

Professional ethics is an application of general moral behavioral norms to a particular vocation or occupation that has been given *professional* recognition. Professional status is usually earned through the trust and confidence that society places in its professionals to act for the betterment of those who partake of the professional's services as opposed to pure self-interests. This means that society expects those who work in a profession to behave differently and follow a different set of standards than nonprofessionals.

There has been vigorous debate in the past over whether pharmacy *is* a profession, primarily because of the business and drug product orientation associated with the practice. Most healthcare practitioners and patients do recognize pharmacy as a profession. Many Gallup research polls of public opinion over the last several years have ranked pharmacists at or near the top of all surveyed occupations for honesty and integrity in their dealings with patients. Pharmacists formed *professional* organizations, such as the American Pharmaceutical Association (APhA) and American Society of Health-System Pharmacists (ASHP), for advancing professional concerns dating from the mid-1800s. This is as opposed to *trade* organizations, such as the National Association of Chain Drugstores (NACDS), whose purpose is to advance the business and profit interests of members. The professional organizations have published codes of ethics that state the standards of professional conduct expected of pharmacists. Nearly every state that licenses pharmacists gives them professional recognition in regulatory and judicial proceedings. As pharmacy practice evolves into more patient-centered activities such as therapeutic disease management and improving therapeutic outcomes, the professional status of pharmacy should become even clearer.

Codes of ethics and standards of practice

One defining characteristic of a profession is the promulgation of a code of ethics. Codes of ethics predate organized government and the licensure laws that now regulate minimum behavioral requirements for healthcare practitioners. Today, codes supplement legal requirements and generally set higher standards of care than those required by law.

Historically, codes of ethics evolved from professional groups as a means of communicating to the public the standards of conduct to which members of the profession are held. Codes also serve to tell members, who voluntarily agree to follow the code, what behavior is expected of each individual within the group. Codes establish moral virtues for a profession and set forth rights and obligations. Depending on the code and group that authored it, standards may be lofty moral goals that members aspire to achieve, or they may be practical expectations for every member to follow. Principles within a code may be generalized vague statements or state specific behavioral requirements. Some professional groups promulgate a code and never attempt to enforce it. In other groups, members may police themselves by imposing sanctions on members who violate provisions in the codes. In these organizations, a peer review or judicial committee may investigate ethics complaints, hold hearings and pass judgment on the behavior of a member. While penalties could range from reprimands to fines or even ostracism from the group, many peer review committees serve an educational function to help members perform better and avoid behavior that conflicts with the values and principles possessed by the group.

Many ethicists and writers critique codes of ethics for their inherent limitations.[3] They tend to be drafted by committees and are therefore a product of negotiation and consensus rather than a well-developed moral philosophy. Principles within a code reflect the values of the committee members and may not represent the views of the whole profession. Codes do not cover every aspect of professional behavior and are rarely specific to particular situations. More often than not, principles are vague and subject to multiple interpretations. There may even be conflicting values within a code or, depending on the circumstances, following a code of ethics guideline might require the practitioner to disobey the law. One of the significant limitations on codes is that they reflect the state of practice and values of a profession at a particular moment in time. If not revised periodically, stoic codes can inhibit professional development or become so archaic in light of changing times that they are ignored. These critiques aside, codes are continuously used by professional groups throughout nearly all professions.

In pharmacy, the APhA Code of Ethics has been widely followed by many state and even other national professional associations. The first APhA code was established in 1852 and was modeled after the 1848 Code of Ethics of the Philadelphia College of Pharmacy.[4] The Code was revised several times to reflect changes in the pharmacy environment. The membership of APhA adopted a dramatic revision of its Code of Ethics for Pharmacists in 1994 (see Table 1). Given that this revision is of recent vintage, most state professional pharmacy organizations have not, as of this writing, revised their codes and are still using the 1981 APhA Code of Ethics as a template.[5] Not all state pharmacy groups follow the APhA Code and will not necessarily be affected by the latest revision.

Several other pharmacy codes provide meaningful insight to the ethics of the adopting organization. In addition, several institutions and business entities adopt a code of ethics or embody moral principles in mission statements or similar published, value-based pronouncements. Furthermore, many institutional organizations such as hospitals and nursing care facilities follow a *Patient's Bill of Rights* of the type published in 1972 by the American Hospital Association.[6] Other pharmacy organizations follow the National Association of Boards of Pharmacy (NABP) *Pharmacy Patient's Bill of Rights* adopted by the NABP in 1992.[7] Some state-based pharmacy technician groups have also adopted codes. For example, the Michigan Society of Pharmacy Technicians (MSPT) adopted a Code of Conduct for its members to follow (see Table 2). The MSPT Code is obviously specific to the activities of pharmacy technicians. While the format of this code mirrors that of the 1981 APhA Code of Ethics, there are differences that should be noted. Depending on the employment situation, pharmacy technicians should determine which, if any, of these various statements will govern their practice at particular locations.

Code of ethics for pharmacists and pharmacy technicians

The American Association of Pharmacy Technicians (AAPT) adopted a Code of Ethics for Pharmacy Technicians (AAPT Code) in 1996 (see Appendix B) that is nearly identical to the 1994 APhA Code of Ethics for Pharmacists (APhA Code) as to the values it contains. Some modifications were made to make it specific to the tasks, obligations and duties of pharmacy technicians. The following discussion is an attempt to provide a brief discussion on the meaning of each section.

Preamble

The AAPT Code begins with the statement that it is "an extension of the ethical standards that guides pharmacists in the delivery of their services." This gives recognition to the obvious link between pharmacists and pharmacy technicians. It suggests that the professional obligations and rights of pharmacy

Table 1 1994 APhA Code of Ethics

American Pharmaceutical Association Code of Ethics for Pharmacists

Adopted by the membership of the American Pharmaceutical Association October 27, 1994.

PREAMBLE

Pharmacists are health professionals who assist individuals in making the best use of medications. This Code, prepared and supported by pharmacists, is intended to state publicly the principles that form the fundamental basis of the roles and responsibilities of pharmacists. These principles, based on moral obligations and virtues, are established to guide pharmacists in relationships with patients, health professionals, and society.

I. A pharmacist respects the covenantal relationship between the patient and pharmacist.

Considering the patient-pharmacist relationship as a covenant means that a pharmacist has moral obligations in response to the gift of trust received from society. In return for this gift, a pharmacist promises to help individuals achieve optimum benefit from their medications, to be committed to their welfare, and to maintain their trust.

II. A pharmacist promotes the good of every patient in a caring, compassionate, and confidential manner.

A pharmacist places concern for the well-being of the patient at the center of professional practice. In doing so, a pharmacist considers needs stated by the patient as well as those defined by health science. A pharmacist is dedicated to protecting the dignity of the patient. With a caring attitude and a compassionate spirit, a pharmacist focuses on serving the patient in a private and confidential manner.

III. A pharmacist respects the autonomy and dignity of each patient.

A pharmacist promotes the right of self-determination and recognizes individual self-worth by encouraging patients to participate in decisions about their health. A pharmacist communicates with patients in terms that are understandable. In all cases, a pharmacist respects personal and cultural differences among patients.

IV. A pharmacist acts with honesty and integrity in professional relationships.

A pharmacist has a duty to tell the truth and to act with conviction of conscience. A pharmacist avoids discriminatory practices, behavior or work conditions that impair professional judgment, and actions that compromise dedication to the best interests of patients.

V. A pharmacist maintains professional competence.

A pharmacist has a duty to maintain knowledge and abilities as new medications, devices, and technologies become available and as health information advances.

VI. A pharmacist respects the values and abilities of colleagues and other health professionals.

When appropriate, a pharmacist asks for the consultation of colleagues or other health professionals or refers the patient. A pharmacist acknowledges that colleagues and other health professionals may differ in the beliefs and values they apply to the care of the patient.

VII. A pharmacist serves individual, community, and societal needs.

The primary obligation of a pharmacist is to individual patients. However, the obligations of a pharmacist may at times extend beyond the individual to the community and society. In these situations, the pharmacist recognizes the responsibilities that accompany these obligations and acts accordingly.

VIII. A pharmacist seeks justice in the distribution of health resources.

When health resources are allocated, a pharmacist is fair and equitable, balancing the needs of patients and society.

Table 2 MSPT Code of Conduct

Michigan Society of Pharmacy Technicians Code of Conduct

PREAMBLE

These principles of conduct are established to guide pharmacy technicians in relationships with pharmacists, pharmacist interns, other health professionals, other pharmacy technicians, patients, and the public.

Al functions requiring professional advice and judgment must be performed by a pharmacist.

A PHARMACY TECHNICIAN has the duty to abide by all rules and regulations pertaining to the practice of pharmacy and the organizational bylaws of the Michigan Society of Pharmacy Technicians.

A PHARMACY TECHNICIAN must perform specifically defined, assigned tasks under the personal charge or direction of a pharmacist.

A PHARMACY TECHNICIAN has the responsibility to protect the health and safety of patients against the incompetent, unethical or illegal practice of any person.

A PHARMACY TECHNICIAN must keep information about patients in strict confidence.

A PHARMACY TECHNICIAN must be courteous in providing service to patients and always attempt to foster a good working relationship with fellow employees and other health professionals.

A PHARMACY TECHNICIAN must be neat and clean in physical appearance and should maintain a positive attitude appropriate to maintaining standards of employment conducive to high quality pharmacy care.

A PHARMACY TECHNICIAN should associate with organizations that have as an objective the development and betterment of pharmacy practice and should contribute time and energy working for the success of these organizations.

technicians do not replace, but supplement, those of the pharmacists with whom they work. The preamble explicitly notes that pharmacy technicians are to apply and support the moral obligations that guide pharmacists. It should be noted that the preambles of both codes indicate that the purpose of each code is to guide pharmacy practitioners in their relationships with three distinct groups: patients, health professionals, and society. As a *guide*, the codes are not to be viewed with the rigorous technicality often associated with statutory interpretation. These codes should be used as a reference point to identify common professional values that will assist in the decision-making process when questions of an ethical dimension are faced.

Section I

APhA Code: ***A pharmacist respects the covenantal relationship between the patient and pharmacist.***

AAPT Code: ***A pharmacy technician respects and supports the relationships of trust between the patient and pharmacist***

The *covenantal relationship* referred to in the APhA Code is an acknowledgment that the relationship between patients and pharmacists is rooted in an implicit contract that goes well beyond the legal obligations of pure contract law. In fact, the implied agreement is more in the nature of a covenant or promise that is based in trust. The explanatory note to this section of the APhA Code states:

> **Considering the patient-pharmacist relationship as a covenant means that a pharmacist has moral obligations in response to the gift of trust received from society. In return for this gift, a pharmacist promises to help individuals achieve optimum benefit from their medications, to be committed to their welfare, and to maintain their trust.**

Note that this relationship is implied or presumed to exist. It is rarely, if ever, expressly stated or written down that pharmacy practitioners are trusted to act for the benefit of patients. Nevertheless, the trust relationship goes to the very heart of the interaction. The AAPT Code expressly refers to the trust relationship and obligates pharmacy technicians to respect and support that relationship between pharmacists and patients.

Section II

APhA Code: ***A pharmacist promotes the good of every patient in a caring, compassionate, and a confidential manner.***

AAPT Code: ***A pharmacy technician supports pharmacists in providing for the patient in a caring, compassionate and confidential manner.***

This section of the codes directs pharmacists and pharmacy technicians to use three values in dealing with patients: 1) that of a caregiver, 2) one who will act with compassion; and 3) one who maintains professional and personal confidences that arise out of the relationship. The explanatory note for this section from the APhA Code states:

> **A pharmacist places concern for the well-being of the patient at the center of professional practice. In doing so, a pharmacist considers needs stated by the patient as well as those defined by health science. A pharmacist is dedicated to protecting the dignity of the patient. With a caring attitude and a compassionate spirit, a pharmacist focuses on serving the patient in a private and confidential manner.**

While the duty to act in a caring and compassionate manner should be obvious to all who practice in a healthcare field, the duty often becomes included in the entanglement of legal requirements governing pharmacy practice. In the introduction to this chapter, an example was given of a commonplace, if not daily, occurrence in most pharmacies. The patient requests refills on expired prescriptions when the physician or other prescriber is unavailable to renew the order. While the law of a majority of states dictates that prescriptions cannot be renewed or refilled without prescriptive authority, compassion and care direct that pharmacists and technicians are not to use the law as a shield against helping the patient. While it is tempting to suggest that good ethical behavior might require that the patient be given a few days of medication and that the law be broken under these circumstances, that is not always the case. Alternative or temporary solutions must be considered to help the patient as necessary to protect health needs. A patient whose health may be threatened by the withholding of medication might be given special consideration. On the other hand, a patient who may be only temporarily inconvenienced if the medication is not received may not be as deserving of the same level of concern. This is an area where professional discretion must be exercised. Furthermore, it must be noted that making exceptions to applicable laws should occur only in extraordinary situations. The exception must never become the rule.

This section of the codes also requires adherence to the duty of confidentiality. Confidentiality as an ethical value has as its roots the principle of autonomy that requires respect for the individual. In this regard, both this section and Section III (discussed later) require pharmacy practitioners to view the individual patient as the single most important priority of the practice. The principle of confidentiality has both legal and moral dimensions. Nearly all states require pharmacies to maintain prescription records in a confidential manner as a matter of law. There are specific exceptions for specific situations. For example, a board of pharmacy (or other licensing agency) inspector may have an absolute right to review all pharmacy records. Police or other law enforcement officers may not have the same rights without a court-authorized search warrant. State laws differ dramatically on these issues making it incumbent of all pharmacy practitioners to know their individual state laws on confidentiality.

However, even with a well-developed knowledge of state law, situations occur where the law is either vague or simply does not address the issues. In the introduction, an example was given of a husband asking for the prescription records of his wife. Many scenarios could be imagined that justify giving out this information, such as income tax preparation or making an insurance claim. Just as many situations could be described where disclosure of the prescription records could be disastrous for the pharmacy practitioner. As was suggested, the couple might be divorcing and the husband is trying to obtain the records to show that his wife is using sedatives or antidepressants to establish that she is an unfit mother for a young child. The husband may suspect that his wife is being treated for an HIV infection and is worried that he may be at risk of exposure. Another area raising concerns about confidentiality occurs when a teenage daughter is taking birth-control pills and a parent asks for the minor's prescription records. Laws on these subjects may be confusing or beyond the scope of knowledge of most pharmacy practitioners. The provisions in the above Codes of Ethics, however, are specific and make no exception for sharing confidential information, even with a spouse or parent. Yet it could also be argued that Section VII of the codes (discussed later) requires pharmacists and technicians to look beyond the confidentiality interests of the individual patient and consider broader societal needs for information sharing. While practitioners may hold widely differing views on the factors justifying breach of confidentiality, discussing the situation with the patient is always better if he or she is a competent decision-maker before records are released. This protects not only the interest of the patient, but also the pharmacy. Breaching confidentiality without appropriate justification could be harmful to the patient in irreparable ways. Furthermore, those involved in making the breach may be exposed to tremendous sanctions.

Often, confidentiality is broken in innocent or unintentional ways. A casual conversation with a friend or even a non-pharmacy coworker where facts and circumstances about an interesting or unusual, but always *unidentified* patient interaction could be the source of an unjustified breach. The friend might know whom you are talking about just by the description. Or worse, might assume the conversation is about someone else. This is one way rumor and gossip begin. These phenomena require everyone to be extremely cautious about disclosing information gained in pharmacy practice. Another common source of unintentional disclosure of prescription information occurs in the pharmacy itself. Many pharmacies leave prescriptions prepared for customer pickups in storage bins in plain view behind the cash register counter with *receipts* that have nearly all the information contained on the prescription. Neighbors and friends of patients may easily read this information to learn what medication is being used. With the ever-increasing prevalence of personal patient counseling in pharmacy, pharmacists and technicians need to make certain that information is discussed in an area free from the often busy pharmacy traffic. These situations require more attention be paid to the legal and ethical obligations of confidentiality.

Section III

APhA Code: ***A pharmacist respects the autonomy and dignity of each patient.***

AAPT Code: ***A pharmacy technician supports pharmacists in the respect of individuality and dignity of each patient.***

As with the value of confidentiality (discussed previously), respect for the dignity and individuality of each patient grows out of the ethical principle of autonomy. Everyone differs, often dramatically, in how we view healthcare decisions and the pursuit of health. As healthcare practitioners, we might disagree with our patients on the course of therapy they have chosen. This section directs that pharmacy practitioners must recognize that patients have their own rights, and we are to assist them in fulfilling those rights as best as possible. The explanatory note to the APhA Code states:

> **A pharmacist promotes the right of self-determination and recognizes individual self-worth by encouraging patients to participate in decisions about their health. A pharmacist communicates with patients in terms that are understandable. In all cases, a pharmacist respects personal and cultural differences among patients.**

This does not mean that pharmacists and technicians are required to participate in every decision that a patient makes. Patients may elect to use certain drugs for abortions or to commit suicide. The codes of ethics and professional standards of care do not address these situations and practitioners are left to make their own judgments whether or not they will participate in the use of prescribed drugs for such purposes. However, practitioners are required to encourage patients to come to their own independent decisions when possible. This, of course, presumes that the patient is a *competent* decision-maker and is able to participate in those decisions. The term *competency* means many different things in different contexts. In the context of health care, it should be understood to mean that the patient is able to understand the risks and benefits of a plan of treatment and is able to provide *informed* consent to pursue the course of action elected. When the individual patient is not competent, a caregiver or someone who has taken on the responsibilities of making decisions for the patient should be consulted and allowed to speak for the patient.

This section also suggests that pharmacists and technicians be sensitive to and respectful of ethnic and cultural differences between people. As with Section IV (below), this section also imposes an ethical prohibition on pharmacy practitioners from discriminating against individuals based on ethnic, cultural, or social classifications. All patients are to be treated with equal dignity and respect without regard to social, educational, or economic status.

In carrying out pharmacy duties, practitioners are directed to speak in terms that patients understand. This does not require pharmacists and technicians to become multi-linguists. Instead, it means that we should avoid technical medical explanations and make certain that information is understood by the individuals who are partaking of pharmacy services.

Section IV

APhA Code: ***A pharmacist acts with honesty and integrity in professional relationships.***
AAPT Code: ***A pharmacy technician supports and promotes honesty and integrity in the profession.***

Pharmacy practitioners enjoy a great deal of knowledge about both the services they render and the patients they serve. Patients should be able to expect that the power that accompanies that knowledge will be used within the highest level of professional honor. Abuse of that power could bring discredit to the pharmacy profession and cause untoward results for patients. The obligation to act with honesty and integrity has tremendous implications for the individual professional person. The APhA Code commentary to this section states:

> **A pharmacist has a duty to tell the truth and to act with conviction of conscience. A pharmacist avoids discriminatory practices, behavior or work conditions that impair professional judgment, and actions that compromise dedication to the best interests of patients.**

"Tell the truth" may sound too simplistic as a basic commandment to be included in a professional code of ethics. Yet it is not always easy, efficient, or safe to tell the truth. It well may be safer to tell a patient presenting a questionable or even obviously forged prescription for a controlled substance that the pharmacy is "out of stock" when that is simply not true. Yet lying is wrong, and there is little wiggle room in the code for twisting the truth for the sake of expediency. When in doubt, technicians should confer with a pharmacist on how to best handle such difficult situations. Withholding essential facts is another form of unacceptable deceit. Failing to disclose a known side effect of a drug to a patient who asks is just as wrong as telling the patient the drug is out of stock. Integrity demands the truth always be told. This is not to say that the disclosure of information that may be difficult to comprehend should be brutal or without compassion. Telling a patient that an oncology drug may cause hair loss or impotency requires a caring attitude and highly developed communication skills if the therapy is to be completed successfully.

Acting with the "conviction of conscience" as a function of personal integrity can also mean making very difficult choices. A patient might want to obtain a prescribed drug for the purpose of committing suicide or causing an abortion. The pharmacy technician or pharmacist knowing this may have a very difficult time complying with the patient's wishes if doing so will violate a personal objection to such behavior. Placing personal values ahead of those of the patient will lead to difficult choices. Yet violating one's own conviction of conscience could be equally troublesome. These are matters where each individual will have to make a decision as to their level of participation, yet ensure appropriate patient care.

Adherence to the notions of integrity and honesty also demand that technicians and pharmacists avoid workplace environments that compromise these values. Filling prescriptions that are not valid, written for unlawful purposes, or are forged may be profitable, but this activity is illegal and unethical. Quitting a job because the individual does not approve of the way the practice of pharmacy is conducted may be a difficult choice, and in some cases, may not be financially viable. Yet continuing to work where there are ongoing unethical practices could prove more harmful in the long run. While Section IV of the code is one of the most basic and straightforward provisions, it is also one of the hardest to follow in everyday practice. The opportunities to twist the truth and bend integrity are common in all occupations including pharmacy. As exemplified by this section, professionals are held to higher personal standards and must be both professionally and personally accountable for their behavior. Following the commandments to be truthful and act with integrity will serve to uphold this notion of professionalism.

Section V

APhA Code: ***A pharmacist maintains professional competence.***
AAPT Code: ***A pharmacy technician maintains competence in their [sic] practice.***

Graduation from a pharmacy program, obtaining a pharmacist's license after passing a board of pharmacy examination or undergoing the training and passing the Pharmacy Technician Certification Examination are all steps necessary to show that pharmacy practitioners have undergone necessary educational requirements. Successful participants are able to demonstrate knowledge-based competencies at a given point in time. Nevertheless, this is not enough to ensure that practitioners remain competent in the face of changing technology and new discoveries in the pharmacy field. Ongoing education and exposure to the latest concepts are required to assure practitioners have the tools and knowledge necessary to ensure patients are receiving optimal care. The APhA explanatory note to this section states:

> **A pharmacist has a duty to maintain knowledge and abilities as new medications, devices, and technologies become available and as health information advances.**

Recognizing the importance of remaining current, for license renewal purposes, nearly all states legally require continuing education for pharmacists. The national Pharmacy Technician Certification Board program for Certified Pharmacy Technicians (CPhTs) also requires continuing education credits be obtained on a regular basis to maintain certification. Life-long learning is a professional obligation.

Section VI

APhA Code: ***A pharmacist respects the values and abilities of colleagues and other health professionals.***

AAPT Code: ***A pharmacy technician respects and values the abilities of pharmacists, colleagues and other health professionals.***

Pharmacists and technicians, though highly-trained individuals, must still frequently consult with other practitioners about a patient's medical condition. A reality of practice is that the vast majority of patients have already seen a physician and obtained a prescription before they access pharmacy services. Pharmacy is not practiced in a vacuum. Physicians, nurses, occupational and physical therapists, other healthcare practitioners, family members, and other caregivers all interact with patients before and after the pharmacy encounter.

Pharmacy practitioners should rely on other health providers for information and opinions about individual patients. Questions frequently arise about the appropriateness of a particular drug therapy and whether other medication might interfere with the safety of another prescribed drug. In these situations, it is necessary to consult with others. The APhA commentary to this section states:

> **When appropriate, a pharmacist asks for the consultation of colleagues or other health professionals or refers the patient. A pharmacist acknowledges that colleagues and other health professionals may differ in the beliefs and values they apply to the care of the patient.**

Occasionally, another health professional will prescribe a course of therapy that a pharmacist or technician believes is less than optimal for a patient. Oftentimes, the differences in opinion are based on different sets of information or beliefs about the patient's condition. When these situations occur, the ethical obligation is to consult with colleagues and other caregivers to determine the best course of action. When confronted by an unusual course of therapy, pharmacists and technicians should recognize that there is a fine line between unconventional medicine and quackery. In some cases, it might be important to refer the patient to another healthcare provider for a second opinion. However, it should also be apparent that healthcare providers do differ in their values and beliefs. These differences must be respected.

Section VII

APhA Code: ***A pharmacist serves individual, community, and societal needs.***

AAPT Code: ***A pharmacy technician, in support of pharmacists, serves the needs of the individuals, community and society.***

The explanatory note to the APhA Code for this section states:

> **The primary obligation of a pharmacist is to individual patients. However, the obligations of a pharmacist may at times extend beyond the individual to the community and society. In these situations, a pharmacist recognizes the responsibilities that accompany these obligations and acts accordingly.**

This section of the codes is relatively new and constitutes a significant departure from prior codes of ethics in pharmacy practice. In many of the older codes, the pharmacist's obligation extends only to the patient. This section indicates, however, that while the patient's interest is still the first priority, the obligations of pharmacy practitioners also reach out into the local community and society in general. This means that when there are conflicts between the interests of a patient and those of the community or society, pharmacists and technicians are to consider the broader implications in resolving the issues. This does not mean that pharmacists or technicians have carte blanche authority to ignore the wishes of an individual patient. The patient is the primary concern. Other individuals may also have rights that must be weighed. Consider the scenario discussed under Section III of the codes where the husband asked for his wife's prescription records because he was concerned that he might be exposed to an HIV infection. Under the older notions of ethical obligations, the principle of confidentiality would suggest that the information could not be disclosed without the spouse's permission. However, withholding the information could potentially lead to a spread of the virus. Depending on how the rights of these individuals are viewed, some may consider it better to break confidentiality and give the husband the information he seeks. This section of the code indicates that the pharmacy practitioners are authorized to at least consider the ramifications of a course of action beyond the interests of just the patient. As the note indicates, this is a serious responsibility that cannot be taken lightly.

Section VIII

APhA Code: ***A pharmacist seeks justice in the distribution of health resources.***

AAPT Code: ***A pharmacy technician supports pharmacists in an efficient and judicious distribution of health resources.***

As the APhA code note indicates:

> **When health resources are allocated, a pharmacist is fair and equitable, balancing the needs of patients and society.**

Consider what happens when a pharmacy is faced with a shortage of a medication, having enough to administer to one patient when two or more patients may benefit from its administration. Considering the needs of one single patient means the others are unable to obtain the medication. Pharmacist practitioners must take into account the needs of all the patients in deciding which patient actually gets the medication. In institutions, an ethics committee may be available to help determine the just course of action. In the community, practitioners have to balance all the needs of society along with the individual patient.

Problem solving

It would be nice if all ethical dilemmas could be solved by reading over the current Code of Ethics for a quick and direct answer. Unfortunately, this is rarely, if ever, the case because everyone puts different weight on the values and principles that are called into question when behavioral conduct is at stake. In the Introduction and in Sections III and VII of the Code, the example of the confidentiality of prescription records between a husband and wife illustrates how difficult conflicts are to resolve. A person who views autonomy as paramount may believe that no circumstances justify a breach of confidentiality. Others who rank the principle of beneficence (doing good) as a higher priority might think the husband's right to the information is more important than the wife's right of confidentiality. In any event, the codes of ethics do not provide a clean, or a *bright line*, answer. As indicated, the codes are only *guidelines* for behavioral standards. They are not ironclad laws. How, then, are these kinds of dilemmas to be resolved? Ultimately, it comes down to a very personal decision by each individual. Technicians and pharmacists should discuss the issues openly and honestly, involving the patient whenever appropriate in an attempt to find a consensus solution.

In trying to resolve ethical dilemmas (i.e., a situation where two or more courses of conduct are available and none is clearly *right* or *wrong*), the goal is to find the *best* or *better* behavior. The process of making the *best* decision is often aided by an analytical framework. Ethicists have developed several methods to assist in problem-solving. The reference section that follows includes many works where the various techniques are described. The following is only one, simple framework, used by this author, to analyze ethical issues and reach a conclusion.

1. ***Does the issue really involve a question of ethical behavior?***
   Many problems confronting pharmacy practitioners involve issues that really do not raise ethical

questions. Whether Medicaid should pay for nonprescription vitamins, the amount of an insurance co-pay or the size of a pharmacy service fee, whether senior citizens should have a Medicare prescription drug benefit, how much drug companies charge for a new biotechnology drug, and the like are *policy* issues that few practitioners will be able to solve. Whether pharmacists should have the right to prescribe or whether pharmacy technicians should have the right to practice independent of pharmacists are *turf* issues that are not easily resolved in the practice setting. The amount of information that must appear on the patient label of a dispensed drug, what information has to appear on a drug receipt, and whether a pharmacist must be physically present in a pharmacy when prescriptions are dispensed are all *legal* questions answered by a legislative body. It will not serve anyone to apply ethical analysis to these kinds of issues. Questions of distribution of scarce drugs, the rights of patients, to how much information about drug therapy, and so on, are more likely solved by ethical analysis. So the first step is to determine whether the issue involves personal behavior or conduct, or whether it involves moral choices where there are two or more kinds or behaviors that are acceptable.

2. ***What are the facts?***

   Many issues are resolved simply by fact clarification. Failure to do fact-finding at an early stage of analyzing a problem will lead to less-than-optimal decision-making. A patient may be prescribed a drug that is clearly contraindicated based on the pharmacy records. Rather than presuming the prescribing physician is a *quack* and that the patient should be referred somewhere else, it may be determined that the patient's condition has changed or that the prescriber is unaware of the contraindication. Simple attention to the facts may avoid having a dilemma at all. On the other hand, if a patient presents a prescription that calls for an obviously lethal dose, a problem could exist. Did the prescriber make a dosing error? What does the patient say? If the patient expresses the desire to terminate his or her own life, an ethical problem exists. Further fact clarification will not solve the dilemma.

3. ***What ethical principles are involved?***

   While there are multiple ways of defining ethical principles, the following five categories are the most frequently encountered in healthcare practice.

   a. **Autonomy**

      The principle of autonomy (respect for individuality and self-determination) is discussed under Section III of the Codes of Ethics as the basis of confidentiality rights and obligations. It is also the principle that underlies the notion of informed consent (the right of an individual to agree to healthcare procedures in advance after being given enough information to make a reasonable conclusion). Often, respecting the patient's wishes requires practitioners to compromise their own values. This may be a source of conflict if issues are not carefully analyzed and handled.

   b. **Beneficence**

      This principle requires practitioners to act for the good of the patient. A closely related concept is altruism, i.e., doing good for others at one's own expense. Much of healthcare ethics is rooted in the Hippocratic Oath centered on *good acts* that benefit patients (see Table 3). While acting in the best interests of patients when rendering health care, practitioners are cautioned to remember that the *best interest* standard should be viewed from the patient's perspective. Otherwise, beneficent actions quickly turn into *paternalism*. The danger of paternalism is that practitioners expect patients to follow directions unquestionably because as we learned as children, our parents know best.

Table 3 The Hippocratic Oath

The Hippocratic Oath

One version, approved by the American Medical Association, is as follows:

You do solemnly swear, each by whatever he or she holds most sacred
That you will be loyal to the Profession of Medicine and just and generous to its members
That you will lead your lives and practice your art in uprightness and honor
That into whatsoever house you shall enter, it shall be for the good of the sick to the utmost of your power, your holding yourselves far aloof from wrong, from corruption, from the tempting of others to vice
That you will exercise your art solely for the cure of your patients, and will give no drug, perform no operation, for a criminal purpose, even if solicited, far less suggest it

That whatsoever you shall see or hear of the lives of men or women which is not fitting to be spoken, you will keep inviolably secret

These things do you swear. Let each bow the head in sign of acquiescence

And now, if you will be true to this, your oath, may prosperity and good repute be ever yours; the opposite, if you shall prove yourselves forsworn.

"Hippocratic Oath," Microsoft® Encarta® Online Encyclopedia 2000

c. **Nonmaleficence**
The principle of nonmaleficence is also found in the Hippocratic Oath under the notion of first, do no harm. This principle requires practitioners to act to avoid harm being done to patients. An example of nonmaleficent behavior would be the refusal to dispense a potentially harmful drug or one that has been prescribed incorrectly.

d. **Justice**
Justice, as the term is used in ethics, means fair and equitable distribution of goods and services. This necessarily means that practitioners must consider the needs of not only individual patients, but also those of other healthcare providers, family members, the community, and society in general. It also requires practitioners to refrain from discriminatory practices despite a patient's social, economic, and ethnic status. Justice concepts are found in Sections IV, VII and VIII of the Codes of Ethics.

e. **Fidelity**
This principle is based on faithfulness and truth telling. It also embodies the idea of keeping express and implied promises. Fidelity is an obligation practitioners have to patients based on the idea that patients trust their healthcare professionals to act in their best interests. It should be noted that many aspects of fidelity are also included in notions of autonomy and beneficence and is not always listed separately. However, special note of the concept should be taken in light of Section I of the current codes of ethics where the covenantal and trust relationships between patients and pharmacy practitioners are given express recognition. In this step, the applicable principles are identified and sorted out from those that do not play a part.

4. ***Which principle should be given higher priority?***
In this step, the implications of the applicable ethical principles are analyzed. For example, consider a situation where a hospital pharmacy receives a call at the end of a fiscal year for a very

expensive drug to treat a heart attack victim. The pharmacy does not have enough drugs to treat the patient for the entire course of therapy required. The prescribing physician indicates that the patient and family want the treatment. No alternatives are available. The patient is indigent and the state Medicaid agency will not pay for the medication. The hospital will absorb the expense if the therapy is provided. The pharmacy has already reached its inventory budget limit for the year and, by ironclad policy of the hospital's administration, cannot buy the drug without special permission from the Board of Directors (not scheduled to meet until next month). The patient is deteriorating rapidly. A supply of the drug is available in a hospital pharmacy across town and it is willing to *lend* the drug if it is assured that it will be *repaid* with other drugs next year. The hospital administration would not have to know about the loan. Should the pharmacy go ahead and take the loan? The answer depends on which ethical principles are involved and which one is given the highest priority. Autonomy, beneficence, and nonmaleficence all suggest that the drug should be dispensed. Notions of justice might require the conclusion that the drug is just too expensive. Fidelity, along with the related ideas of honesty and integrity, might prohibit obtaining the drug due to the hospital budgetary policy. How the issue is resolved will depend on the relative ranking each principle is given.

5. ***What rights and duties are involved?***
   If the prior four steps have been applied properly and it still cannot be determined what course of action is most appropriate, sorting out the applicable rights and duties of the parties involved may be useful. There is no single definition of *rights* or *duties* just as there is no good test of whether a *right* or *duty* exists. Rights should be thought of as justifiable claims. The justification may be a natural or social expectation of certain behavior or it may be embodied in a legal entitlement. In health care, rights are often considered to have a moral basis. For every right that does exist, a corresponding duty or obligation of certain behavior is created. While pharmacy practitioners may also have rights, such as the right to exercise professional discretion without interference, more often attention is given to the duties towards the patients who partake of services. Determining the applicable rights and duties in an ethical conflict may be useful in determining the best course of action. It is usually at this point where codes of ethics are consulted for guidance on the standards of practice that govern the profession.

Conclusion

Professional ethics in pharmacy practice creates rights and responsibilities for its practitioners. The best interests of patients form the cornerstones of ethical healthcare behavior. Complex and difficult dilemmas may be resolved through solid analysis of the principles involved. The current codes of ethics for pharmacists and pharmacy technicians provide guidelines and standards that are useful in resolving conflicts.

References

1. Weinstein, Bruce, Ethical Issues in Pharmacy, Pharmacy Practice and the Law, Abood and Brushwood, Aspen, 1994, p. 311.
2. Lawrence, John, Argument for Action: Ethics and Professional Conduct, Ashgate Publishing, Brookfield, VT, 1999, p. 5.
3. Buerki, Robert A., and Vottero, Louis D., Ethical Responsibility in Pharmacy Practice, American Institute of the History of Pharmacy, Madison, WI, 1994, pp. 40-43.
4. Id. p. 40.
5. Id. pp. 159-160.
6. Id. pp. 166-167.
7. Id. pp. 168-169.

Bibliography

Brushwood David B., Vivian, Jesse C., Ethical Perspectives: Guidelines for Dealing with Ethics in Pharmacy Practice, The Upjohn Co., Kalamazoo, MI, 1988.

Buerki, Robert A., Editor, Teaching and Learning Strategies in Pharmacy Ethics, 2nd Edition, Special Issue of *Journal of Pharmacy Teaching*, Vol. 6, No. 1/2, 1997.

Buerki, Robert A, Vottero, Louis D., Ethical Responsibility in Pharmacy Practice, American Institute of the History of Pharmacy, Madison, WI, 1994.

Haddad, Amy Marie, Buerki, Robert A., Editors, Ethical Dimensions of Pharmaceutical Care, Pharmaceutical Products Press, Binghamton, NY, 1996.

Haddad, Amy Marie, Teaching and Leaning Strategies in Pharmacy Ethics, 2nd Edition, Pharmaceutical Products Press, Binghamton, NY, 1997.

Lawrence, John, Argument for Action: Ethics and Professional Conduct, Ashgate Publishing, Brookfield, VT, 1999.

Mongagle, John F., Thomasma, David C., Health Care Ethics: Critical Issues for the 21st Century, Aspen Publications, Gaithersberg, MD, 1998.

Purtilo, R., Ethical Dimensions in the Health Professions, 3rd Edition, W. B. Saunders, Philadelphia, PA, 1999.

Smith, M., Strauss, S.B., John H., Alberts, K., Pharmacy Ethics, Pharmaceutical Products Press, Binghamton, NY, 1991.

Weinstein, Bruce, "Ethical Issues in Pharmacy," *Pharmacy Practice and the Law*, Abood and Brushwood, Aspen, 1994.

About the author

Jesse C. Vivian received his bachelor's of science and juris doctor degrees from the University of Michigan College of Pharmacy and Wayne State University Law School. He teaches pharmacy jurisprudence, pharmacy ethics and healthcare policy in the Department of Pharmacy Practice at Wayne State University. Vivian is a past president of the American Society for Pharmacy Law and serves as general counsel to the Michigan Pharmacists Association. He is a frequent lecturer and author of several texts and articles dealing with pharmacy law and ethics. Further information about Vivian is available at http://wizard.pharm.wayne.edu/jcv/.

Self-assessment questions

1. Standards of professional conduct expected by members of a professional organization are most frequently found in the organization's:
   a. Code of Ethics.
   b. Standards of Practice.
   c. Policy and Procedural Manual.
   d. Rules and Regulations.

2. Which of the following is true regarding the principles found in a typical code of ethics?
   a. They are ironclad laws mandating prescribed behavior.
   b. They provide clear right and wrong decisions for each situation.
   c. They are only guidelines for behavioral standards.
   d. They eliminate personal discretion in deciding how to resolve ethical conflicts.

3. The principle that requires practitioners to act for the good of the patient is:
   a. justice.
   b. beneficence.
   c. nonmaleficence.
   d. fidelity.

4. The principle that requires practitioners act to avoid harm being done to the patient is:
   a. justice.
   b. beneficence.
   c. nonmaleficence.
   d. autonomy.

5. An ethical dilemma is a situation where:
   a. there is only one right answer.
   b. two or more alternative behaviors may be acceptable.
   c. the law requires morally unacceptable conduct.
   d. it is impossible to know what the right answer is.

6. The purpose of a professional organization is to:
   a. advance the financial and personal interests of the individual members.
   b. advance the professional interests of the group.
   c. advocate policy changes for society.
   d. enact legal standards of care.

7. The first problem-solving step in analyzing a dilemma is to:
   a. determine if the issue involves an ethical question.
   b. determine and rank the relative importance of the ethical issues.
   c. obtain qualified legal advice.
   d. determine your own personal values.

8. As an ethical principle, fidelity is best defined as:
   a. do no harm.
   b. the ability to act as a parental authority.
   c. do good.
   d. act truthfully, with integrity and keep express and implied promises.

9. The duty to maintain a patient's confidentiality is derived from which ethical principle?
   a. Justice
   b. Nonmaleficence
   c. Beneficence
   d. Autonomy

10. Altruism means:
    a. respect for the individual.
    b. acting truthfully and with integrity.
    c. doing no harm.
    d. acting for the benefit of another even at some cost to yourself.

Part VI: Calculations

CHAPTER
32

CALCULATIONS

Tony Michienzi, R.Ph., and Stephen T. Smith, M.S.

Learning objectives

Upon completion of this chapter, the technician should be able to do the following:

- Determine the flow rate of an intravenous (IV) solution when given the total volume, total time of administration, and the drops delivered per milliliter (ml) by the administration set.
- Calculate the volumes needed of two solutions of different strengths in order to produce a new solution of a specific strength.
- Determine the final strength of a diluted solution when given the original strength, the volume, and the final volume.
- Calculate a child's dose of medication when given the weight of the child and the normal pediatric dose.
- Define the word *markup.*
- Define the term *net profit.*
- Define the word *turnover.*

Introduction

Nearly every aspect of drug preparation or drug dispensing requires a consideration of numbers or calculations because each dose of medication contains an exact amount of active ingredient. A decimal point can mean the difference between a correct dose and a serious overdose or underdose. Therefore, accuracy of calculations, correct interpretation of numeric symbols and Latin abbreviations, and complete comprehension of concepts are important.

A review of basic arithmetic is essential to simplify and intensify the pharmacy technician's understanding of more advanced concepts related to pharmacy. Regardless of the pharmacy technician's background, he or she needs a basic knowledge of elementary arithmetic and algebra and must understand the importance of accuracy in the mechanical operations of mathematics.

Estimation

Accuracy in pharmacy calculation is critical. A misplaced demical point can have disastrous results. Using estimation as a methodology can reveal incorrect answers. Pharmacists and pharmacy technicians can estimate the answer to a problem *prior* to attempting to solve for the answer. Estimation serves as a guide to determine the reasonableness of the final result. All problems follow this procedure: (1) *estimate,* (2) *compute,* and (3) *check.*

Estimation is basically simple. The numbers in a given problem are mentally rounded up (to a slightly larger number) or rounded down (to a slightly smaller number), each containing fewer *significant* numbers. For example, 38 may be rounded up to 40, and 518 may be rounded down to 500. Thus, the product of 38 x 518 can be mentally estimated as 40 x 500, or approximately 20,000. The resulting estimate is known to be slightly greater or smaller than the actual result, but it is close enough to eliminate either 2,000 or 200,000 as a possible answer if a decimal point is misplaced.

Common fractions

A common fraction consists of three parts: (1) the **denominator**—the number below the fraction line that tells the number of parts into which a quantity is divided, (2) the **numerator**—the number above the fraction line that tells how many of those parts are used, (3) the **fraction line,** that separates the denominator from the numerator. Thus, 2/3 means that 2 of 3 parts are used.

Four basic types of fractions

Proper Fraction: The numerator is smaller than the denominator, such as 3/4. The value is less than one.

Improper fraction: The numerator is larger than or equal to the denominator, such as 3/2. The value is greater than one. The improper fraction must be reduced by dividing the numerator by the denominator.

$$\frac{3}{2} = 3 \div 2 = 1\frac{1}{2}$$

Simple fraction: A proper fraction is reduced to its lowest terms. 9/12 is a proper fraction that, on reduction, equals 3/4, a simple fraction that cannot be reduced.

$$\frac{9}{12} = \frac{3 \times 3}{3 \times 4} = \frac{3}{4}$$

Complex fraction: The numerator and the denominator are both fractions. The complex fraction is simplified by dividing the numerator by the denominator.

$$\frac{1/2}{3/4} = 1/2 \div 3/4 = 1/2 \times 4/3 = 4/6 = \frac{\not{2} \times 2}{\not{2} \times 3} = 2/3$$

Calculations with fractions

When calculating with fractions, the pharmacy technician must understand four basic rules.

> ***Rule 1:*** Multiplying the numerator *increases* the value of the fraction; multiplying the denominator *decreases* the value of the fraction. The value of a fraction does not change if both the numerator and the denominator are multiplied by the same number. The following three examples will illustrate these three previous statements with the fraction 2/3 as the base fraction.

$$\frac{2 \times 2}{3} = \frac{4}{3}$$ 4/3 is greater than 2/3

$$\frac{2}{3 \times 2} = \frac{2}{6} = \frac{1}{3}$$ 1/3 is less than 2/3

$$\frac{2 \times 2}{3 \times 2} = \frac{4}{6} = \frac{2}{3}$$ The value is unchanged.

Rule 2: Dividing the numerator *decreases* the value of the fraction. Dividing the denominator *increases* the value of the fraction. The value of a fraction does not change if both the numerator and the denominator are divided by the same number. This is shown with three examples below, with 4/16 as the base fraction.

$$\frac{4 \div 2}{16} = \frac{2}{16}$$ 2/16 is less than 4/16

$$\frac{4}{16 \div 2} = \frac{4}{8}$$ 4/8 is greater than 4/16

$$\frac{4 \div 2}{16 \div 2} = \frac{2}{8}$$ 2/8 equals 4/16

Rule 3: Change all mixed numbers to improper fractions before performing any calculations. To convert a mixed number to an improper fraction, multiply the whole number by the denominator to obtain the product and then add the numerator to the product. Write the new number as the numerator over the old denominator.

$$1\ 2/3 = \frac{3}{3} + \frac{2}{3} = \frac{5}{3}$$ note that 1 is equal to 3/3

Rule 4: Express all whole numbers as fractions with "1" as the denominator. To multiply a fraction by a whole number, consider the whole number as a fraction where the whole number is the numerator and 1 is the denominator.

$$\frac{5}{8} \times 16 = \frac{5}{8} \times \frac{16}{1} = \frac{80}{8} = 10$$

Remember to apply these four rules to be able to add, subtract, divide and multiply fractions properly and correctly.

Reduction of fractions

To reduce a fraction to simplest terms, divide the numerator and the denominator by the largest multiple that is common to both terms. Let us begin with the unreduced fraction 8/12.

$$\frac{8 \div 4}{12 \div 4} = \frac{2}{3}$$ 4 is the largest number that divides both 8 and 12 evenly

Addition and subtraction of fractions

To add or subtract fractions, change all fractions to a common denominator, and then add or subtract the numerators.

$$\frac{3}{4} + \frac{5}{6} + \frac{7}{12}$$

To be able to add these fractions, our first step is to find a common denominator. To do this, find the lowest number that all of denominators are evenly divided into. In this case, all three denominators (4, 6, and 12) can be multiplied by whole numbers to achieve a common denominator of 12. Therefore, all three fractions can be rewritten as:

$$\frac{9}{12} + \frac{10}{12} + \frac{7}{12}$$

Now that we have a common denominator, we can simply add the numerators to the answer

$$\frac{26}{12}$$

which can be reduced to $\frac{13}{6}$

and changed to 2 1/6

Subtraction of fractions is achieved in the same way. Take the fractions, find a common denominator, and then subtract the second numerator from the first numerator.

$$\frac{15}{32} - \frac{3}{8} = \frac{15}{32} - \frac{12}{32} = \frac{3}{32}$$

Multiplication of Fractions

To multiply fractions, multiply the numerators to get a new numerator, and multiply the denominators to get a new denominator.

$$\frac{5}{8} \times \frac{4}{25} = \frac{20}{200} = \frac{1}{10}$$

Division of Fractions

To divide fractions, invert the divisor and multiply.

$$\frac{3}{4} \div \frac{1}{8} = \frac{3}{4} \times \frac{8}{1} = \frac{24}{4} = 6$$

Cancellation

Cancellation may be used in multiplying fractions. The numerator of one fraction may be reduced by the denominator of another fraction. Any term in the numerator and in the denominator is considered as 1 and can be cancelled without changing the value of the fraction.

$$\frac{5}{8} \times \frac{4}{25} = \frac{\cancel{5}^{1}}{\cancel{8}_{2}} \times \frac{\cancel{4}^{1}}{\cancel{25}_{5}} = \frac{1}{10}$$

$$\frac{5}{8} \div \frac{3}{16} = \frac{5}{\cancel{8}_{1}} \times \frac{\cancel{16}^{2}}{3} = \frac{10}{3} = 3\ 1/3$$

$$\frac{2 \times 3 \times 7}{5 \times 11 \times 2} = \frac{\cancel{2} \times 3 \times 7}{5 \times 11 \times \cancel{2}} = \frac{3 \times 7}{5 \times 11} = \frac{21}{55}$$

Decimal Fractions

Decimal fractions are fractions with denominators of 10, or any multiple of 10 (100, 1,000, 10,000, etc.). Decimal fractions differ from common fractions by signifying the denominator with a decimal point placed at the left of the numerator. Therefore, 1/10 is written 0.1, 65/100 is written 0.65, and 12/1000 is written 0.012. To avoid possible error, always write one zero to the left of the decimal if there are no other numbers. For example, 0.19 is more clearly read than .19.

The value of the denominator is determined by the number of digits at the right of the decimal point. Decimal fractions are written as whole numbers, qualified by the position of the decimal point, and they may be subtracted, multiplied, and divided in much the same way as a whole number.

Moving a decimal point one position to the right multiplies a number by 10. For example, 65.35 becomes 653.5 (65.35 x 10 = 653.5). Moving the decimal point one position to the left divides a number by 10. For example 65.35 becomes 6.535 (65.35 ÷ 10 = 6.535). Each position is 10 times the position to the right and one-tenth the position to the left.

Multiplication and division of decimal fractions with common fractions

When multiplying or dividing decimal and common fractions, convert all terms to the same system; that is, use all common fractions or all decimal fractions. Calculate the multiplication of decimal fractions as with whole numbers. To determine the position of the decimal point, count the total number of decimal places in the numbers multiplied. From right to left, count the same number of places, adding zeros as necessary to make the correct number of decimal spaces.

```
0.465 x 0.032 =        0.465
                     x 0.032
                         930
                       1395
                       000
                      14880
                     6 5 4 3 2 1
              =     0.014880
```

A total of six decimal places are needed, but there are only five places available; therefore a zero must be added in front of the answer to calculate the required six spaces.

Dividing decimals requires that the divisor is a whole number. Convert the divisor to a whole number by moving the decimal point to the right. To maintain an equal equation, move the decimal of the divendant an equal number of places to the right.

0.6535 ÷ 0.005	=	6.535 ÷ 0.05	=	65.35 ÷ 0.5	=	653.5 ÷ 5
		(1 place right)		(2 places right)		(3 places right)

The numbers are now ready to be divided, and the decimal has already been properly placed in the correct position for the answer.

```
   130.7
5)653.5
  5
  15
  15
   03
    0
    35
    35
     0
```

Converting decimal fractions to common fractions

Decimal fractions are fractions with denominators of 10 or multiples of 10. A decimal fraction with one digit to the right of the decimal point is expressed in "tenths." For example, 0.6 is also written 6/10. If the decimal fraction has two digits to the right of the decimal point, it is expressed as "hundredths." For example, 0.25 is also written 25/100. The number 0.25 is read as "twenty-five hundredths," but is also read as "zero point two five," or "point two five."

Percentage

Percentage is a way of expressing fractions with denominators of 100. Percentage is always referred to as total parts per 100. To express percent as a common fraction, place the number over 100, remove the percent sign (%), and reduce to lowest terms (see problem *a* below). To express a common fraction as a percent, multiply the common fraction by 100 and add the percent sign (see problem *b* below). **Remember:** To calculate percent, multiply by 100; to remove percent, divide by 100.

40% = 40/100 = 2/5

1/3 = 1/3 x 100 = 1/3 x 100/1 = 100/3 = 33 1/3%

Sample percentage problems

To determine the amount of an active ingredient when the percent strength is given, change the percent strength to a decimal fraction, and multiply the decimal fraction by the total.

a. What is 20% of 80?
Change 20% to 20/100 = 0.20, then multiply.
80 x 0.20 = 16

To determine the percent strength of an active ingredient when the weight is given, divide the weight of the active ingredient by the total weight and multiply by 100, and add the percent sign to change the decimal fraction to a percent.

b. What is the percent strength of salicyclic acid if 3 grams are mixed with petrolatum for a total volume of 30 grams?

$$\frac{\text{Active ingredient}}{\text{Total quantity}} = \frac{3 \text{ grams}}{30 \text{ grams}} \times 100 = \frac{300}{30} = 10\%$$

Arabic and Roman numerals

Arabic numerals are the nine digits (1, 2, 3, 4, 5, 6, 7, 8, and 9) and the cipher (0). In pharmacy, Roman numerals are important when used to designate prescription quantities when ingredients are measured by the common, or apothecary system. Roman numerals are used only for recording quantities and are usually expressed as capital letters. They are not used in calculations.

Other Roman numerals are expressed by various arrangements of these basic numerals. To interpret Roman numerals, add smaller or equal numerals to the right of the basic numeral. Conversely, subtract a smaller numeral occurring to the left of a larger numeral. A smaller numeral occurring between two larger numerals is subtracted from the sum of the two larger numerals. Add or subtract any other numeral in the combination according to its placement. No more than three of the same Roman numerals are written together, as a rule. Forty could be written XXXX, but is is more easily written as XL.

Table 1 Most commonly used Roman numerals

I	=	1
V	=	5
X	=	10
L	=	50
C	=	100
D	=	500
M	=	1000

Sample problems in Roman numerals

a. Add smaller or equal numerals to the right of the basic numeral

III = 1 + 1 + 1 = 3
VII = 5 + 1 + 1 = 7
LX = 50 + 10 = 60
CXII = 100 + 10 + 1 + 1 = 112

b. Subtract a smaller numeral occurring to the left of a larger numeral

IX = 10 - 1 = 9
XLII = (50 - 10) + 1 + 1 = 42

c. Add or subtract any other numeral in the combination according to its placement.

XIV = (10 + 5) - 1 = 14
XLIX = (50 - 10) + (10 - 1) = 49
XCIV = (100 - 10) + (5 - 1) = 94

Ratio and proportion

A *ratio* is the comparison of the relationship between two like quantities. That is, a ratio expresses the relation between two numbers as a part of the whole. The ratio 1:2 is read as "one part to two parts" or simply as "one to two." If both terms of a ratio are multiplied or divided by the same number, the value is unchanged. For example, 1:5 is equivalent to 4:20.

A *proportion* is the expression of an equality between two terms. The proportion a/b = c/d is read: "a is to b, as c is to d." The relationship between a and b is compared to the relationship between c and d. The equation is a statement that two terms are equal. They are joined by the sign of equality (=).

The daily application of any type of mathematics is not based on a group of figures nicely arranged into numerators and denominators, and separated by an equality sign. Instead, the pharmacist and pharmacy technician observe certain facts, know others, and evaluate the data available to discover the information actually needed is unknown. The next step is to examine the known facts and determine whether that information can be assembled in the terms needed for the missing information. This type of situation, often called a word problem, is the practical application of certain fundamentals of arithmetic and algebra to the specialized art of pharmacy. It is important to assure that the proportion compares the same kind of relationship or the equality is destroyed. In most cases, the derived equation can be classified as one of several basic types as follows.

$A = B \times C$

On rearranging, this equation can be expressed as

$C = \frac{A}{B}$ *or* $B = \frac{A}{C}$

in which two facts are known and a third fact must be calculated.

$A \times B = C \times D$

Since the equation contains four terms, there are numerous ways of rearranging the terms while still maintaining equality. Of the four terms in the equation, three are given or may be deduced by reasoning, and the unknown fourth term is calculated.

$A = \frac{C \times D}{B}$ $B = \frac{C \times D}{A}$ $\frac{A}{C} = \frac{D}{B}$ $\frac{B}{C} = \frac{D}{A}$ $C = \frac{A \times B}{D}$ $D = \frac{A \times B}{C}$

Sample proportion problems

a. Determine the value of C.

$$\frac{\text{2 tablets}}{\text{30 grams}} = \frac{\text{C}}{\text{60 grams}}$$

$$\text{2 tablets x 60 grams} = \text{30 grams x C}$$

$$\text{120 tablets-grams} = \text{30 grams C}$$

$$\frac{\text{120 tablets-}\cancel{\text{grams}}}{\text{30 }\cancel{\text{grams}}} = \text{C}$$

$$\text{4 tablets} = \text{C}$$

b. If 100 grams of an ointment contains 4 grams of drug, how many grams of ointment contains 1 gram of drug?

$$\frac{\text{4 grams drug}}{\text{100 grams ointment}} = \frac{\text{1 grams drug}}{\text{D}}$$

$$\text{100 grams x 1 grams} = \text{4 grams x D}$$

$$\text{100 grams-grams} = \text{4 grams D}$$

$$\frac{\text{100 grams-}\cancel{\text{grams}}}{\text{4 }\cancel{\text{grams}}} = \text{D}$$

$$\text{25 grams} = \text{D}$$

c. Using the previous example, determine how many grams of ointment contains 500mg of drug. It is imperative to change units to grams or to milligrams.

$$\text{500mg} = \text{0.5gm}$$

$$\frac{\text{4 grams drug}}{\text{100 grams ointment}} = \frac{\text{0.5 grams drug}}{\text{D}}$$

$$\text{100 grams x 0.5 grams} = \text{4 grams x D}$$

$$\text{50 grams-grams} = \text{4 grams D}$$

$$\frac{\text{50 grams-}\cancel{\text{grams}}}{\text{4 }\cancel{\text{grams}}} = \text{D}$$

$$\text{12.5 grams} = \text{D}$$

The fraction cancellation rule states that any term in both numerator and denominator is considered "1" and can be cancelled without changing the value of the fraction. This also applies to proportion equalities where like numbers and units of measurements can be cancelled without altering the equality. The following is an alternate way to solve sample proportion problem c.

$$\frac{4 \text{ grams drug}}{100 \text{ grams ointment}} = \frac{500\text{mg drug}}{D}$$

$$100\text{gm} \times 500\text{mg} = 4\text{gm} \times \frac{1{,}000\text{mg}}{\text{gm}} \times D$$

$$50{,}000\text{mg-gm} = \frac{4{,}000\text{mg-}\cancel{\text{gm}}\ D}{\cancel{\text{gm}}}$$

$$50{,}000\text{mg-gm} = 4{,}000\text{mg } D$$

$$\frac{50{,}000\cancel{\text{mg}}\text{-gm}}{4{,}000\cancel{\text{mg}}} = \frac{\cancel{4{,}000\text{mg}}\ D}{\cancel{4{,}000\text{mg}}}$$

$$12.5\text{gm} = D$$

Using 1,000mg = 1gm equality maintains the comparison of like units of measurements necessary to calculate a correct answer. No change in the equality occurs because 1,000mg/1gm is the same as "1." (Remember, any number over itself is equal to 1.) Multiplying one side of the equation by "1" does not change the value of the equation. Units of measurement are multiplied and divided as integers and all rules of arithmetic are followed. Units cancel out, leaving comparison of like units. If the pharmacy technician takes care to assure equality is maintained and all units cancel, the correct answer is always calculated.

Weights and measures

All matter has two properties. It has mass, or weight, and it has bulk, or volume. Most calculations in pharmacy are based on these properties. The metric system of weights and measures attempts to standardize the language describing these properties and their relationship to each other. Standardization has not been complete, and it is sometimes necessary to interpret information given in the avoirdupois, apothecary, and household systems of measure. Certain drugs, some hormones and vitamins for instance, are labeled in units. These are drugs that cannot be analyzed by chemical means and are standardized according to their effects on laboratory animals.

Metric system primary units

The metric system is based on the measure of length called the meter. However, each table of the metric system contains a definitive unit. These units are called primary units and are as follows:

1) Meter—length
2) Liter—volume
3) Gram—mass (weight)

To simplify measuring, each primary unit is subdivided into 1,000, 100, and 10 smaller parts. Units larger than the primary units are given in multiples of 10, 100, and 1,000. All units differ from each

Table 2 Metric system primary units

Prefixes		Suffixes (primary units)
kilo-	(1,000)	-meter
hecto-	(100)	-liter
deka-	(10)	-gram
deci-	(0.1)	
centi-	(0.01)	
milli-	(0.001)	
micro-	(0.000001)	

other by some power of 10. Multiples of the primary units are expressed by adding Latin prefixes to the name of the primary unit.

The metric tables of length, mass, and volume may be learned as one common table. Then each table may be distinguished from the others by the substitution of the suitable primary units. The prefixes are the same in each table. The suffixes (primary units) are different for each table, but they are the same throughout any one table. Prescriptions that are written in the metric system always have the amounts in Arabic numerals, and decimal fractions, not common fractions, are used to indicate fractional quantities.

Table 3 Metric system terms for length, volume, and weight

Prefixes	**Suffixes**	**Prefixes**	**Suffixes**
If the unit is this,		***...then it is equal to this:***	
1,000 micro-	(-meter, -liter, -gram)	= 1 milli-	(-meter, -liter, -gram)
10 milli-	(-meter, -liter, -gram)	= 1 centi-	(-meter, -liter, -gram)
10 centi-	(-meter, -liter, -gram)	= 1 deci-	(-meter, -liter, -gram)
10 deci-	(-meter, -liter, -gram)	= 1 meter, liter or gram	
	10 meters, liters, grams	= 1 deka-	(-meter, -liter, -gram)
10 deka-	(-meter, -liter, -gram)	= 1 hecto-	(-meter, -liter, -gram)
10 hecto-	(-meter, -liter, -gram)	= 1 kilo-	(-meter, -liter, -gram)

Apothecary system

The units of apothecary weight and volume have been adapted to the needs of pharmacy without any particular regard for uniformity. The units of the apothecary system have no simple, consistent relationship to each other, as do those of the metric system. Even though the apothecary system is not official, some physicians still use this system, especially grains. ***Scruples and minims are rarely used!***

Apothecary weight
20 grains = 1 scruple
3 scruples = 1 dram (ʒ) = 60 grains
8 drams = 1 ounce (℥) = 480 grains
12 ounces = 1 pound (℔.) = 5,760 grains

Apothecary fluid measure
60 minims (♏) = 1 fluid dram
8 fluid drams (**flʒ**) = 1 fluid ounce (fl. oz.) = 480 minims
16 fluid ounces (**fl℥**) = 1 pint (pt.)
2 pints = 1 quart (qt.) = 32 fl. oz.
4 quarts (8 pt.) = 1 gallon (cong.) = 128 fl. oz.

Avoirdupois system

The avoirdupois system of weight is often used in commerce. Pharmaceutically, it is sometimes used in buying and selling drugs and chemicals.

Avoirdupois weight
437.5 grains (gr.) = 1 ounce (oz.)
16 ounces = 1 pound (lb.)
7,000 grains = 1 pound

Conversion between systems

Apothecary units of weight converted to metric system
15.432 grains = 1 gram
1 grain = 64.8 milligrams
1 ounce = 31.1 grams
1 pound = 373.2 grams

Apothecary units of volume converted to metric system
16.23 minims = 1 milliliter
1 fluid ounce = 29.57 milliliters
1 pint = 473.2 milliliters
1 gallon = 3,785.3 milliliters

Avoirdupois units of weight converted to metric system
1 ounce = 437.5 grains = 28.35 grams
1 pound = 7,000 grains = 453.6 grams
2.2 pounds = 1 kilogram

Household units converted to approximate metric system
Although household units are shown here, *they are by no means exact,* but they are used in measurement in the community pharmacy on a daily basis for their practicality and ease of use.

1 teaspoonful (tsp.) = 5 milliliters
1 tablespoonful (tbs., tbsp.) = 15 milliliters
1 fluid ounce = 30 milliliters
1 pint = 16 fluid ounces = 480 milliliters
1 quart = 2 pints = 32 fluid ounces = 960 milliliters
1 gallon = 4 quarts = 128 fluid ounces = 3,840 milliliters

Also

1 ounce = 30 grams
16 ounces = 1 pound = 454 grams
2.2 pounds = 1,000 grams = 1 kilogram

Conversion to the next integer (whole number)
Conversion (sometimes known as "rounding-off") to the next whole number (or integer) is acceptable in actual pharmacy practice for reasons of convenience and consistency with commercially manufactured products. The following conversions are acceptable and do not compromise dosage accuracy:
1 gram = 15 grains
1 grain = 65 milligrams
1 ounce = 30 grams
1 fluid ounce = 30 milliliters
1 pint = 480 milliliters

Dosage calculations

The pharmacist and pharmacy technician need a thorough knowledge of the previously mentioned systems of weights and measures to correctly calculate and prepare medications. Determining the number of doses, the quantity to dispense, or the quantity of an ingredient are everyday calculations in all pharmacy practice settings.

Sample dosage problems

$$\text{Number of doses} = \frac{\text{Total amount}}{\text{Size of each dose}}$$

a. How many doses are contained in 5 grams, if the dosage is 25mg?

$$\text{Number of doses} = \frac{5\text{gm}}{25\text{mg}} \times \frac{1{,}000\text{mg}}{1\text{gm}}$$

$$\text{Number of doses} = \frac{5{,}000\text{mg}}{25\text{mg}}$$

$$\text{Number of doses} = 200$$

b. How many 15ml doses are contained in 480ml of a medication?

$$\text{Number of doses} = \frac{480\text{ml}}{15\text{ml}}$$

$$\text{Number of doses} = 32$$

Rearranging the dosage equations provides two other useful equations

$$\text{Size of each dose} = \frac{\text{Total amount}}{\text{Number of doses}}$$

$$\text{Total amount} = \text{Number of doses} \times \text{Size of each dose}$$

c. What dosage is given if a total of 40 grams of medicine is divided into 20 equal doses?

$$\text{Size of each dose} = \frac{40\text{gm}}{20\text{ doses}}$$

$$\text{Size of each dose} = \frac{2\text{gm}}{\text{dose}}$$

d. Calculate the amount of elixir needed to dispense 14 doses of 25ml each?

$$\text{Total amount} = 14\text{ doses} \times \frac{25\text{ml}}{\text{dose}}$$

$$\text{Total amount} = 350\text{ml}$$

$$\text{Quantity of each dose} = \frac{\text{Total quantity}}{\text{Number of doses}}$$

$$\frac{\text{Quantity of each dose}}{\text{Size of each dose}} = \frac{\text{Total quantity}}{\text{Total amount}}$$

e. How much codeine is needed to prepare 20 doses of a 15mg/dose preparation?

$$\frac{15\text{mg}}{\text{dose}} = \frac{\text{Total amount}}{20 \text{ doses}}$$

$$20 \text{ doses} \times \frac{15\text{mg}}{\text{dose}} = \frac{\text{Total amount} \times 20 \text{ doses}}{20 \text{ doses}}$$

300mg = Total amount
or 0.3gm

f. How much codeine is needed to prepare 120ml of a 15mg/ml concentration?

$$\frac{15\text{mg}}{\text{ml}} = \frac{\text{Total quantity}}{120\text{ml}}$$

$$120\text{ml} \times \frac{15\text{mg}}{\text{ml}} = \frac{\text{Total quantity}}{120\text{ml}} \times 120\text{ml}$$

1,800mg = Total quantity
or 1.8gm

Calculation of children's doses and adult dosages based on body mass or weight

The average doses of drugs given in the United States Pharmacopeia and the National Formulary (USP/NF) are for adults and generally suitable for a 70kg (154lb) individual (remember that 2.2 pounds is equal to 1 kilogram and 1 pound is equal to 454 grams). Since children cannot tolerate adult doses of drugs, it is necessary to have some standard method to calculate safe doses of drugs for children of various sizes and ages. The determination of drug dosage for young patients on the basis of body weight is considered more dependable than that based strictly on age. The dosage of a number of drug substances is based on body weight and is frequently expressed on a milligram (drug) per kilogram (body mass) basis.

Reducing and enlarging formulas

Pharmacists and pharmacy technicians may be asked to prepare pharmaceuticals from a specific recipe or formula. Most manufacturing formulas are based on a quantity of 100gm or 1,000ml. The pharmacist and pharmacy technician may need to make a smaller or larger quantity and, therefore, must reduce or enlarge the formula. The desired amount of ingredient is calculated by using the following proportion.

$$\frac{\text{Total amount in formula}}{\text{Total amount desired}} = \frac{\text{Quantity in formula}}{\text{Quantity in amount desired}}$$

Rearranging this proportion, we see that

$$\text{Quantity in amount desired} = \frac{\text{Total amount desired}}{\text{Total amount formula}} \times \text{Quantity in formula}$$

To calculate the factor to multiply each formula quantity, determine the relationship of the final amount to the amount of formula. If 50gm is desired from a 1,000gm formula, use the factor to multiply each formula quantity by 0.05 or 50/1,000. If a gallon (3,785ml) is needed from a 1,000ml formula, the factor is 3.785 or 3,785/1,000. Multiply each ingredient of the formula by the factor to determine the required amount of each ingredient for the final total.

Sample reducing/enlarging formula problems

a. Calculate the amounts to make 1 gallon of Compound Tincture Benzoin from the following formula.

Benzoin	100gm	x 3.785	=	378.5gm
Aloe	20gm	x 3.785	=	75.7gm
Storax	80gm	x 3.785	=	302.8gm
Tolu Balsam	40gm	x 3.785	=	151.4gm

Alcohol, to make 1,000ml qs to 3,785mls

(The factor 3.785 [3,785ml/1,000ml is used] to calculate each ingredient.)

b. Calculate the quantities of each ingredient to make 480ml of Calamine Lotion from the following formula.

Calamine	80gm	x 0.48	=	38.4gm
Zinc Oxide	80gm	x 0.48	=	38.4gm
Glycerin	20ml	x 0.48	=	9.6ml
Bentonite Magma	250ml	x 0.48	=	120ml

Calcium Hydroxide Solution to make 1,000ml qs to 480ml

(The factor 0.48 [480ml/1,000ml] is used to calculate each ingredient.)

Percentage preparations

Weight-in-weight (w/w) percentage means parts by weight of the total mixture by weight. Percent weight-in-weight expresses the number of grams (gm) of a drug or active ingredient in 100 grams of a mixture (grams/grams).

Volume-in-volume (v/v) percentage means parts by volume of the total mixture. Percentage volume in volume expresses the number of milliliters (ml) of a drug or active ingredient in 100 milliliters (ml) of a mixture and is usually used for mixtures of liquids in liquids.

Weight-in-volume (w/v) percentage means parts by weight in parts by volume. Percent weight in volume expresses the number of grams (gm) of a drug or active ingredient in 100 milliliters (ml) of a mixture.

Ratio strength (1:N) is one part by weight or volume in "N" parts by weight (mass) or volume. A 1:200 ratio strength can be 1gm solid to 200ml solid or 1ml liquid to 200ml liquid or 1gm solid to 200ml liquid. Conversion of percentage strengths and ratio strengths to mg/ml is commonplace in the patient care setting. This conversion produces a concentration (mg/ml) that is easily understood by all health-care professionals.

Sample percentage/ratio strength problems

a. If 2,000gm of ointment contains 75gm of hydrocortisone, what is the percentage strength weight/weight (w/w) of the ointment?

$$\frac{75\text{gm}}{2{,}000\text{gm}} = \frac{X\ \%}{100\%}$$

$$75 \times 100 = 2{,}000X$$

$$\frac{7{,}500}{2{,}000} = \frac{2{,}000X}{2{,}000}$$

$$3.75\% = X$$

b. If 8ml of phenol is added to 480ml of lotion, what is the percentage (v/v) of phenol in the lotion?

$$\frac{8ml}{480ml} = \frac{X\%}{100\%}$$

$$8 \times 100 = 480X$$

$$\frac{800}{480} = \frac{480X}{480}$$

$$1.66\% = X$$

c. If 1.2gm of menthol is added to 480ml of lotion, what is the percentage weight/volume (w/v) of menthol in the lotion?

$$\frac{1.2gm}{480ml} = \frac{X\%}{100\%}$$

$$1.2 \times 100 = 480X$$

$$\frac{120}{480} = \frac{480X}{480}$$

$$0.25\% = X$$

d. How many grams of zinc chloride are needed to make 2,500ml of a 1:50 solution?

$$\frac{1gm}{50ml} = \frac{X\ gm}{2500ml}$$

$$2{,}500 = 50X$$

$$\frac{2{,}500}{50} = \frac{50X}{50}$$

$$50gm = X$$

e. What is the mg/ml concentration of a 1:2,500 solution?

$$\frac{1gm}{2{,}500ml} = \frac{X\ mg}{1ml}$$

$$1gm \times 1ml \times \frac{1{,}000mg}{gm} = 2{,}500X\ mg\text{-}ml$$

$$1{,}000 = 2{,}500X$$

$$\frac{1{,}000}{2{,}500} = \frac{2{,}500X}{2{,}500}$$

$$0.4mg/ml = X$$

f. Convert 15% to mg/ml.

(Remember: 15% actually means 15gm/100ml or 15gm/100gm, depending on the compound being described)

$$\frac{15gm}{100ml} = \frac{X\ mg}{1ml}$$

$$15gm \times 1ml \times \frac{1{,}000mg}{gm} = 100X\ mg\text{-}ml$$

$$15{,}000 = 100X$$

$$\frac{15{,}000}{100} = \frac{100X}{100}$$

$$150mg/ml = X$$

Pharmaceutical calculations using dilution and concentration

The formula for dilution and concentration may be expressed in terms of ratio and proportion. Verbally, the equation may be expressed, "The final total volume is to the initial volume as the initial strength is to the final strength." The initial and final strength may be expressed as a percent strength or as a ratio strength. Ratio strength is defined as one part active ingredient contained in a designated number of parts of the total preparation. Ratio strength is represented as 1/X. Mathematically, the equation may be expressed as

$$\frac{\text{Final total volume}}{\text{Initial volume}} = \frac{\text{Initial strength}}{\text{Final strength}}$$

This is derived directly from the initial strength and initial volume of the product is equal to the final total volume and the final strength of the product.

Example
If 500ml of a 15% solution are diluted to 1,500ml, what will be (a) the percent strength, and (b) the ratio strength of the final product?

Answer
1. Determine pertinent data and set up equation.
2. 1,500ml is the final total volume.
3. 500ml is the initial volume.
4. 15% is the initial percent strength.
Let X equal the unknown final percent strength.

The equation is as follows:

$$\frac{\text{(final total volume) } 1{,}500ml}{\text{(initial volume) } 500ml} = \frac{15\%\text{ (initial strength)}}{X\ \%\text{ (final strength)}}$$

Cross multiply to determine the unknown percent strength (X = 5%).
To determine the ratio strength, express the percent strength as a common fraction and reduce to 1/X.

$$5\% = \frac{5}{100} = \frac{1}{20}$$

Exception: The exception to this method for computing ratio strength occurs if the final percent strength is less than 1%.

Example 0.5%

Express 0.5% as a common fraction and multiply it by a number equal to "1" that will raise the value of the numerator to a whole number. Then, reduce this fraction to 1/X.

$$0.5\% = \frac{0.5}{100} = \frac{0.5}{100} \times \frac{2}{2} = \frac{1}{200}$$

A ratio may also be expressed as 1:X. Therefore, 1:10,000 is the same as 1/10,000. Conversely, to change a ratio to a percent strength, multiply the ratio by 100%.

1/20 = 1/20 x 100% = 100%/20 = 5%

Pharmaceutical calculations using alligation

Alligation is a method used for calculating the average value of a mixture obtained by combining known quantities of two or more substances with known values. Alligation is often expanded to include calculations that determine the volume amount of each of the components combined to make a given amount of a different strength solution. It is done in the following manner.

1. Draw a "tic-tac-toe" pattern.
2. Enter the percent strength of the stronger solution (A) used in the upper left-hand box.
3. Enter the percent strength of the weaker solution (B) used in the lower left-hand box.
4. Enter the desired percent strength of the desired solution (C) in the center box.
5. Let x equal the unknown volume of solution A needed to obtain the finished solution.
6. Let x equal the unknown volume of solution B needed to obtain the finished solution.

Table of alligation formula

Stronger Solution A		**X (C-B)** (desired volume of A)
	Strength of C **Desired Solution**	
Weaker Solution B		**Y (A-C)** (desired volume of B)

Sample alligation problem

a. What proportions of 95% alcohol and 50% alcohol are mixed to make 70% alcohol?

A **95%**		**X** **20**	=	$\frac{\mathbf{20}}{\mathbf{(20+25)}}$
	C **70%**			
B **50%**		**Y** **25**	=	$\frac{\mathbf{25}}{\mathbf{(20+25)}}$

Procedure

1. Subtract B from C to solve for X. Subtract C from A to solve for Y.
2. X = 20 parts and Y = 25 parts. Therefore, we now have a total of X+Y parts or 20+25 parts = 45 parts, of which 20/45 = X and 25/45 = Y. Therefore, the ratio amount of 95% alcohol is equal to X as defined earlier (20/45), and the ratio amount of 50% alcohol is equal to Y (25/45). The addition of these two ratios will make up the 70% alcohol.

As in the previous example, the two ratios are 20/45 for X and 25/45 for Y. This example, however, can be expanded to include a desired volume amount.

b. How much 95% alcohol and how much 50% alcohol are needed to make 450ml of 70% alcohol?

$$\frac{20 \text{ parts}}{45 \text{ parts}} + \frac{25 \text{ parts}}{45 \text{ parts}}$$

To solve for volume of 95% alcohol

$$\frac{20 \text{ parts (95\% alcohol)}}{45 \text{ parts (total parts in mixture)}} \times 450\text{ml (total final volume)}$$

$$= \frac{4 \text{ parts}}{9 \text{ parts}} \times 450\text{ml} = \frac{1{,}800}{9} = 200\text{ml of 95\% alcohol}$$

To solve for volume of 50% alcohol

$$\frac{25 \text{ parts (50\% alcohol)}}{45 \text{ parts (total parts in mixture)}} \times 450\text{ml (total final volume)}$$

$$= \frac{5 \text{ parts}}{9 \text{ parts}} \times 450\text{ml} = \frac{2{,}250}{9} = 250\text{ml of 50\% alcohol}$$

Note: If you add 200ml and 250ml, the final volume is the total 450ml. This step serves as an excellent check of your calculations.

This same problem can be completed using dilution and concentration equation and solving for the unknown.

Remember: Initial volume x Initial strength of each ingredient = Final total volume x Final strength

c. Let the volume of the 95% alcohol be xml and the volume of the 50% alcohol be (450ml - x), where 450ml is the total volume as given in the problem.

95% (X) + 50% (450ml-X) = 70% (450ml)

0.95X + 0.5 (450ml-X) = 0.7(450ml)

0.95X + 225ml – 0.5x = 315ml

0.45X = 90ml

x = 200ml, which is equal to the amount of 95% alcohol and remembering that 450ml-x is equal to the amount of the 50% alcohol or 250ml.

Therefore, whichever method one chooses, the correct answer is achieved. The choice is yours as to how you complete alligation exercises.

Flow rate calculations

Large volume parenteral solutions are most often administered over a long period of time. Solutions drip slowly into a vein by gravity flow or through an infusion device. Prescribers specify a rate of flow in milliliters per minute, drops per minute, amount of drug in milligrams per hour, or duration of time for the total volume of solution. Pharmacists and pharmacy technicians calculate flow rates to verify correct dosages and infusion times.

$$\frac{\text{ml of solution x number of drops/ml}}{\text{minutes of administration}} = \text{drops/minute}$$

Sample flow rate problems

a. Determine the flow rate to be used to infuse 1,000ml of dextrose 5% in water over 8 hours if the set delivers 10 drops per ml.

$$\frac{\text{1,000ml x 10 drops/ml}}{\text{8 hours x 60 minutes/hour}} = \frac{\text{10,000 drops}}{\text{480 minutes}} = \text{20.8 or 21 drops/minute}$$

Or, you can solve the problem by setting up equation to end with desired units in the numerator and denominator.

$$\frac{\text{1,000ml}}{\text{8 hr}} \times \frac{\text{1 hr}}{\text{60 min}} \times \frac{\text{10 drops}}{\text{1ml}} = \frac{\text{20.8 drops}}{\text{minute}} = \text{21 drops/minute}$$

b. Determine the infusion time of 500ml of 0.9% sodium chloride if an infusion set delivering 20 drops/ml is set at 42 drops/minute.

$$\text{500ml} \times \frac{\text{20 drops}}{\text{ml}} \times \frac{\text{1 min}}{\text{42 drops}} \times \frac{\text{1 hr}}{\text{60 min}} = \frac{10{,}000}{2{,}520} = \text{3.96 or 4 hours}$$

Specific gravity

Specific gravity is the ratio of the mass of a substance compared to the mass of an equal volume of a reference substance. Generally, water is used as the reference substance for liquids and solids; hydrogen or sometimes air is the reference substance for gases. Specific gravity is determined by dividing the mass of a given substance by the mass of an equal volume of the reference substance. Therefore, if 100ml of chloroform weighs 147.5gm and 100ml of water weighs 100gm, the specific gravity is:

$$\frac{\text{weight of 100ml of chloroform}}{\text{weight of 100ml of water}} = \frac{\text{147.5gm}}{\text{100gm}} = 1.475$$

Sample specific gravity problems

a. Determine the specific gravity if 150ml of a substance weighs 165gm.

$$\frac{\text{weight of 150ml of substance}}{\text{weight of 150ml of water}} = \frac{\text{165gm}}{\text{150gm}} = 1.1$$

b. Determine the weight of 100ml of a alcohol with a specific gravity of 0.815.

$$\frac{\text{weight of 100ml of alcohol}}{\text{weight of 100ml of water}} = 0.815$$

$$= \frac{\text{X gm}}{\text{100gm}} = 0.815 \times 100 = \text{81.5gm}$$

Milliequivalents

A chemical unit, the milliequivalent (mEq), is used to express the concentration of electrolytes in a solution. Electrolytes are substances that when placed in solution have varying degrees of dissociation, or breaking up into smaller constituents. A milliequivalent weight is 1/1,000 of an equivalent weight, is related to the total number of ionic charges in solution, and takes into account the valence charge of the ions in that solution. Milliequivalents are most often used with electrolyte replacement solutions such as potassium chloride (KCl) or sodium chloride (NaCl). This is important because electrolyte replacement replenishes chemicals that are necessary for the electrical activity of nerve conduction and muscle contraction. An equivalent weight of potassium chloride is obtained by dividing the atomic weight (39gm) by the valence or charge (1+) = 39gm; 1 mEq of K+ is 39gms/1,000 = 0.039gm = 39mg K+. Although rarely called upon to calculate the number of milliequivalents in a specific weight of chemical, it is important to know the relationship between weight and valence (charge) of the chemical.

Sample milliequivalent problems

a. An elixir contains 20mEq of potassium chloride/5ml. If a daily dose of 60mEq of potassium chloride is needed, how manyml of potassium chloride are needed to provide 10 days of therapy?

$$\frac{60\text{mEq KCl}}{\text{day}} \times \frac{5\text{ml}}{20\text{mEq KCl}} = \frac{15\text{ml}}{\text{day}}$$

$$\frac{15\text{ml}}{\text{day}} \times 10 \text{ days} = 150\text{ml}$$

b. You must add 45mEq NaCl to an intravenous solution. If the stock solution of NaCl injection contains 2.5mEq/2ml, how manyml of NaCl are needed?

$$45\text{mEq NaCl} \times \frac{2\text{ml}}{2.5\text{mEq NaCl}} = 36\text{ml}$$

Millimoles

A millimole (mM) weight is 1/1,000 of a molecular weight. Millimoles are generally used to express replacement solutions of multivalent ions like phosphate. Depending on the pH of the surrounding solution, phosphate ions can carry different charges. Therefore, their milliequivalent (mEq) value changes based on the pH. To accurately measure the amount of phosphate ion, it is best to measure replacement on molecular weight. A molecular weight for monobasic phosphate (HPO_4) is 96gm. Therefore, 1mM of phosphate ion is 96 gram/1,000 = 0.096gm = 96mg phosphate.

Sample millimole problems

a. A physician prescribed replacing 18mM of phosphate ion in a IV solution. If the injectable solution contains 45mM of phosphate in 15ml, how manyml of phosphate are needed?

$$18\text{mM phosphate} \times \frac{15\text{ml}}{45\text{mM phosphate}} = 6\text{ml}$$

b. An injectable solution contains phosphate ion in a concentration of 3mM/1ml. If a patient requires a daily dose of 21mM of phosphate, how manyml of phosphate injection is needed to provide 10 days of therapy?

$$21\text{mM phosphate} \times \frac{1\text{ml}}{3\text{mM phosphate}} = 7\text{ml}$$

$$7\text{ml} \times 10 \text{ days} = 70\text{ml}$$

Temperature conversion

The Fahrenheit thermometer is most commonly used in the United States; however, the Celsius or Centigrade thermometer is becoming increasingly popular and is the standard method of measuring temperature in the remainder of the world. A pharmacist or pharmacy technician may be asked to convert a temperature from one scale of measurement to another. Two formulas express the relationship between the Fahrenheit and Celsius temperature scales:

°F = 32 + 9/5 C°
°C = 5/9 (F° - 32)

Table 3 Temperatures that are common and their conversion to Fahrenheit

	Celsius temperature	Fahrenheit temperature
Water freezes	0° C	32° F
Normal room temperature	20° C	68° F
Normal body temperature	37° C	98.6° F
Boiling point of water	100° C	212° F

Sample temperature conversion problems

a. Convert 15° C to Fahrenheit
°F = 32 + (9/5 x 15)
°F = 32 + 27
°F = 59°

b. Convert 98.6° F to Celsius
°C = 5/9 (98.6 -32)
°C = 5/9 (66.6)
°C = 37°

Reconstitution of powdered drugs

Some drugs are available in the pharmacy in powdered or crystalline form to allow them a longer shelf life. A liquid such as sterile water or saline must be added to prepare these powdered drugs for administration or dispensing; it is usually added immediately before administration to the patient. When a liquid is added to the powdered drug in preparation for administration, the procedure is referred to as a **reconstitution** of the drug. The liquid added is called a *solvent* or a *diluent*. Most injectable or oral powdered drugs are accompanied by printed reconstitution information provided by the manufacturer and packaged with each container. The directions for reconstitution of a drug usually tell precisely how much liquid must be added to obtain the desired final concentration.

Sample powder reconstitution problems

a. An antibiotic oral suspension states, "Add 180ml of distilled water; each 5ml contains 500mg." If the bottle contains 40 doses of 5ml each, what is the volume of the dry powder?

$$40 \text{ doses} \times \frac{5\text{ml}}{\text{dose}} = 200\text{ml final volume}$$

200ml volume - 180ml water = 20ml powder

Note: Regardless of the weight or mass of the dry powder, it still occupies a fixed volume and that volume is determined by measuring the difference between the amount of solvent added (in this case distilled water) and the volume of the final preparation.

b. A 2,000,000 unit vial of penicillin G potassium contains 500,000 units/ml when reconstituted with 3.2ml of water for injection. What is the volume of the dry powder?

$$2{,}000{,}000 \text{ units} \times \frac{\text{ml}}{500{,}000 \text{ units}} = 4\text{ml of final volume}$$

$$4\text{ml final volume} - 3.2\text{ml water} = 0.8\text{ml powder}$$

Extemporaneous compounding

Pharmacists and pharmacy technicians often prepare prescriptions with drugs that are only available in tablets or capsules. To compound the prescription, the pharmacist must determine the amount of drug needed from that tablet or capsule and obtain the correct number of tablets or capsules.

Sample extemporaneous compounding problems

a. How many 30mg potassium permanganate tablets are needed for the following prescription?

Rx: Potassium Permanganate Solution 1:5,000
Dispense: 600ml

$$1{:}5{,}000 = \frac{1\text{gm}}{5{,}000\text{ml}} = \frac{1{,}000\text{mg}}{5{,}000\text{ml}}$$

$$\frac{1{,}000\text{mg}}{5{,}000\text{ml}} = \frac{x\text{ mg}}{600\text{ml}}$$

$$600\text{ml} \times 1{,}000\text{mg} = X\text{ mg} \times 5{,}000\text{ml}$$

$$\frac{600{,}000}{5{,}000} = \frac{5{,}000X}{5{,}000}$$

$$120\text{mg} = x$$

$$120\text{mg} \times \frac{\text{tablet}}{30\text{mg}} = 4 \text{ tablets}$$

b. How many 150mg clindamycin capsules are required for the following prescription?

Rx: Clindamycin 3% Topical Solution
Alcohol qs 60ml
Dispense: 60ml

$$3\% = \frac{3\text{gm}}{100\text{ml}} = \frac{3{,}000\text{mg}}{100\text{ml}}$$

$$\frac{3{,}000\text{mg}}{100\text{ml}} = \frac{X\text{ mg}}{60\text{ml}}$$

$$3{,}000 \times 60 = 100X$$

$$\frac{180{,}000}{100} = X$$

$$1{,}800\text{mg} = X$$

$$1{,}800\text{mg} \times \frac{\text{capsule}}{150\text{mg}} = 12 \text{ capsules}$$

Commercial cost calculations

The pharmacy's *cost* of acquisition, or the figure included on the invoice, is usually the total cost of all items of one kind received. The cost of a single item may be calculated by dividing the cost by the number of items received. For example, if a case of 24 bottles of antacid lists an invoice cost of $12, each bottle of antacid costs 50 cents. This is one example of cost, but other factors may enter into the actual price of an item.

Commercial markup calculations

Markup is defined as the difference between the cost of an article and its selling price. This difference may also be known as gross profit. It is a confusing term and must be qualified to determine its true meaning. Unless specifically stated as percent markup, markup means the actual amount in dollars and cents that the cost of an item was increased to determine a selling price. For example, if the selling price of a bottle of antacid is $1.50 and the cost is $0.50, the markup is $1.00.

Commercial selling price

The *commercial selling price* figure is always 100 percent of the amount received for the sale of an item, and it is the sum of the cost of the article plus the amount of gross profit. The selling price is usually figured directly from the cost.

Selling price = Cost + Gross profit (markup)

Gross profit

It was previously stated that markup is sometimes referred to as *gross profit*. This is the difference in dollars and cents between the cost of an article and its selling price. Gross profit is the sum of the overhead and the net profit as explained below.

Gross profit (markup) = Selling price - Cost

Percent markup

Percent markup is always based on cost. The amount of markup and the amount of gross profit is the same ($1.00, in the aforementioned example), but percent markup is always based on *cost*, not selling price. Percent markup indicates the percent that the cost is increased to determine a selling price.

$$\text{Percent markup} = \frac{\text{Markup (actual dollar amount)}}{\text{Cost}} \times 100\%$$

For example, the percent markup on the $1.50 bottle of antacid is 200%.

$$\text{Percent markup} = \frac{\$1.00}{0.50} \times 100\% = 2 \times 100\% = 200\%$$

Percent gross profit

The term percent markup is used occasionally when *percent gross profit* is intended, but this is incorrect. *Percent gross profit* is always based on the *selling price*, not the cost.

$$\text{Percent gross profit} = \frac{\text{Markup (actual dollar amount)}}{\text{Selling price}} \times 100\%$$

For example, the percent gross profit on the $1.50 bottle of antacid is 66 2/3%.

$$\text{Percent gross profit} = \frac{\$1.00}{\$1.50} \times 100\% = 0.666 \times 100\% = 66\ 2/3\%$$

Overhead

Overhead is a very important item used in figuring the actual profit realized from a business. It includes all of the operating costs of the business, and it must be considered in determining the net profit that the business realizes. Overhead includes salaries, rent, utilities, freight, interest on investment, uncollected accounts, taxes, insurance, and all other specific and incidental expenses. The overhead plus the net profit equals the gross profit. The percent of the overhead is based on the gross sales.

Net profit

The net profit is calculated by deducting the sum of the cost of an article plus the overhead from the selling price. The percent of the net profit is based on the selling price.

Turnover

This is inventory terminology that represents the number of times that a specified amount of merchandise is sold in a given length of time, usually one year.

Inventory

Inventory is an itemized statement of all the merchandise on hand, with its value listed at cost.

Depreciation

Depreciation is an amount representing loss in the sale value of an item. Many drug items depreciate little within a length of time; however, sundry items often become obsolete or shopworn and lose their original retail value. Equipment and fixtures depreciate regularly, and this amount is considered with other operating costs.

Gross sales

All money received for goods sold within a given period of time is known as gross sales.

Determination of a prescription price

Though there are many methods of determining a prescription price, or the price that the patient pays for the medication, they are all based on the patient not having a third party payor involved in paying the pharmacy for a portion or all of the prescription. When a third party payor is involved in the payment of a prescription, the equation becomes much more complex and will vary with every contract upon which the pharmacy and third party plan agree. Further discussion of this matter follows later.

For the cash-paying customer, which in the past two decades has dwindled to a very small percentage, there are basically three methods by which the pharmacist decides a fair price for the consumer and a good return on investment to ensure a profitable pharmacy, together with providing good service to the community.

1. *Percent markup*—This is the simplest method where the selling price is determined directly from and added to the cost of the ingredients. Therefore:

   Cost of ingredients + (Cost of ingredients x % Markup) = Final prescription price

   Note that the pharmacy may choose to have a different percent markup based on the cost of the ingredients or some other criteria. That is, there may be a percent markup for so-called expensive medications and a higher percent markup for lower priced medications, two different markups for branded and generic drugs, or whatever other variable the pharmacy may choose.

2. *Percent markup plus a professional (dispensing) fee*—Here a small percent markup plus a professional fee is added to the cost of the ingredients. In this case the dispensing or professional fee is added to every prescription regardless of the cost of the ingredients and is determined based on the cost of the container, label, computer leasing, overhead and depreciation, and professional services, which could include after hours service, delivery services, etc.

   Cost of ingredients + (Cost of ingredients x % Markup) + Professional fee = Final price

3. Professional fee method—In this method, a professional or dispensing fee is only used without regard to a percent markup.

   Cost of ingredient + Dispensing Fee = Final prescription price

Third party plans—As discussed earlier, more and more patients have prescription benefits provided by private or government insurance programs. These insurers are called *third party insurance payors* because in addition to the pharmacist and patient, they are a *third party* involved in the financial transaction related to the prescription. The formulae or equations used to determine the payment structure are placed in a contract that is agreed upon by the pharmacy and the third party payor. Whichever equation is used, these plans ensure that a pharmacy will inevitably decrease its reimbursement for a prescription and thereby see a decrease in gross profits and net profits. It is sometimes possible for a pharmacy to accept a plan that actually has no profit or even has a loss. When accepting such plans, the pharmacy is counting on the fact that it sells many other services and has a diversified array of products that carry much higher gross profits, and assumes that the patient will purchase a product in addition to the prescription that will increase profits for the store as a whole.

Sample commercial problems

a. A pharmacist sells a bottle of medication for $4.24, realizing a gross profit of 60% on the cost. Calculate the cost of the medication. *Selling price = Cost + Gross profit.*

$$\$4.24 = X + 60\%X$$

$$\$4.24 = 1X + 0.6X$$

$$\$4.24 = 1.6X$$

$$\$2.65 = X$$

b. Determine the correct selling price for 100 capsules of antacid at a cost of $9.74 if the percent gross profit is 25% (markup of 25% on selling price). *Selling price = Cost + Gross profit.*

$$X = \$9.74 + 25\%X$$

$$1X = \$9.74 + 0.25X$$

$$1X - 0.25X = \$9.74$$

$$0.75X = \$9.74$$

$$X = \$9.74/0.75 = \$12.99$$

c. Determine the correct selling price for 100 capsules of antacid at a cost of \$9.74 if the percent markup is 25% (markup of 25% on cost). *Selling price = Cost + Gross profit.*

X = \$9.74 + (25% x \$9.74)

X = \$9.74 + (0.25 x \$9.74)

X = \$9.74 + \$2.44

X = \$12.18

Conclusion

Calculations are used every day within the pharmacy. The pharmacy technician who can accurately perform the various mathematical calculations discussed in this chapter can serve as an invaluable aide to the pharmacist with respect to the distributive functions and operations of a pharmacy.

Acknowledgment

The authors and publisher wish to acknowledge Denise Hultz, CPhT, for her extensive contributions to this chapter.

About the authors

Tony Michienzi received his bachelor's of science in physiology from the University of Western Ontario in London, Ontario, Canada, in 1989. He received his bachelor's degree in pharmacy from Ferris State University College of Pharmacy in 1992. Michienzi worked for a small chain in Ontario and then for Walgreens in Florida, and now in Grand Rapids, Michigan. He has been an adjunct faculty member for Ferris State University for five years and enjoys giving back to future pharmacists. Michienzi was asked by Walgreens in 1997 to help guide the review sessions for pharmacy technicians and store managers who wanted to become certified pharmacy technicians.

Stephen T. Smith is an original member of the MPA Pharmacy Certified Technician (PCT) Task Force started in 1978. He has held various positions on the PCT Board of Examiners over many years. He has also served as a question item writer for the national Pharmacy Technician Certification Board examination. Smith obtained his bachelor's degree in pharmacy from the University of Michigan in Ann Arbor in 1979 and his master's degree in pharmacy in 1988 from Wayne State University in Detroit, Michigan. He currently works for Owen Healthcare and serves as the director of pharmacy at Crittenton Hospital in Rochester, Michigan. He holds membership in the American Society of Health-System Pharmacists, the Michigan Pharmacists Association, the Michigan Society of Health-System Pharmacists, and the Southeastern Michigan Society of Health-System Pharmacists. Smith has a long history of service in pharmacy professional organizations, having served as a member on several task forces and committees and as an officer and board member.

Self-assessment questions

Fractions

1. Define the following:
   a. Proper fraction____________________

   b. Improper fraction____________________

2. Which of the following are examples of an improper fraction?

a.	7/8	f.	5/4
b.	5/6	g.	4/5
c.	9/7	h.	4/3
d.	1/1	i.	2/2
e.	2/3	j.	9/8

3. Briefly explain why the following is an incorrectly expressed fraction.
   2 grains
   7 ounces

Mixed numbers and improper fractions

1. What is a mixed number?

2. Change the following mixed numbers to improper fractions.
   a. 3 3/4
   b. 2 1/2
   c. 4 1/4
   d. 1 1/3
   e. 5 1/2
   f. 8 1/2
   g. 7 1/8
   h. 12 2/3
   i. 7 1/2
   j. 5 3/4
   k. 3 1/3
   l. 20 1/3

3. Change the following improper fractions to mixed numbers.
   a. 15/4
   b. 21/4
   c. 8/3
   d. 29/4
   e. 24/5
   f. 35/3
   g. 16/5
   h. 7/6
   i. 34/5
   j. 16/3
   k. 35/4
   l. 31/2

Adding fractions with like denominators

1. Add the following fractions, and when necessary, reduce to the lowest possible terms.
   a. 1/8 + 3/8 =
   b. 1/4 + 1/4 =
   c. 1/6 + 1/6 =
   d. 1/3 + 1/3 =
   e. 5/6 + 5/6 =
   f. 1/5 + 2/5 =
   g. 1/2 + 1/2 =
   h. 2/7 + 3/7 =
   i. 3/8 +3/8 =
   j. 2/3 + 1/3 + 1/3 =
   k. 1/4 + 1/4 +1/4 =
   l. 1/10 + 3/10 + 7/10 =

2. For the present, disregard the terminology (grains) used in these sample problems and concentrate only on the fractions.
   a. 1/2 grain + 1/2 grain =
   b. 1/3 grain + 1/3 grain =
   c. 1/4 grain + 1/4 grain =
   d. 1/8 grain + 1/8 grain =
   e. 1/32 grain + 1/32 grain =
   f. 1/64 + 1/64 =
   g. You have two tablets of a drug and each tablet is 1/6 grain. If the two tablets are

given together, how many grains of the drug are given?____________________

Adding fractions with unlike denominators

1. Add the following fractions and, when necessary, reduce to the lowest possible terms.
   a. 2/3 + 1/4 =____________________
   b. 1/5 + 1/4 =____________________
   c. 1/3 + 1/6 =____________________
   d. 1/2 +1/3 = ____________________
   e. 2/3 + 1/8 =____________________
   f. 4/9 + 1/5 =____________________
   g. 1/3 + 1/5 =____________________
   h. 1/4 + 2/5 = ____________________
   i. 1/5 + 3/10 = ____________________
   j. 2/7 + 1/3 =____________________
   k. 1/32 + 1/64 = ____________________

2. Add the following fractions and change improper fractions to a mixed number.
   a. 1/2 + 2/3 =____________________
   b. 2/3 + 5/6 =____________________
   c. 1/3 + 8/9 =____________________
   d. 4/5 + 2/3 =____________________
   e. 3/8 + 9/10 =____________________
   f. 6/7 + 2/3 =____________________
   g. 10/11 + 1/3 =____________________

3. Add the following mixed numbers or fractions and mixed numbers.
   a. 2 1/2 + 2 1/2 = ____________________
   b. 1 2/3 + 3/4 = ____________________
   c. 2 2/5 + 4 1/2 = ____________________
   d. 3 1/3 + 2 1/3 = ____________________
   e. 5 1/2 + 1/8 = ____________________
   f. 7 3/4 + 7 1/2 = ____________________
   g. 4 1/4 + 2/3 = ____________________

4. Again, disregard the terminology (grains) used in these sample problems and concentrate on the fractions and mixed numbers.
   a. 7 1/2 grains + 7 1/2 grains = __________
   b. 3 3/4 grains + 3 3/4 grains = __________
   c. 1 1/2 grains + 3 1/4 grains = __________
   d. 1 1/2 grains + 1 1/2 grains = __________
   e. 1 2/3 grains + 1/2 grain = __________
   f. 1/4 grain + 1/2 grain =__________

Comparison of fractions

1. Which is the larger fraction?
   a. 1/3 or 2/3? ____________________
   b. 5/6 or 1/6? ____________________
   c. 1/4 or 3/4? ____________________
   d. 3/9 or 5/9? ____________________
   e. 2/5 or 3/5? ____________________
   f. 2/3 or 1/10? ____________________
   g. 1/4 or 1/2? ____________________
   h. 3/4 or 5/8? ____________________
   i. 2/5 or 5/9? ____________________
   j. 2/3 or 1/2? ____________________
   k. 5/16 or 3/8? ____________________
   l. 2/3 or 3/5? ____________________

Multiplying fractions

1. Multiply the following fractions and, when necessary, reduce to the lowest possible terms.
   a. 1/8 x 1/4 =____________________
   b. 1/2 x 1/2 =____________________
   c. 1/3 x 2/3 =____________________
   d. 1/2 x 2/3 =____________________
   e. 3/5 x 1/3 =____________________
   f. 7/9 x 1/3 =____________________
   g. 4/5 x 4/5 =____________________
   h. 4/8 x 3/6 =____________________
   i. 10/12 x 2/3 =____________________
   j. 3/4 x 1/4 =____________________

2. Multiply the following fractions and whole numbers. When necessary, change the improper fraction of the answer to a mixed number and reduce to lowest terms.
   a. 5 x 1/8 =____________________
   b. 4 x 2/3 =____________________
   c. 1 x 1/2 =____________________

d. 3 x 1/4 = ______

e. 5 x 1/2 = ______

f. 7 x l/3 = ______

g. 2 x 3/10 = ______

h. 7 x 2/16 = ______

i. 3 x 2/3 = ______

j. 4 x 1/4 = ______

k. 7 x 6/7 = ______

l. 2 x 1/2 = ______

3. Mr. Burke receives 1/3 of the usual dose of a medicine. Mr. Herman receives 1/6 of the usual dose of the same medicine. Which patient received the larger dose?

______

4. Which is the largest dose, morphine grain 1/4 or morphine grain 1/6? ______

5. If Mrs. Novak received two times her usual dose of medicine, phenobarbital grain 1/4, how many grains did she receive?

______

6. Two patients receive 500ml of a dietary supplement. Mrs. Klein drank two thirds of her supplement, and Mrs. Cleary drank one half of hers. Which patient drank more?

______

7. Multiply the following whole and mixed numbers and, when necessary, reduce to the lowest possible terms.

a. 3 x 2 1/2 = ______

b. 4 x 3 1/2 = ______

c. 6 x 1 1/2 = ______

d. 5 x 5 1/4 = ______

e. 2 x 4 1/4 = ______

f. 1 x 3 1/3 = ______

g. 7 x 2 1/4 = ______

h. 3 x 4 5/8 = ______

8. Multiply the following mixed numbers and, when necessary, reduce to the lowest possible terms.

a. 2 1/2 x 3 1/4 = ______

b. 3 1/2 x 3 1/2 = ______

c. 4 1/4 x 5 1/8 = ______

d. 1 1/2 x 5 6/7 = ______

e. 2 1/4 x 4 1/4 = ______

f. 5 1/4 x 2 1/8 = ______

g. 1 2/3 x 3 1/5 = ______

h. 2 1/6 x 4 1/8 = ______

9. Mrs. Graham is seen in the emergency department, and the physician tells you that she took five times her usual dose of medicine, that is grains 1 1/2. How many grains did Mrs. Graham take? ______

10. Mr. Shields tells you that he took three times the dose of a drug that his physician prescribed. If the dose is grains 3 3/4, how many grains did he take? ______

Dividing Fractions

1. Divide the following fractions and, when necessary, reduce to the lowest possible terms.

a. 1/8 ÷ 1/4 = ______

b. 1/3 ÷ 1/2 = ______

c. 1/4 ÷ 1/6 = ______

d. 1/5 ÷ 1/12 = ______

e. 1/10 ÷ 1/2 = ______

f. 1/7 ÷ 2/3 = ______

g. 2/3 ÷ 1/3 = ______

h. 4/5 ÷ 1/5 = ______

i. 2/3 ÷ 1/8 = ______

j. 2/5 ÷ 4/6 = ______

k. 3/7 ÷ 2/3 = ______

l. 5/6 ÷ 2/3 = ______

m. 1/100 ÷ 1/1,000 = ______

n. 1/250 ÷ 1/2 = ______

o. 1/100 ÷ 1/2 = ______

p. 1/100 ÷ 1/200 = ______

2. Divide the following fractions and mixed numbers and, when necessary, reduce to the lowest possible terms.

a. 2 1/3 ÷ 1/4 = ______

b. 2 1/2 ÷ 1/2 = ______

c. 1/2 ÷ 2 1/4 = ______

d. 1 1/2 ÷ 1/3 = ______

e. 1/3 ÷ 1 1/4 = ______

f. 3 5/8 ÷ 4/5 = ______

g. 2/3 ÷ 5 3/8 = ______________

h. 1/5 ÷ 2 2/3 = ______________

3. Divide the following whole numbers and fractions and, when necessary, reduce to the lowest possible terms.

a. 2 ÷ 2 2/3 = ______________

b. 1/4 ÷ 2 = ______________

c. 4 ÷ 1/4 = ______________

d. 1/3 ÷ 2 = ______________

e. 2/3 ÷ 2 = ______________

f. 6 ÷ 1/4 = ______________

g. 1/32 ÷ 2 = ______________

h. 1/2 ÷ 2 = ______________

i. 1/16 ÷ 2 = ______________

j. 1/8 ÷ 2 = ______________

4. Divide the following whole numbers and mixed numbers and, when necessary, reduce to the lowest possible terms.

a. 4 ÷ 2 2/3 = ______________

b. 2 ÷ 1 1/2 = ______________

c. 6 ÷ 2 1/4 = ______________

d. 3 1/3 ÷ 4 = ______________

e. 2 1/2 ÷ 2 = ______________

f. 4 1/2 ÷ 5 = ______________

Ratios

1. Write the following both as a ratio and as a fraction. When necessary, reduce to the lowest possible terms.

	Ratio	Fraction
a. one part to ten parts		
b. two parts to fifteen parts		
c. five parts to twenty-five parts		
d. one part to one hundred parts		
e. two parts to five hundred parts		

2. Write the following ratios as fractions.

a. 1:1,000 ______________

b. 1:50 ______________

c. 1:6 ______________

d. 2:3 ______________

e. 1:20 ______________

3. Express the following fractions as ratios.

a. 1/4 = ______________

b. 1/150 = ______________

c. 1/32 = ______________

d. 5/8 = ______________

e. 1/5,000 = ______________

4. If one solution is labeled 1/4 strength and another labeled 1/2 strength, which solution is the stronger?

____

5. If a solution is labeled 1:5,000, is it stronger or weaker than a solution labeled 1:500?

____

6. If one drug is grain 1/100 and another grain 1/250, which is the stronger drug?

____

7. If one drug is grain 1/64 and another grain 1/32, which is the weaker drug?

____

Percent

1. Change each of the following percents to a fraction and, when necessary, reduce to the lowest possible terms.

a. 25% = ______________

b. 50% = ______________

c. 37% = ______________

d. 75% = ______________

e. 41% = ______________

f. 22% = ______________

g. 84% = ______________

h. 90% = ______________

2. Change each of the following fractions to a percent.

a. 4/5 = ______________

b. 1/2 = ______________

c. 2/3 = ______________

d. 5/8 = ____________

e. 2/5 = ____________

f. 1/7 = ____________

g. 3/8 = ____________

h. 1/4 = ____________

i. 1/6 = ____________

j. 1/10 = ____________

3. Change each of the following ratios to a percent.

a. 1:500 = ____________

b. 1:100 = ____________

c. 1:1,000 = ____________

d. 1:8 = ____________

e. 1:25 = ____________

f. 1:5,000 = ____________

g. 1:4 = ____________

h. 1:10 = ____________

i. 1:2,000 = ____________

j. 1:200 = ____________

4. Change each of the following percents to a ratio.

a. 5% = ____________

b. 25% = ____________

c. 30% = ____________

d. 80% = ____________

e. 1% = ____________

f. 0.3% = ____________

g. 8% = ____________

h. 12% = ____________

5. Mrs. Conrad has a solution applied to a leg ulcer. The bottle is labeled 1:250. What is the percentage of the solution?

____

6. A solution used for bladder irrigations is labeled 1:4,000. What is the percentage of the solution?

____

7. Mr. Jennings has an irrigating solution labeled 10%. Express this percent as a ratio.

____

Proportions

1. Solve the following problems for X.

a. 5:10 :: 10:x X = ____________

b. 3/x = 5/20 X = ____________

c. 2:6 as x:9 X = ____________

d. 1:7 :: 10:x X = ____________

e. 15/1 = 30/x X = ____________

f. 6:12 :: x:144 X = ____________

2. Set up and solve the following proportions.

a. If a man takes 15 hours to pick all the corn planted on one acre, how many acres can he pick in 30 hours?
Proportion: ____________
Solution: X = ____________

b. Using the same figures but substituting medical terminology, if 15 grains is equal to 1 gram, how many grams are in 30 grains?
Proportion: ____________
Solution: X = ____________

c. If 2.2 pounds equals 1 kilogram, how many pounds are in 40 kilograms?
Proportion: ____________
Solution: X = ____________

d. If 1 milligram equals 1/60 grain, how many grains are in 6 milligrams?
Proportion: ____________
Solution: X = ____________

Decimals

1. Write the following as decimals.

a. nine tenths ____________

b. four hundredths ____________

c. five and four tenths ____________

d. one tenth ____________

e. two hundredths ____________

f. one thousandth ____________

2. Write out the following decimals.

a. 0.4 is read as ____________

b. 0.75 is read as ____________

c. 1.6 is read as ____________

d. 5.58 is read as ____________

e. 7.755 is read as ____________

3. Add the following decimals.
   a. 2.25 + 5.86 = ____________
   b. 3.75 + 0.66 = ____________
   c. 1.75 + 2.25 = ____________
   d. 23.65 + 0.56 = ____________
   e. 475.45 + 4.66 = ____________
   f. 62.32 + 0.007 = ____________
   g. 5.63 + 4.24 + 3.1 = ____________
   h. 66.2 + 0.25 + 1.755 = ____________
   i. 4.004 + 2.1 + 34.6 = ____________
4. Subtract the following decimals.
   a. 5.5 – 3.4 = ____________
   b. 68.07 – 14.6 = ____________
   c. 1.77 – 0.015 = ____________
   d. 7.75 – 3.875 = ____________
   e. 7.5 – 3.75 = ____________
5. Multiply the following whole numbers and decimals.
   a. 5 x 0.5 = ____________
   b. 25 x 0.1 = ____________
   c. 2 x 2.25 = ____________
   d. 15 x 1.4 = ____________
   e. 500 x 0.25 = ____________
   f. 3 x 0.75 = ____________
   g. 4 x 1.35 = ____________
6. Multiply the following decimals.
   a. 2.75 x 0.5 = ____________
   b. 4.4 x 1.2 = ____________
   c. 2.5 x 2.5 = ____________
   d. 6.25 x 1.15 = ____________
   e. 7.5 x 2.5 = ____________
   f. 1.5 x 1.5 = ____________
   g. 5.46 x 2.17 = ____________
   h. 1.5 x 3.5 = ____________
7. Divide the following decimals.
   a. 0.65 ÷ 0.3 = ____________
   b. 0.7 ÷ 0.2 = ____________
   c. 1.42 ÷ 6.2 = ____________
   d. 4 ÷ 0.75 = ____________
   e. 6 ÷ 2.2 = ____________
   f. 5 ÷ 5.5 = ____________
   g. 4.4 ÷ 3 = ____________
   h. 3.6 ÷ 2 = ____________
8. Change each of the following decimals to a fraction and, when necessary, reduce to the lowest possible terms.
   a. 0.2 = ____________
   b. 0.65 = ____________
   c. 0.87 = ____________
   d. 0.5 = ____________
   e. 0.68 = ____________

MATHEMATICS OF PHARMACOLOGY

Systems of measurements

1. Name the two systems of weights and measurement used in pharmacology.

   ____

   ____
2. The unit of weight in the metric system is ____________
3. The unit of volume in the metric system is ____________
4. The unit of linear measurement in the metric system is ____________
5. The unit of weight in the apothecary system is ____________
6. The unit of volume in the apothecary system is ____________
7. The following are metric measurements. Give the *approximate* apothecary equivalents of the following.

Metric weight	**Apothecary weight**
a. 1 milligram	____________
b. 65 milligrams	____________
c. 1 gram	____________
d. 30 grams	____________
e. 1 kilogram	____________

Metric volume	Apothecary volume
f. 1 milliliter	______
g. 30 milliliters	______
h. 480 milliliters	______
i. 960 milliliters	______

8. Give the abbreviations or symbols for the following.
   a. milligram ______
   b. grains ______
   c. kilogram ______
   d. microgram ______
   e. gram ______
   f. ounce ______
   g. ounce (symbol) ______
   h. minims (symbol) ______
   i. dram (symbol) ______
   j. milliliter ______

9. Convert from apothecary to metric systems, or metric to apothecary, using proportion and equivalents. Use abbreviations when labeling the answer.
   a. 30 grains to grams______
   b. 4.4 pounds to kilograms______
   c. 66 pounds to kilograms ______
   d. 2 milligrams to grains______
   e. 8 minims to milliliters______
   f. 1 quart to liters ______
   g. 2 fluid ounces to milliliters ______
   h. 1 1/2 grains to grams ______
   i. 1 quart to milliliters ______
   j. 0.3 milligrams to grains ______
   k. 1/100 grain to milligrams______
   l. 1 milligram to micrograms______
   m. 1/4 grain to milligrams ______
   n. 10 milligrams to grains ______
   o. 16 minims to milliliters ______
   p. 2 grains to milligrams______
   q. 500 milliliters to pints______
   r. 1/200 grain to milligrams______
   s. 1/8 grain to milligrams ______
   t. 60 milliliters to fluid ounces ______
   u. 30 minims to milliliters ______
   v. 60 grains to grams______
   w. 1/60 grain to milligrams______
   x. 0.8 milligrams to grains ______
   y. 140 pounds to kilograms ______
   z. 8 milliliters to fluid drams ______
   aa. 45 minims to milliliters ______
   bb. 1.5 milliliters to minims ______
   cc. 0.1 milligram to grains______
   dd. 4 milliliters to minims______
   ee. 55 kilograms to pounds ______

10. Convert the following metric system measurements to the designated equivalent. Use abbreviations in labeling the answer.
   a. 2,000 milliliters to liters ______
   b. 60 milligrams to grams ______
   c. 1.5 grams to milligrams ______
   d. 0.1 gram to milligrams ______
   e. 3,000 milliliters to liters ______
   f. 0.5 gram to milligrams ______
   g. 750 milligrams to grams______
   h. 2,000 micrograms to milligrams______
   i. 0.2 milligrams to micrograms ______
   j. 500 milliliters to liters______
   k. 1,500 milliliters to liters ______
   l. 500 milligrams to grams______
   m. 2.5 grams to milligrams ______
   n. 100 milligrams to grams______
   o. 500 micrograms to milligrams______

Oral dosages of drugs

1. Find the correct dosage of the following solid oral preparations. Label each answer (tablets, capsules, etc.).
   a. codeine sulfate 30mg tablets; give 60mg.
   ______

b. codeine sulfate 15mg tablets; give 1gr. ______

c. ampicillin 250mg capsules; give 0.5gm. ______

d. phenobarbital 15mg tablets; give 1/4gr. ______

e. cephalexin 250mg capsules; give 0.25gm. ______

f. papaverine hydrochloride 100mg tablets; give 1 1/2gr. ______

g. secobarbital sodium 1 1/2 grain capsules; give 100mg. ______

h. methimazole 5mg tablets; give 15mg. ______

i. glutethimide 0.5gm tablets; give 500mg. ______

j. mephobarbital 100mg tablets; give 50mg. ______

k. warfarin 2.5mg tablets; give 5mg. ______

l. If the total daily dose of a drug is 0.9 grams and the drug is given in three equally divided doses each day, what is the amount of each dose in milligrams? ______

m. If the dose of a drug is 10mg for each kilogram of body weight, what is the dose for an adult weighing 132 pounds? ______

n. If the dose of a drug is 2.5mg for each kilogram of body weight, what is the dose for a child weighing 44 pounds? ______

o. The daily dose of a drug is 1 gram and is divided into four equal doses. How many milligrams are in each dose? ______

p. If a drug is available as 250mg tablets and 0.5 grams are given BID, how many tablets are given each day? ______

2. Find the correct dosage of the following liquid oral preparations. Label each answer.
   a. erythromycin ethylsuccinate syrup 100mg in 2.5ml; give 200mg. ______
   b. clindamycin solution 300mg in 1ml; give 600mg. ______
   c. ampicillin suspension 125mg in 5ml; give 250mg. ______
   d. potassium chloride 20% solution with 40mEq (milliequivalents) in 15ml; give 20mEq. ______
   e. nalidixic acid suspension 250mg in 5ml; give 125mg. ______
   f. If a dose of a drug is one teaspoonful for 60 pounds of body weight, how many teaspoonfuls are given to a child weighing 30 pounds? ______
   g. How many milliliters are in a teaspoonful? ______
   h. If a patient receives 1/2 ounce of Gelusil®, how many milliliters is he receiving? ______
   i. John weighs 60 pounds. He receives 3mg per pound of a drug per day. How many milligrams does he receive each day? ______
   j. If the daily dose of John's drug is divided into two equal doses, how many milligrams are in each dose? ______
   k. If the drug John receives is supplied as 60mg in 5ml, how many milliliters are given for each dose? ______

Parenteral dosages of drugs

1. Determine the correct dosage of the following parenteral preparations. These problems also illustrate some of the labeling and writing variations that may be encouraged in hospital practice. Label each answer.
   a. meperidine 50mg in 1ml; give 75mg. ______
   b. diazepam 10mg/2ml; give 5mg. ______
   c. atropine sulfate 0.3mg in 1ml; give 1/200 grain. ______
   d. kanamycin sulfate 75mg per 2ml; give 37.5mg. ______
   e. butorphanol tartrate 2mg per ml; give 1mg. ______
   f. digoxin 0.5mg in 2ml; give 0.25mg. ______
   g. digoxin 0.5mg in 2ml; give 0.125mg. ______
   h. hydralazine hydrochoride 20mg per ml; give 40mg. ______

i. morphine sulfate 10mg in 1ml; give 1/4 grain. ______

j. deferoxamine mesylate 500mg per 2ml; give 0.5gm. ______

k. tolazoline hydrochloride 10ml vial labeled 1ml/25mg; give 50mg.

______

l. fentanyl 0.05mg/ml; give 0.1mg.

______

m. penicillin G procaine 300,000 units per ml; give 150,000 units.

______

n. mithramycin 500mcg/ml with dose based on patient's weight at 25mcg/kg. How many milliliters are needed for a patient weighing 110 pounds?

______

o. what dose in micrograms is administered to a 110-pound patient?

______

p. scopolamine 0.3mg per ml; give 1/400 grains. ______

q. phentolamine 5mg/ml; give 2mg.

______

r. hydromorphone hydrochloride 2mg per ml; give 1/60 grain. ______

s. lidocaine 20mg/ml; give 15mg.

______

t. cimetidine hydrochloride 300mg per 2ml; give 0.3 grams. ______

u. colchicine 1mg in 2ml; give 0.5mg.

______

v. penicillin G procaine 600,000 units/ml; give 300,000 units.

______

w. heparin sodium 2,500 units/ml; give 5,000 units. ______

x. A U-40 insulin syringe is calibrated to measure 40 units per ml. How many milliliters of solution is in the syringe when the 20-unit mark is reached?

______

y. cephalothin 1 gram/10ml; give 500mg.

______

z. meperidine 50mg/ml; give 0.1 gram.

______

2. The following preparations require reconstitution before parenteral administration. The directions for reconstitution are usually printed on the vial. Determine the volume for the following dosages. Label each answer.

a. nafcillin sodium powder; add 1.8ml sterile water to 500mg vial to make 2ml; give 0.25gm. ______

b. nafcillin sodium powder; add 6.6ml sterile water to 2.0gm vial to make 8ml; give 500mg. ______

c. penicillin G sodium is labeled: 5,000,000 units per vial; may be diluted with 23ml, 18ml, 8ml, 3ml to provide 200,000 units, 250,000 units, 500,000 units or 1,000,000 units per ml, respectively.

(1) If you dilute the vial containing 5,000,000 units with 23ml and each milliliter contains 200,000 units, how much liquid is in the vial?

______

(2) If you now withdraw 400,000 units of penicillin G sodium from the vial, how many milliliters are in the syringe?

______

3. Hypodermic tablets are used for parenteral injection. Determine the number of tablets dissolved and the amount of solution administered for the following problems. Remember to specify if you use milliliters or minims in the answer.

a. Morphine sulfate 10mg as hypodermic tablets; give 1/6gr. Dissolve ______ tablet(s) in ______

b. Atropine sulfate 0.4mg as hypodermic tablets; give 0.6mg. Dissolve ______ tablet(s) in ______

Temperatures

1. Convert the following temperatures written in Fahrenheit to Celsius.

a. 98.6° F = ______

b. 100° F = ______

c. 101° F = ______

d. 101.4° F = ______

e. 97° F = ______

f. 101.6° F = ______

g. 100.8° F = ______

h. 99° F = ______

2. Convert the following Celsius temperatures to Fahrenheit temperatures.

a. 36.2° C = ______

b. 30° C = ______

c. 38.4° C = ______

d. 38° C = ______

e. 32° C = ______

f. 38.1° C = ______

g. 37.3° C = ______

h. 39° C = ______

Solutions

1. Solve the following problem about solutions from liquid drugs, using proportion or D/H x quantity desired = amount of solute.
   a. A 1:2,000 solution is available. How much of this solution is needed to make 1,000ml of a 1:4,000 solution?

      ______
   b. How much solute is required to make 200ml of a 50% solution from a 100% solution? ______
   c. How much of a 10% solution is needed to prepare 100ml of a 7% solution?

      ______
   d. How much of a 20% solution is needed to prepare 500ml of a 10% solution?

      ______

2. Solve the following problem about solutions using the same formula in Question #1.
   a. How many 10 grain tablets are required to make 1,000ml of a 1:1,000 solution?

      ______
   b. If 5 grams are dissolved in 100ml of solution, what is the percentage of the solution? ______
   c. If you have 200ml of a 10% solution, how many grams of the drug are in this solution? ______

3. Solve the following problem about ratio of a solution.
   a. What is the ratio of a 20% solution?

      ______
   b. What is the ratio of a 10% solution?

      ______
   c. What is the ratio of a 2% solution?

      ______
   d. What is the ratio of a 50% solution?

      ______

4. Solve the following problem about percentage of a solution.
   a. If 9 grams are dissolved in 1,000ml of solution, what is the percentage of this solution?______
   b. If 500ml contains 0.5 grams, what is the percentage of the solution?______
   c. What is the percentage of a 1:4,000 solution?______
   d. What is the percentage of a 1:25 solution?______

Additional story problems

1. Mr. Brown's usual dose of the medication is 5 1/2 grains. Today, he takes three times the usual dose. How many grains has he taken today?

   ______
2. Miss Tucker is still experiencing pain with her usual dose of 5 grains of analgesic. Her doctor says she can increase the dose by 1 1/2 times for one week. What is the new dose?

   ______
3. If an ointment is labeled 1:30 and another is labeled 1:45, which ointment is stronger?

   ______
4. If one solution is labeled 3/4 strength and another is labeled 5/8 strength, which is the stronger solution? ______
5. If a cough syrup has 10mg of active ingredients per 5ml, how many teaspoons are needed to get 30mg of an active ingredient?______
6. If a drug is labeled 1gm/10ml, how many mls are needed for a dose of 500mg? ______
7. If an injectable drug is labeled 4mg/ml and the dose needed is 12mg, how many mls are needed? How many mls would be needed for a dose of 3mg? ______
8. If an injectable drug is labeled 500mcg/2ml and 0.125mcg is the dose, how many mls are needed? ______
9. If an injectable drug is labeled 500mcg/5ml and 750mcg is the dose, how many mls are needed?

   ______
10. A drug comes in 325mg tablets, and the patient needs a dose of 10 grains. How many tablet(s) are needed per dose? ______
11. The drug is available in tablets of 5mg each. How many tablets are needed for one dose of 0.015gm? ______
12. The daily dose for a medication is 2.4gm. The drug is available in 400mg tablets. How many tablets are needed for a one-day supply?

    ______

13. If the physician orders 0.1gm of a certain drug and the label on the bottle reads 100mg per tablet, how many tablets does the patient receive? ______________________

14. A child is given a 2.5ml dropperful of erythrocin drops four times daily. He is receiving _____ cc medication daily. If each 2.5ml contains 100mg of medication, he receives _____ gm of the drug daily.

15. A patient needs a dose of 0.2 gm of medication. The pharmacy has tablets of 50mg, 100mg, and 200mg each. What is the best dose for the patient? __________ tablets ___________ mg.

16. How many tablet(s) does a patient need for a dose of 3mg if the tablets are labeled 1/20gr?

    ____

17. If a patient takes a 0.5gm of antibiotic three times daily, her total daily dose is ________ mg.

18. You need to add 40 units of insulin to an intravenous solution from a bottle of insulin 100 units/ml. You will need to use ________ml(s) of insulin.

19. The strength of Domeboro® solution needed is 1:40. If the Domeboro® directions recommend one tablet in each quart of water for a strength of 1:40, how many tablet(s) are needed in a liter of water for the desired strength?

    ____

20. The label on an injectable medication reads "store at a temperature of 4° to 9° Celsius." The thermometer in the pharmacy refrigerator reads 41° Fahrenheit. Is it the appropriate temperature for storing this medication? ______________

Part VII: Appendices

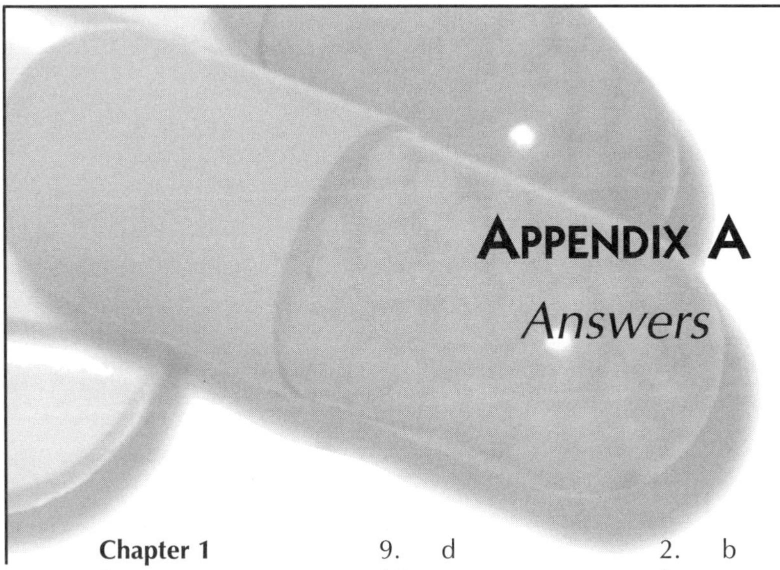

Appendix A
Answers

Chapter 1
1. c
2. c
3. b
4. a
5. d
6. b
7. d
8. d
9. c
10. b

Chapter 2
1. d
2. c
3. b
4. c
5. b

Chapter 3
1. d
2. c
3. a
4. c
5. b

Chapter 4
1. b
2. c
3. a
4. d
5. b
6. a
7. a
8. c
9. d
10. c

Chapter 5
1. a
2. c
3. d
4. b
5. a

Chapter 6
1. a
2. c
3. d
4. d
5. a
6. d
7. d
8. b
9. b
10. c

Chapter 7
1. d
2. c
3. d
4. a
5. b
6. a
7. b
8. c
9. c
10. d

Chapter 8
1. d
2. b
3. a
4. b
5. d
6. b
7. d
8. a
9. c
10. d
11. b
12. b
13. c
14. a
15. d

Chapter 9
1. c
2. c
3. b
4. c
5. a
6. c
7. a
8. d
9. c
10. d

Chapter 10
1. d
2. a
3. c
4. b
5. a.
6. a
7. c
8. b
9. b
10. b

Chapter 11
1. c
2. b
3. b
4. c
5. d
6. a
7. d
8. a
9. b
10. c

Chapter 12
1. a
2. b
3. c
4. a
5. d
6. c
7. d
8. d
9. b
10. a

Chapter 13
1. b
2. c
3. a
4. d
5. b
6. d
7. d
8. b

9. b
10. c

Chapter 14
1. b
2. c
3. a
4. b
5. a
6. b
7. c
8. a
9. b
10. d

Chapter 15
1. a
2. b
3. c
4. c
5. a
6. b
7. a
8. d
9. d
10. b

Chapter 16
1. c
2. b
3. b
4. a
5. d
6. b
7. a
8. b
9. d
10. c

Chapter 17
1. b
2. a
3. d
4. b
5. c
6. c
7. c
8. a
9. c
10. d

Chapter 18
1. c
2. d
3. a
4. c
5. a
6. b
7. a
8. d
9. a
10. d

Chapter 19
1. d
2. c
3. b
4. b
5. c
6. b
7. a
8. b
9. c
10. d

Chapter 20
1. b
2. c
3. c
4. d
5. b
6. c
7. a
8. a
9. c
10. c
11. a
12. a
13. c
14. c
15. c

Chapter 21
1. d
2. c
3. c
4. d
5. b
6. a
7. b
8. d
9. b
10. a

Chapter 22
1. a
2. c
3. b
4. c
5. c
6. a
7. d
8. a
9. b
10. c

Chapter 23
1. b
2. b
3. d
4. b
5. d
6. b
7. d
8. c
9. c
10. d

Chapter 24
1. d
2. b
3. a
4. b
5. a
6. b
7. d
8. d
9. c
10. d

Chapter 25
1. c
2. a
3. d
4. d
5. b
6. c
7. a
8. b
9. a
10. b

Chapter 26
1. b
2. b
3. b
4. c
5. c
6. d
7. a
8. d
9. c
10. d

Chapter 27
1. c
2. a
3. d
4. a
5. c
6. b
7. d
8. b
9. c
10. c

Chapter 28
1. d
2. b
3. a
4. a
5. d
6. c
7. b
8. b
9. a
10. a

Chapter 29
1. c
2. d
3. a
4. a
5. c

Chapter 30
1. a
2. c

3. c
4. b
5. a
6. b
7. a
8. d
9. a
10. b
11. d
12. d
13. d
14. a
15. b

Chapter 31

1. a
2. c
3. b
4. c
5. b
6. b
7. a
8. d
9. d
10. d

Chapter 32

Fractions

1. a. Part of a whole number; any number less than a whole number.
   b. A fraction having a numerator larger than or equal to the denominator.
2. c, d, f, h, and j
3. The numerator and denominator must be of like entities.

Mixed numbers and improper fractions

1. A whole number plus a proper fraction.
2. a. 15/4
   b. 5/2
   c. 17/4
   d. 4/3
   e. 11/2
   f. 17/2
   g. 57/8
   h. 38/3
   i. 15/2
   j. 23/4
   k. 10/3
   l. 61/3
3. a. 3 3/4
   b. 5 1/4
   c. 2 2/3
   d. 7 1/4
   e. 4 4/5
   f. 11 2/3
   g. 3 1/5
   h. 1 1/6
   i. 6 4/5
   j. 5 1/3
   k. 8 3/4
   l. 15 1/2

Adding fractions with like denominators

1. a. 1/2
   b. 1/2
   c. 1/3
   d. 2/3
   e. 1 2/3
   f. 3/5
   g. 1
   h. 5/7
   i. 3/4
   j. 4/3 or 1 1/3
   k. 3/4
   l. 11/10 or 1 1/10
2. a. 1 grain
   b. 2/3 grain
   c. 1/2 grain
   d. 1/4 grain
   e. 1/16 grain
   f. 1/32 grain
   g. 1/3 grain

Adding fractions with unlike denominators

1. a. 11/12
   b. 9/20
   c. 1/2
   d. 5/6
   e. 19/24
   f. 29/45
   g. 8/15
   h. 13/20
   i. 1/2
   j. 13/21
   k. 3/64

2. a. 1 1/6
   b. 1 1/2
   c. 1 2/9
   d. 1 7/15
   e. 1 11/40
   f. 1 11/21
   g. 1 8/33
3. a. 5
   b. 2 5/12
   c. 6 9/10
   d. 5 2/3
   e. 5 5/8
   f. 15 1/4
   g. 4 11/12
4. a. 15 grains
   b. 7 1/2 grains
   c. 4 3/4 grains
   d. 3 grains
   e. 2 1/6 grains
   f. 3/4 grain

Comparison of fractions

1. a. 2/3
   b. 5/6
   c. 3/4
   d. 5/9
   e. 3/5
   f. 2/3
   g. 1/2
   h. 3/4
   i. 5/9
   j. 2/3
   k. 3/8
   l. 2/3

Multiplying fractions

1. a. 1/32
   b. 1/4
   c. 2/9
   d. 1/3
   e. 1/5
   f. 7/27
   g. 16/25
   h. 1/4
   i. 5/9
   j. 3/16

2. a. 5/8
   b. 8/3 or 2 2/3
   c. 1/2
   d. 3/4
   e. 5/2 or 2 1/2
   f. 7/3 or 2 1/3
   g. 3/5
   h. 7/8
   i. 2
   j. 1
   k. 6
   l. 1
3. Mr. Burke
4. grain 1/4
5. grain 1/2
6. Mrs. Klein
7. a. 7 1/2
   b. 14
   c. 9
   d. 26 1/4
   e. 8 1/2
   f. 3 1/3
   g. 15 3/4
   h. 13 7/8
8. a. 8 1/8
   b. 12 1/4
   c. 21 25/32
   d. 8 11/14
   e. 9 9/16
   f. 11 5/32
   g. 5 1/3
   h. 8 15/16
9. 7 1/2 grains
10. 11 1/4 grains

Dividing fractions

1. a. 1/2
   b. 2/3
   c. 1 1/2
   d. 2 2/5
   e. 1/5
   f. 3/14
   g. 2
   h. 4
   i. 5 1/3
   j. 3/5
   k. 9/14
   l. 1 1/4
   m. 10
   n. 1/125
   o. 1/50
   p. 2

2. a. 9 1/3
   b. 5
   c. 2/9
   d. 4 1/2
   e. 4/15
   f. 4 17/32
   g. 16/129
   h. 3/40
3. a. 3/4
   b. 1/8
   c. 16
   d. 1/6
   e. 1/3
   f. 24
   g. 1/64
   h. 1/4
   i. 1/32
   j. 1/16
4. a. 1 1/2
   b. 1 1/3
   c. 2 2/3
   d. 5/6
   e. 1 1/4
   f. 9/10

Ratios

1. a. 1:10; 1/10
   b. 2:15, 2/15
   c. 1:5, 1/5
   d. 1:100, 1/100
   e. 1:250, 1/250
2. a. 1/1,000
   b. 1/50
   c. 1/6
   d. 2/3
   e. 1/20
3. a. 1 part is to 4 parts or 1:4
   b. 1 part is to 150 parts or 1:150
   c. 1 part is to 32 parts or 1:32
   d. 5 parts is to 8 parts or 5:8
   e. 1 part is to 5,000 parts or 1:5,000
4. 1/2 strength
5. weaker
6. grain 1/100
7. grain 1/64

Percent

1. a. 1/4
   b. 1/2
   c. 37/100
   d. 3/4
   e. 41/100
   f. 11/50
   g. 21/25
   h. 9/10
2. a. 80%
   b. 50%
   c. 66 2/3%
   d. 62 1/2%
   e. 40%
   f. 14 2/7%
   g. 37 1/2%
   h. 25%
   i. 16 2/3%
   j. 10%
3. a. 0.2%
   b. 1%
   c. 0.1%
   d. 12.5%
   e. 4%
   f. 0.02%
   g. 25%
   h. 10%
   i. 0.05%
   j. 0.5%
4. a. 1:20
   b. 1:4
   c. 3:10
   d. 4:5
   e. 1:100
   f. 3:1000
   g. 2:25
   h. 3:25
5. 0.4%
6. 0.025%
7. 1:10

Proportions

1. a. 20
   b. 12
   c. 3
   d. 70
   e. 2
   f. 72
2. a. Proportion: 15 hours:1 acre :: 30 hours:x acres
   Solution: $x = 2$ acres

- b. Proportion: 15 grains:1 gram :: 30 grains:*x* grams
  Solution: *x* = 2 grams
- c. Proportion: 2.2 pounds:1 kilogram :: *x* pounds:40 kilograms
  Solution: *x* = 88 pounds
- d. Proportion: 1 milligram:1/60 grain :: 6 milligrams:*x* grains
  Solution: *x* = 1/10 grain

Decimals

1. a. 0.9
   b. 0.04
   c. 5.4
   d. 0.1
   e. 0.02
   f. 0.001
2. a. four tenths
   b. seventy-five hundredths
   c. one and six tenths
   d. five and fifty-eight hundredths
   e. seven and seven hundred fifty-five thousandths
3. a. 8.11
   b. 4.41
   c. 4
   d. 24.21
   e. 480.11
   f. 62.327
   g. 12.97
   h. 68.205
   i. 40.704
4. a. 2.1
   b. 53.47
   c. 1.755
   d. 3.875
   e. 3.75
5. a. 2.5
   b. 2.5
   c. 4.5
   d. 21
   e. 125
   f. 2.25
   g. 5.4
6. a. 1.375
   b. 5.28
   c. 6.25
   d. 7.1875
   e. 18.75
   f. 2.25
   g. 11.8482
   h. 5.25
7. a. 2.167
   b. 3.5
   c. 0.229
   d. 5.33
   e. 2.727
   f. 0.909
   g. 1.467
   h. 1.8
8. a. 1/5
   b. 13/20
   c. 87/100
   d. 1/2
   e. 17/25

MATHEMATICS OF PHARMACOLOGY

Systems of measurement

1. apothecary and metric
2. gram
3. liter
4. meter
5. grain
6. minim
7. a. 1/65 grain
   b. 1 grain
   c. 15 grains
   d. 1 ounce
   e. 2.2 pounds
   f. 16 minims
   g. 1 fluid ounce
   h. 1 pint
   i. 1 quart
8. a. mg
   b. gr
   c. kg
   d. mcg
   e. gm
   f. oz
   g. ℥
   h. ♍
   i. ʒ
   j. ml
9. a. 2gm (or 1.95gm)
   b. 2 kg
   c. 30 kg

d. gr. 1/30 (or 0.03gr)
e. 0.5ml
f. 1 liter
g. 60ml
h. 0.1gm (or 0.097gm)
i. 960ml (or 1,000ml)
j. gr. 1/200 (or 0.03 gr)
k. 0.65mg (or 0.6mg)
l. 1000 mcg
m. 16.2mg
n. gr 1/6 (or 1/6 gr)
o. 1ml
p. 130mg
q. 1 pt
r. 0.325mg
s. 8.125mg
t. 2 fl℥ (or 2 fl. oz.)
u. 1.85ml
v. 4gm (or 3.89gm.)
w. 1mg
x. gr 1/80 (or 0.0125gr)
y. 63.6 kg
z. 2.16 flʒ
aa. 2.77ml
bb. 24.35 ♍
cc. gr 1/600 (or 0.00154gr)
dd. 64.92 ♍
ee. 121 lb

10. a. 2 liters
b. 0.06gm
c. 1500mg
d. 100mg
e. 3 liters
f. 500mg
g. 0.75gm
h. 2mg
i. 200 mcg
j. 0.5 liter
k. 1.5 liters
l. 0.5gm
m. 2500mg
n. 0.1gm
o. 0.5mg

Oral dosages of drugs

1. a. 2 tablets
b. 4 tablets
c. 2 capsules
d. 1 tablet
e. 1 capsule
f. 1 tablet
g. 1 capsule
h. 3 tablets
i. 1 tablet
j. 1/2 tablet
k. 2 tablets
l. 300mg
m. 600mg
n. 50mg
o. 250mg
p. 4 tablets

2. a. 5ml
b. 2ml
c. 10ml
d. 7.5ml
e. 2.5ml
f. 1/2 teaspoonful or 2.5ml
g. 5ml
h. 15ml
i. 180mg
j. 90mg
k. 7.5ml

Parenteral dosages of drugs

1. a. 1.5ml
b. 1ml
c. 1ml
d. 1ml
e. 0.5ml
f. 1ml
g. 0.5ml
h. 2ml
i. 1.5ml
j. 2ml
k. 2ml
l. 2ml
m. 0.5ml
n. 2.5ml
o. 1250 mcg
p. 0.5ml
q. 0.4ml
r. 0.5ml
s. 0.75ml
t. 2ml
u. 1ml
v. 0.5ml
w. 2ml
x. 0.5ml

y. 5ml
z. 2ml

2. a. 1ml
   b. 2ml
   c. (1) 25ml
   (2) 2ml

3. a. 1 tablet in 1ml (or 16♍) and give 1ml (Note: the answer may vary for this type of problem; 1 tablet could be dissolved in any amount from 0.5 - 2ml [8-32 ♍] and the entire amount given.)
   b. 2 tablets in 2ml and give 1.5ml (Note: 2 tablets could be dissolved in any amount from 0.75-2.0ml [12-32 ♍]; proportion can be used to determine your answer if you selected an amount other than 2ml.)

Temperatures

1. a. 37° C
   b. 37.7° C
   c. 38.3° C
   d. 38.5° C
   e. 36.1° C
   f. 38.7° C
   g. 38.2° C
   h. 37.2° C
2. a. 97.2° F
   b. 86° F
   c. 101.1° F
   d. 100.4° F
   e. 89.6° F
   f. 100.6° F
   g. 99.1° F
   h. 102.2° F

Solutions

1. a. 500ml
   b. 100ml
   c. 70ml
   d. 250ml
2. a. 1 1/2 tablets
   b. 5%
   c. 20gm
3. a. 1:5
   b. 1:10
   c. 1:50
   d. 1:2
4. a. 0.9%
   b. 0.1%
   c. 0.025%
   d. 4%

Additional story problems

1. 16 1/2 grains
2. 7.5 grains
3. 1:30
4. 3/4 strength
5. 3 teaspoons
6. 5ml
7. 3ml, 0.75ml
8. 0.5ml
9. 7.5ml
10. 2 tablets
11. 3 tablets
12. 6 tablets
13. one tablet
14. 10, 0.4
15. one, 200
16. one
17. 1,500
18. 0.4
19. one
20. yes, 41° F = 5° C

APPENDIX B

American Association of Pharmacy Technicians, Inc. Code of Ethics for Pharmacy Technicians

Preamble

Pharmacy Technicians are healthcare professionals who assist pharmacists in providing the best possible care for patients. The principles of this code, which apply to pharmacy technicians working in any and all settings, are based on the application and support of the moral obligations that guide the pharmacy profession in relationships with patients, healthcare professionals and society.

Principles

I. **A** pharmacy technician's first consideration is to ensure the health and safety of the patient, and to use knowledge and skills to the best of his/her ability in serving others.

II. **A** pharmacy technician supports and promotes honesty and integrity in the profession, which includes a duty to observe the law, maintain the highest moral and ethical conduct at all times and uphold the ethical principles of the profession.

III. **A** pharmacy technician assists and supports the pharmacist in the safe, efficacious and cost effective distribution of health services and healthcare resources.

IV. **A** pharmacy technician respects and values the abilities of pharmacists, colleagues and other healthcare professionals.

V. **A** pharmacy technician maintains competency in his/her practice, and continually enhances his/her professional knowledge and expertise.

VI. **A** pharmacy technician respects and supports the patient's individuality, dignity and confidentiality.

VII. **A** pharmacy technician respects the confidentiality of a patient's records and discloses pertinent information only with proper authorization.

VIII. **A** pharmacy technician never assists in the dispensing, promoting or distribution of medications or medical devices that are not of good quality or do not meet the standards required by law.

IX. **A** pharmacy technician does not engage in any activity that will discredit the profession, and will expose, without fear or favor, illegal or unethical conduct in the profession.

X. **A** pharmacy technician associates with and engages in the support of organizations which promote the profession of pharmacy through the utilization and enhancement of pharmacy technicians.

Approved by the AAPT Board of Directors
January 7, 1996

APPENDIX C

Associations and Organizations

Pharmacy organizations

American Association of Colleges of Pharmacy
1426 Prince Street, Alexandria, VA 22314-2841
(703) 739-2330; FAX (703) 836-8982
www.aacp.org

The American Council on Pharmaceutical Education
311 W. Superior Street, Suite 512, Chicago, IL 60610
(312) 664-3575; FAX (312) 664-4652, (312) 664-7008
www.acpe-accredit.org

American Hospital Association
One N. Franklin, Chicago, IL 60606
(312) 422-3000; FAX (312) 422-4796
www.aha.org

American Pharmaceutical Association
2215 Constitution Avenue, NW, Washington, DC 20037-2985
1-800-237-APhA; (202) 628-4410; FAX (202) 783-2351
www.aphanet.org

American Society for Parenteral and Enteral Nutrition
8630 Fenton Street, Suite 412, Silver Spring, MD 20910
(301) 587-6315
www.nutritioncare.org

American Society for Pharmacy Law
P.O. Box 7163, Auburn, CA 95604-7163
FAX (916) 823-5259
www.aspl.org

American Society of Consultant Pharmacists
1321 Duke Street, Alexandria, VA 22314-3563
1-800-355-2727, (703) 739-1300; FAX 1-800-220-1321, (703) 739-1321
www.ascp.com

American Society of Health-System Pharmacists
7272 Wisconsin Avenue, Bethesda, MD 20814
(301) 657-3000; FAX (301) 657-8817, (301) 652-8278
www.ashp.com

Joint Commission on Accreditation of Health Care Organizations
One Renaissance Boulevard, Oakbrook Terrace, IL 60181
(630) 792-5000; FAX (630) 792-5005
www.jcaho.org

National Association of Boards of Pharmacy
700 Busse Highway, Park Ridge, IL 60068
(847) 698-6227; FAX (847) 698-0124
www.nabp.net

National Association of Chain Drug Stores
413 North Lee Street, P.O. Box 1417-D49, Alexandria, VA 22313-1480
(703) 549-3001; FAX (703) 836-4869
www.nacds.org

National Community Pharmacists Association (formerly NARD)
205 Daingerfield Road, Alexandria, VA 22314
(703) 683-8200; FAX (703) 683-3619
www.ncpanet.org

National Council for Prescription Drug Programs, Inc.
4201 N. 24th Street, #365, Phoenix, AZ 85016-6268
(602) 957-9105; FAX (602) 955-0749
www.ncpdp.org

National Council on Patient Information and Education
4915 St. Elmo Ave., Suite 505, Bethesda, MD 20814-6053
(301) 656-8565; FAX (301) 656-4464
www.talkaboutrx.org

National Pharmaceutical Council
1894 Preston White Drive, Reston, VA 20191
(703) 620-6390; FAX (703) 476-0904
www.npcnow.org

National Wholesale Druggists' Association
1821 Michael Faraday Drive, Suite 400, Reston, VA 20190-5348
(703) 787-0000; FAX (703) 787-6930
www.nwda.org

Pharmaceutical Manufacturers Association
1100 15th Street, NW, Washington, DC 20005
(202) 835-3400; FAX (202) 785-4834
www.phrma.org

Technician organizations

American Association of Pharmacy Technicians
P.O. Box 1447, 620 S. Elm, Greensboro, NC 27402
(336) 275-1700; FAX (336) 275-7222
www.pharmacytechnician.com

National Pharmacy Technician Association
P.O. Box 683148, Houston, TX 77268-3148
1-888-247-8700; FAX (281) 895-7320
www.pharmacytechnician.org

Pharmacy Technician Certification Board
2215 Constitution Avenue, NW, Washington, DC 20037-2985
(202) 429-7576; FAX (202) 429-7596
www.ptcb.org

Pharmacy Technician Educators Council
1426 Prince Street, Alexandria, VA 22314
(703) 683-9493
www.mbnet.mb.ca/ptec

APPENDIX D

Resources for More Information

Government agencies

Drug Enforcement Administration, regional offices

www.usdoj.gov/dea/

Atlanta division *(Georgia, North Carolina, South Carolina, Tennessee)*: (404) 331-4401

Boston division *(Connecticut, Massachusetts, Maine, New Hampshire, Rhode Island, Vermont)*: (617) 557-2100

Caribbean division *(Barbados, Dominican Republic, Haiti, Jamaica, Netherlands Antilles, Puerto Rico, Virgin Islands)*: (787) 775-1815

Chicago division *(Illinois, Indiana, Minnesota, North Dakota, Wisconsin)*: (312) 353-7875

Dallas division *(Oklahoma, Texas)*: (214) 640-0801

Denver division *(Colorado, New Mexico, Utah, Wyoming)*: (303) 705-7300

Detroit division *(Kentucky, Michigan, Ohio)*: (313) 234-4000

Houston division *(Texas)*: (713) 639-3000

Los Angeles division *(California, Hawaii, Guam, Nevada)*: (213) 894-2650

Miami division *(Bahamas, Florida)*: (305) 590-4870

Newark division *(New Jersey)*: (973) 273-5000

New Orleans division *(Alabama, Arkansas, Louisiana, Mississippi)*: (504) 840-1100

New York division *(New York)*: (212) 337-3900

Philadelphia division *(Delaware, Pennsylvania)*: (215) 861-3474

Phoenix division *(Arizona)*: (602) 664-5600

San Diego division *(California)*: (858) 616-4100

San Francisco division *(California)*: (415) 436-7900

Seattle division *(Alaska, Idaho, Montana, Oregon, Washington)*: (206) 553-5443

St. Louis division *(Iowa, Illinois, Kansas, Missouri, Nebraska, South Dakota)*: (314) 538-4600

Washington, D.C. division *(District of Columbia, Maryland, Virginia, West Virginia)*: (202) 305-8500

U.S. Food & Drug Administration, general information

www.fda.gov

(888) INFO-FDA or (888) 463-6332

U.S. Food & Drug Administration's MEDWATCH program

www.fda.gov/medwatch/index.html

(800) FDA-1088; FAX (800) FDA-0178

Publications for further research or study

Pharmacy Certified Technician Workbook, Michigan Pharmacists Association. To order, call the Michigan Pharmacists Association: (517) 484-1466.
Handbook of Federal Drug Law, Nielsen J.R., Lea & Febiger, 1992.
Handbook of Non-Prescription Drugs, American Pharmaceutical Association, 2000.
Manual for Pharmacy Technicians, American Society of Health-System Pharmacists, 1998.
Pharmaceutical Calculations, Stoklosa M. and Ansel H., Lea & Febiger, 1996.
Pharmacy Practice and the Law, Abood R.R. and Brushwood D.B., Aspen Publishers, 1994.
Pharmacy Technician Certification: Quick-Study Guide, American Pharmaceutical Association, 1999.
Pharmacy Technician Workbook: A Self-Instructional Approach, American Society of Health-System Pharmacists, 1994.
Training Manual for Intravenous Admixture Personnel, Hunt M., PreceptPress, 1995.

State Boards of Pharmacy

Alabama	(205) 967-0130
Alaska	(907) 465-2589
Arizona	(602) 255-5125
Arkansas	(501) 682-0190
California	(916) 445-5014
Colorado	(303) 894-7750
Connecticut	(860) 713-6070
Delaware	(302) 739-4798
District of Columbia	(202) 442-9200
Florida	(850) 414-2969
Georgia	(912) 207-1686
Hawaii	(808) 586-2698
Idaho	(208) 334-2356
Illinois	(217) 785-8159
Indiana	(317) 232-1140
Iowa	(515) 281-5944
Kansas	(785) 296-4056
Kentucky	(502) 573-1580
Louisiana	(225) 925-6496
Maine	(207) 624-8625
Maryland	(410) 764-4755
Massachusetts	(617) 727-9953
Michigan	(517) 373-9102
Minnesota	(612) 617-2201
Mississippi	(601) 354-6750
Missouri	(573) 751-0091
Montana	(406) 444-3737
Nebraska	(402) 471-2115
Nevada	(775) 850-1440
New Hampshire	(603) 271-2350
New Jersey	(973) 504-6450
New Mexico	(505) 841-9102
New York	(518) 474-3848
North Carolina	(919) 942-4454
North Dakota	(701) 328-9535
Ohio	(614) 466-4143
Oklahoma	(405) 521-3815
Oregon	(503) 731-4032
Pennsylvania	(717) 783-7157
Puerto Rico	(787) 725-8161
Rhode Island	(401) 222-2837
South Carolina	(803) 896-4700
South Dakota	(605) 362-2737
Tennessee	(615) 741-2718
Texas	(512) 305-8000
Utah	(801) 530-6633
Vermont	(802) 828-6767
Virginia	(804) 662-9911
Virgin Islands	(340) 774-0117
Washington	(360) 753-6834
West Virginia	(304) 558-0558
Wisconsin	(608) 266-2812
Wyoming	(307) 234-0294

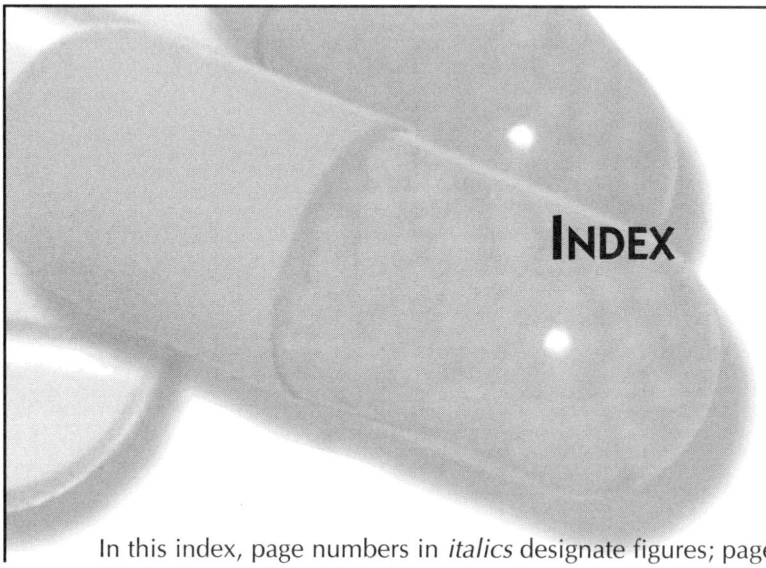

INDEX

In this index, page numbers in *italics* designate figures; page numbers followed by the letter "t" designate tables. *See also* cross-references designate related topics or more detailed topic breakdowns. Drugs significantly discussed are listed by generic name.